Sure Success in Pharmacology for Nursing Students

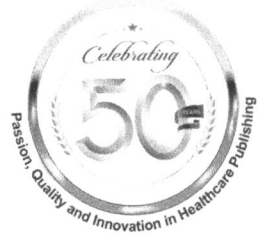

Sure Success in Pharmacology for Nursing Students

(As per INC Syllabus)

P Nirmala MD PhD (Pharma)
Professor and Head
Department of Pharmacology
Rajah Muthiah Medical College
Annamalai University
Tamil Nadu, India

Foreword
A Mangaiarkkarasi

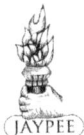

JAYPEE BROTHERS MEDICAL PUBLISHERS
The Health Sciences Publisher
New Delhi | London | Panama

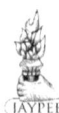

Jaypee Brothers Medical Publishers (P) Ltd

Headquarters
Jaypee Brothers Medical Publishers (P) Ltd
4838/24, Ansari Road, Daryaganj
New Delhi 110 002, India
Phone: +91-11-43574357
Fax: +91-11-43574314
Email: jaypee@jaypeebrothers.com

Overseas Offices

J.P. Medical Ltd
83 Victoria Street, London
SW1H 0HW (UK)
Phone: +44 20 3170 8910
Fax: +44 (0)20 3008 6180
Email: info@jpmedpub.com

Jaypee-Highlights Medical Publishers Inc
City of Knowledge, Bld. 235, 2nd Floor, Clayton
Panama City, Panama
Phone: +1 507-301-0496
Fax: +1 507-301-0499
Email: cservice@jphmedical.com

Jaypee Brothers Medical Publishers (P) Ltd
17/1-B Babar Road, Block-B, Shyamoli
Mohammadpur, Dhaka-1207
Bangladesh
Mobile: +08801912003485
Email: jaypeedhaka@gmail.com

Jaypee Brothers Medical Publishers (P) Ltd
Bhotahity, Kathmandu
Nepal
Phone: +977-9741283608
Email: kathmandu@jaypeebrothers.com

Website: www.jaypeebrothers.com
Website: www.jaypeedigital.com

© 2019, Jaypee Brothers Medical Publishers

The views and opinions expressed in this book are solely those of the original contributor(s)/author(s) and do not necessarily represent those of editor(s) of the book.

All rights reserved. No part of this publication may be reproduced, stored or transmitted in any form or by any means, electronic, mechanical, photocopying, recording or otherwise, without the prior permission in writing of the publishers.

All brand names and product names used in this book are trade names, service marks, trademarks or registered trademarks of their respective owners. The publisher is not associated with any product or vendor mentioned in this book.

Medical knowledge and practice change constantly. This book is designed to provide accurate, authoritative information about the subject matter in question. However, readers are advised to check the most current information available on procedures included and check information from the manufacturer of each product to be administered, to verify the recommended dose, formula, method and duration of administration, adverse effects and contraindications. It is the responsibility of the practitioner to take all appropriate safety precautions. Neither the publisher nor the author(s)/editor(s) assume any liability for any injury and/or damage to persons or property arising from or related to use of material in this book.

This book is sold on the understanding that the publisher is not engaged in providing professional medical services. If such advice or services are required, the services of a competent medical professional should be sought.

Every effort has been made where necessary to contact holders of copyright to obtain permission to reproduce copyright material. If any have been inadvertently overlooked, the publisher will be pleased to make the necessary arrangements at the first opportunity. The **CD/DVD-ROM** (if any) provided in the sealed envelope with this book is complimentary and free of cost. **Not meant for sale.**

Inquiries for bulk sales may be solicited at: jaypee@jaypeebrothers.com

Sure Success in Pharmacology for Nursing Students

First Edition: **2019**

ISBN: 978-93-5270-527-6

Dedicated to

My parents Mr K Parthasarathy and Mrs Kasthuri Parthasarathy, in-laws Mr P Padmanabhan and Mrs Vatsala Padmanabhan, husband Dr P Ashok Kumar, son and daughter-in-law, Dr A Naren Kumar and Dr S Abhinaya.

Foreword

It is my pleasure and privilege to write the Foreword for the book *Sure Success in Pharmacology for Nursing Students.* I had the privilege to work with Professor Dr Nirmala during the years between 2004 and 2008 who is very much interested in educating the medical professionals and research activities including guiding the PhD students.

The book has been written in simple, precise, concise and coherent, in well-organized and systematized way of all drug class and individual drugs emphasizing explanations wherever possible. Best attempt has been made to explore the basic concept of drugs and elementary principles in simple language and as much as possible the basic intellectual level of readership. It is hoped that this book will provide useful information to nursing students as well as to other students from different linguistic and schooling backgrounds. I hope that this book will offer nursing students enough exposure to the subject matter and enable to equip them in their success.

This book also highlights the awareness of roles and responsibilities of nursing students in diverse health discipline during their patient care.

This book has been prepared according to the syllabus of Indian Nursing Council. The nursing students will find it as a 'textbook' for their examination. I am much pleased to recommend this book for the nursing health personnel and congratulate the professor for her excellent work.

A Mangaiarkkarasi MD
Professor and Head
Department of Pharmacology
Sri Venkateshwaraa Medical College
Hospital and Research Centre
Puducherry, India

Preface

A basic knowledge of pharmacology is essential for nursing students as they provide bedside care to patients. Although many textbooks deal elaborately about pharmacodynamics, pharmacokinetics, routes of administration, doses, side effects, therapeutic indications and contraindications, none have been presented in a concise format focusing on exam preparation. This book is written from exam point of view and provides details about therapeutic agents in a precise manner. It also deals in detail about the need for monitoring the emergence of important side effects that are required to be reported to the attending physician, the manner of administration of drugs and procedures to be followed while the patient is on medication, thereby providing better clinical knowledge to nursing students and greater perspective towards nursing responsibilities in therapeutics. This book will help the students to understand the concept more easily.

This book focuses on the main aspects required for a sure success in examination. It focuses mainly on the salient features of each drug and will help students to present the answers neatly. However, it also deals elaborately about nursing responsibilities during therapy and emphasizes on vital issues such as drug storage, mode of drug administration and monitoring the important adverse effect. It will impart adequate clinical knowledge to the nursing students and will enable them to provide a better bedside care.

P Nirmala

Acknowledgments

I would like to express my sincere gratitude to our honorable Vice Chancellor Prof S Manian, our respected Registrar Prof K Arumugam for permitting the publishing of this book.

My whole-hearted thanks to Dr P Rajkumar, Dean, Faculty of Medicine for allowing me to publish this book.

I profoundly thank my friend Dr A Mangaiarkkarasi, Professor and Head, Department of Pharmacology, Sri Venkateshwaraa Medical College Hospital and Research Centre, Puducherry, India, for writing the foreword of this book.

Syllabus

PHARMACOLOGY

Placement: Second Year   **Time:** Theory - 45 Hours

Course Description
This course in designed to enable students to acquire understanding pharmacodynamics, pharmacokinetics, principles of therapeutics and nursing implications.

Total Hours: 45

Unit No.	Section
Unit I **Learning Objectives** • Describe pharmacodynamics, pharmacokinetics, classification and the principles of drug administration. **Introduction to Pharmacology** • Definitions • Sources • Terminology used • Types: Classification • Pharmacodynamics: Actions, therapeutic • Adverse, toxic • Pharmacokinetics: Absorption, distribution, metabolism, interaction, excretion • Review: Routes and principles of administration of drugs • Indian pharmacopoeia: Legal issues • Rational use of drugs • Principles of therapeutics **Teaching Learning Activities** • Lecture Discussion **Assessment Methods** • Short Answers • Objective Type	I
Unit II **Learning Objectives** • Explain chemotherapy of specific infections and infestations and nurse's responsibilities. **Chemotherapy** Pharmacology of commonly used: • Penicillin • Cephalosporins	XI

Unit No.	Section
• Aminoglycosides • Macrolide and broad-spectrum antibiotics • Sulfonamides • Quinolones • Antiamoebic • Antimalarials • Anthelmintics • Antiscabies agents • Antiviral and antifungal agents • Antitubercular drugs • Antileprosy drugs • Anticancer drugs • Immunosuppresants: Composition, action, dosage, route, indications, contraindications, drug interactions, side effects, adverse effects, toxicity and role of nurse **Teaching Learning Activities** • Lecture Discussion • Drug study presentation **Assessment Methods** • Short Answers • Objective Type	
Unit III **Learning Objectives** • Describe Antiseptics, disinfectants, insecticides, and nurse's responsibilities. **Pharmacology of Commonly used Antiseptic, Disinfectants and Insecticides** • Antiseptics: Composition, action, dosage, route, indications, contraindications, drug interactions, side effects, adverse effects, toxicity and role of nurse • Disinfectants • Insecticides **Teaching Learning Activities** • Lecture Discussion • Drug study/presentation **Assessment Methods** • Short Answers • Objective Type	XII
Unit IV **Learning Objectives** • Describe drugs action on gastrointestinal system and nurse's responsibilities. **Drugs Acting on GI System** Pharmacology of commonly used: • Antiemetics • Emetics • Purgatives • Antacids	IX

Unit No.	Section
• Cholinergic • Anticholinergics • Fluid and electrolyte • Antidiarrheals • Histamines: Composition, action, dosage, route, indications, contraindications, drug interactions, side effects, adverse effects, toxicity and role of nurse **Teaching Learning Activities** • Lecture Discussion • Drug study/presentation **Assessment Methods** • Short Answers • Objective Type	
Unit V **Learning Objectives** • Describe the drug used on respiratory systems and nurse's responsibilities. **Drugs used on Respiratory Systems** Pharmacology of commonly used: • Antiasthmatics • Mucolytics • Decongestants • Expectorants • Antitussives • Bronchodilators • Bronchoconstrictors • Anthistamines composition, action, dosage, route, indications, contraindications, drug interactions, side effects, adverse effects, toxicity and role of nurse **Teaching Learning Activities** • Lecture Discussion • Drug study/presentation **Assessment Methods** • Short Answers • Objective Type	X

Unit VI
Learning Objectives
• Describe drugs used on urinary system and nurse's responsibilities.
Drugs used on Urinary System
Pharmacology of commonly used:
• Diuretics and antidiuretics
• Urinary antiseptics:
  – Cholinergic and anticholinergics
  – Acidifiers and alkalanizers: Composition, action, dosage, route, indications, contraindications, drug interactions, side effects, adverse effects, toxicity and role of nurse
	XI

Unit No.	Section
Teaching Learning Activities • Lecture Discussion • Drug study/presentation **Assessment Methods** • Short Answers • Objective Type	
Unit VII **Learning Objectives** • Describe drugs used in dead diction, emergency, deficiency of vitamins and minerals. **Miscellaneous** • Drugs used in deaddiction • Drugs used in CPR and emergency • Vitamins and minerals • Immunosuppresants • Antidotes • Antivenom • Vaccines and sera **Teaching Learning Activities** • Lecture Discussion • Drug study/presentation **Assessment Methods** • Short Answers • Objective Type	XII
Unit VIII **Learning Objectives** • Describe drugs and on skin and mucous membranes and nurse's responsibilities. **Drugs used on Skin and Mucous Membranes** • Topical applications for skin, eye, ear, nose and buccal cavity Antipruritics: Composition, action, dosage, route, indications, contraindications, drug interactions, side effects, adverse effects, toxicity and role of nurse **Teaching Learning Activities** • Lecture Discussion • Drug study/presentation **Assessment Methods** • Short Answers • Objective Type	XII
Unit IX **Learning Objectives** • Describe drugs used on nervous systems and nurse's responsibilities. **Drugs acting on Nervous system** Basic and applied pharmacology of commonly used: • Analgesics and Anesthetics • Analgesics: – Nonsteroidal anti-inflammatory drugs (NSAIDs)	IV

Unit No.	Section

- Antipyretics
- Hypnotics and sedatives
- Opioids
- Non-opioids
- Tranquilizers
- General and local anesthetics
- Gases
- Oxygen
- Nitrous oxide
- Carbon-dioxide
• Cholinergic and anticholinergics:
  - Muscle relaxants
  - Major tranquilizers
  - Antipsychotics
  - Antidepressants
  - Anticonvulsants
  - Adrenergics
  - Noradrenergic
  - Mood stabilizers
  - Acetylcholine
  - Stimulants: Composition, action, dosage, route, indications, contra-indications, drug interactions, side effects, adverse effects, toxicity and role of nurse
	II

Unit X **Learning Objectives** • Describe drugs used on cardiovascular systems and nurse's responsibilities. **Cardiovascular drugs** • Hematinics • Cardiotonics • Antianginals • Antihypertensives and vasodilators • Antiarrhythmics • Plasma expanders • Coagulants and anticoagulants • Antiplatelets and thrombolytics • Hypolipidernics: Composition, action, dosage, route, indications, contraindications, drug interactions, side effects, adverse effects, toxicity and role of nurse **Teaching Learning Activities** • Lecture Discussion • Drug study/presentation **Assessment Methods** • Short Answers • Objective Type	VI and VII

Unit No.	Section
Unit XI **Learning Objectives** - Describe drugs used for hormonal disorders and supplementation, contraception and medical termination of pregnancy and nurse's responsibilities. **Drugs used for hormonal disorders and supplementation, contraception and medical termination of pregnancy** - Insulins and oral hypoglycemics - Thyroid supplements and suppressants - Steroids, Anabolics - Uterine stimulants and relaxants - Oral contraceptives - Other estrogen-progestrone preparations - Corticotrophine and Gonadotropines - Adrenaline - Prostoglandins - Calcitonins - Calcium salts - Calcium regulators: Composition, action, dosages, route, indications, contraindications, drug interactions, side effects, adverse effects, toxicity and role of nurse **Teaching Learning Activities** - Lecture Discussion - Drug study/presentation **Assessment Methods** - Short Answers - Objective Type	VIII
Unit XII **Learning Objectives** - Demonstrate awareness of the common drugs used in alternative system of medicine. **Introduction to drugs used in alternative systems of medicines** - Ayurveda, Homeopathy, Unani and Siddha, etc. **Teaching Learning Activities** - Lecture Discussion - Drug study/presentation **Assessment Methods** - Short Answers - Objective Type	XIII

Contents

Section I: General Pharmacology

1. Source of Drugs — 3
2. Routes of Drug Administration — 4
3. Pharmacokinetics — 10
4. Pharmacodynamics — 17
5. Adverse Drug Reactions — 20
6. Factors Modifying Drug Action — 26
7. Legal Aspects in Nursing Practice — 28

Section II: Autonomic Nervous System

8. Cholinergics — 33
9. Anticholinergics — 41
10. Adrenergic Agonists — 46
11. Alpha Blockers — 59
12. Beta Blockers — 64
13. Skeletal Muscle Relaxants — 74
14. Ganglionic Stimulants and Blockers — 79
15. Local Anesthetics — 81

Section III: Autacoids

16. Antihistamines — 89
17. Serotonin Agonists and Antagonists — 92
18. Lipid Derived Autacoids — 96

Section IV: Central Nervous System

19. Ethyl Alcohol — 101
20. General Anesthetics — 105
21. Sedatives and Hypnotics — 116
22. Antiepileptic Drugs — 121
23. Drugs in Neurodegenerative Disorders — 133
24. Opioid Analgesics — 139

Section V: Psychopharmacology

25.	Pharmacotherapy of Depression and Anxiety	151
26.	Pharmacotherapy of Psychosis and Mania	157
27.	Drug Addiction	166

Section VI: Cardiovascular System

28.	Antianginal Drugs	169
29.	Diuretics	180
30.	Drugs in Heart Failure	188
31.	Antihypertensive Drugs	195
32.	Antiarrhythmic Agents	209

Section VII: Blood

33.	Coagulants	223
34.	Anticoagulants	227
35.	Fibrinolytic Drugs	235
36.	Antiplatelet Agents	238
37.	Hypolipidemic Drugs	242
38.	Treatment of Shock	248
39.	Iron Deficiency Anemia	254
40.	Megaloblastic Anemia and Hematopoietic Growth Factors	257

Section VIII: Hormones and Hormone Antagonists

41.	Growth Hormone, Prolactin, Gonadotropins and GnRH Agonists	263
42.	Thyroid Hormone and Antithyroid Drugs	271
43.	Corticosteroids	278
44.	Insulin and Oral Hypoglycemic Drugs	283
45.	Estrogens and Progestins	291
46.	Hormonal Contraceptives	300
47.	Androgens	305
48.	Agents Involved in Bone Turnover	311
49.	Uterine Stimulants and Relaxants	318

Section IX: Gastrointestinal System

50. Drugs in Peptic Ulcer and GERD — 325
51. Antiemetic Drugs — 333
52. Drugs in Constipation, Diarrhea and Other GIT Conditions — 338

Section X: Respiratory System

53. Pharmacotherapy of Bronchial Asthma — 359
54. COPD, Mucolytics, Expectorants and Treatment of Cough — 367

Section XI: Chemotherapy

55. Introduction to Chemotherapeutic Agents — 373
56. Sulfonamides, Trimethoprim and Co-trimoxazole — 376
57. Quinolones — 381
58. Beta-Lactam Antibiotics — 387
59. Aminoglycosides — 399
60. Broad Spectrum Antibiotics — 403
61. Macrolides and Ketolides — 407
62. Miscellaneous Antibiotics — 411
63. Urinary Antiseptics and Chemotherapy of Urinary Tract Infection — 418
64. Chemotherapy of Sexually Transmitted Diseases — 421
65. Chemotherapy of Tuberculosis — 423
66. Chemotherapy of Leprosy — 430
67. Chemotherapy of Worm Infestation — 433
68. Chemotherapy of Filariasis — 438
69. Antimalarial Drugs — 440
70. Chemotherapy of Amebiasis — 447
71. Chemotherapy of Other Protozoal Infection — 451
72. Chemotherapy of Fungal Infection — 456
73. Anti Non-Retroviral Agents — 467
74. HIV Infection and Antiretroviral Agents — 478
75. Anticancer Drugs — 492
76. Immunosuppressants — 515

Section XII: Miscellaneous Topics

77.	Nonsteroidal Anti-Inflammatory Drugs (NSAIDs)	519
78.	Pharmacotherapy of Rheumatoid Arthritis	528
79.	Pharmacotherapy of Gout	531
80.	Chelating Agents	536
81.	Antiseptics, Disinfectants and Ectoparasiticides	540
82.	Drugs Acting on Skin and Mucous Membrane	544

Section XIII: Alternative Systems of Medicine

83.	Ayurveda, Siddha, Homeopathy and Unani Medicine	549

Index   555

SECTION I

General Pharmacology

- Source of Drugs
- Routes of Drug Administration
- Pharmacokinetics
- Pharmacodynamics
- Adverse Drug Reactions
- Factors Modifying Drug Action
- Legal Aspects in Nursing Practice

Source of Drugs

I. **NATURAL / PLANT SOURCE**
   A. **Alkaloid:** Morphine, atropine
   B. **Glycoside:** Digoxin, digitoxin
   C. **Gum:** Gum acacia, gum tragacanth
   D. **Tannin:** Tincture catechu

II. **OIL**
   A. **Fixed oil:** Olive oil, castor oil
   B. **Mineral oil:** Liquid paraffin
   C. **Volatile oil:** Oil of peppermint, oil of wintergreen

III. **RESIN: Tincture benzoin**

IV. **OLEORESIN: Mixture of resin and volatile oil**

V. **OTHER NATURAL PRODUCTS**
   A. **Flavonoid:** Quercetin
   B. **Retinoid:** Tretinoin
   C. **Phytoestrogen:** Soy product, genistein

VI. **ANIMAL: Heparin, insulin**

VII. **MICROORGANISMS: Penicillin, streptomycin**

VIII. **SYNTHETIC: Benzodiazepines, barbiturates**

IX. **BIOLOGICAL SUBSTANCES: Monoclonal antibodies**

CHAPTER 2

Routes of Drug Administration

TOPICAL OR LOCAL APPLICATION
- The action of a drug is restricted to the site of its application.
- Paste, lotion, ointment, liniment, powder, eye and ear drops are used topically.
- These are applied on skin, mucous membrane, eye and ear.
- Vaginal pessary and rectal suppository are applied topically.
- Analgesic ointment, antibiotic eye or ear drops, antifungal powder can also be applied locally.
- They may get absorbed causing systemic toxicity.

ORAL OR ENTERIC ROUTE
- It is a common mode of drug administration.
- Solid as well as liquid formulation can be administered through this route.
- The absorption of a drug from intestine is more than its absorption from stomach.
- This is due to the large surface area of the intestine.
- Tablet, capsule, syrup, spansule, mixture and emulsion can be administered orally.

Advantages
- It is a convenient and safe route.
- It does not require assistance.
- It improves patient compliance as it is easy and painless to administer.
- It does not require sterilization.
- It is economical.

Disadvantages
- The onset of action is slow and cannot be used in emergency.
- The bioavailability is low, if drugs are incompletely absorbed.
- It is ineffective in patients with nausea and vomiting.
- Bitter drugs are difficult to administer orally.

- Drugs that undergo high first pass metabolism are less effective through this route.
- Drugs with high molecular weight are not absorbed.
- It is unsuitable for drugs destroyed by gastric juice.
- Such drugs should be given in enteric coated form.

ENTERIC COATED PILLS
Drugs are coated with cellulose acetate phthalate.

Advantages
- Enteric coated tablet is not destroyed by gastric juice.
- It does not cause gastric irritation.

Disadvantages
If the coating is thick, it may not dissolve and the drug will be incompletely absorbed.

SUBLINGUAL ROUTE
The drug placed under the tongue dissolves and is absorbed through sublingual veins.

Advantages
- The absorption is rapid.
- The onset of action is quick.
- Sublingual route of administration bypasses the first pass metabolism.
- The effect of the drug can be quickly terminated by spitting the tablet.
- Glyceryl trinitrate and buprenorphine are given through this route.

Disadvantages
- Only nonirritant drugs can be administered through this route.
- The drugs can cause stinging sensation.
- Mucosal ulceration can occur.

RECTAL ROUTE
Suppository and enema are administered through this route.

Advantages
- This route of administration avoids first pass metabolism.
- It is more convenient for pediatric and geriatric age group.

- It can be administered to patients with nausea and vomiting.
- Diazepam and paraldehyde can be administered through this route.

Disadvantages
- The absorption of drug is incomplete.
- Irritant drugs can cause mucosal ulcer.

INHALATIONAL ROUTE
- Metered dose aerosol (MDI) – Salbutamol
- Nebulizer – Salbutamol
- Dry powder – Salbutamol
- Gas – Nitrous oxide

Advantages
- The onset of action is quick.
- The termination of effect is rapid.
- The drug enters alveoli and passes quickly into systemic circulation.
- General anesthetics and salbutamol are administered through this route.

Disadvantages
- Systemic toxicity is possible.
- Drugs can cause nasal mucosal ulceration.
- The absorption is irregular.
- Irritant drugs cannot be administered.

PARENTERAL ROUTE
Advantages
- Drugs can be administered in unconscious and in uncooperative patients.
- It is effective even in patients with nausea and vomiting.
- The onset of action is quick.
- The bioavailability is high.
- Gastric irritation is avoided.

Disadvantages
- Self medication is not possible.
- It is painful and costly.
- Hence, it may interfere with patient compliance.

- Needles should be sterilized before injection.
- Once injected, the drug cannot be withdrawn.
- It can cause injury to adjacent nerves and arteries.

INTRADERMAL ROUTE
- The drug is injected into the skin layer.
- This route is employed in testing drug allergy and for BCG vaccination.
- It is often painful and only small quantities can be administered.

SUBCUTANEOUS ROUTE
- The drug is injected into the subcutaneous pad of fat.
- Insulin and depot hormone preparation are administered through this route.

Advantages
- The absorption is delayed.
- Hence, the action is sustained.

Disadvantages
- The absorption can be irregular.
- Irritant drugs cannot be administered through this route.

INTRAMUSCULAR ROUTE
- The drug is injected into skeletal muscles of hand and gluteal region.
- Even oily solution and suspension can be administered through this route.

Advantages
- The absorption is rapid due to rich blood supply of muscles.
- The bioavailability is higher than oral route of administration.

Disadvantages
- This route can be painful.
- Injury to nerves and muscles can occur.

INTRAVENOUS ROUTE
Advantages
- 100% bioavailability.
- The onset of action is rapid.

- Large volume can be administered.
- Titration of dose is feasible.
- So, easier to maintain uniform plasma concentration.

Disadvantages
- IV infusion should be slow, to prevent toxicity of drugs.
- Once infused, effect of the drug cannot be reversed.
- Self administration is not possible as special assistance is necessary.
- Irritant drugs can cause phlebitis.
- Extravasation of drugs can result in sloughing and necrosis.

INTRA-ARTERIAL ROUTE
Advantages
- Action of the drug can be localized to a particular organ or tissue.
- This route is also used for diagnostic purposes such as angiogram.
- Anticancer drug mechlorethamine is administered through this route.

Disadvantages
Administration of drugs through this route is difficult and requires expertise.

INTRATHECAL ROUTE
- The drugs are injected into CSF in lumbar space for spinal anesthesia.
- Local anesthetics can be administered through this route.
- Drugs for brain tumor or acute CNS infection are given through this route.
- The drugs can also be injected into epidural space.
- Opioid analgesic fentanyl is administered through epidural route.
- Continuous administration is possible through the catheter placed in epidural space.

INTRAPERITONEAL ROUTE
- This route has larger surface area for absorption.
- Hence large volume can be administered.
- It is also used for peritoneal dialysis.

INTRAOSSEOUS ROUTE
- Drugs are administered into joint space.
- Corticosteroids are administered through this route in arthritis.

DERMOJET
Transcutaneous administration of drugs.

TRANSDERMAL ROUTE
- Drug is released from the adhesive unit placed on skin.
- Scopolamine is available as transdermal application for motion sickness.

Nursing Responsibilities
- Patient should be erect during oral administration of drugs.
- Patient should be advised to drink at least 150 mL of water after swallowing a tablet or a capsule.
- Extended release or sustained release preparations should not be crushed before use.
- Hands should be washed before and after injecting drugs and latex gloves should be used while handling blood and its products.
- The site of injection should be cleaned with antiseptic swab before injecting drugs.
- Needle and syringe should be disposed after each injection and new set should be used each time.
- IM injection should not be given into gluteus maximus muscle in a child who is yet to start walking, as it is very thin in this age group.
- Before starting intravenous infusion, patency of infusion line should be checked.
- The infusion site should be visible for verifying extravasation.
- For intramuscular injection, the skin should be pulled taut and needle injected at 90°, plunger withdrawn slightly to rule out the presence of needle inside blood vessels.
- Z track method prevents leakage of drugs into subcutaneous tissue.
- To avoid needle stick injuries, needle should not be bent or manipulated after use but should be recapped using single handed scoop technique.
- Needle, syringe and broken ampoules should be discarded immediately after use.

CHAPTER 3

Pharmacokinetics

Pharmacokinetics includes absorption, distribution, metabolism and excretion of drugs. It determines the plasma concentration of a drug.

TRANSPORT OF DRUGS
- Lipophilic and hydrophilic drugs can be absorbed through passive diffusion.
- Solute carrier (SLC) and ATP binding cascade (ABC) are drug transporters which help in drug transport.
- Anionic and cationic transporters permit for both influx and efflux of drugs.
- Transmembrane transport can be either through facilitated transport or through active transport.
- Active transport of drugs requires energy.
- Carrier protein facilitates transport of drugs against electrical gradient.
- Drugs also pass through ionic channels.
- They are also transported through endocytosis and pinocytosis.
- Most lipid soluble drugs are absorbed through passive diffusion.

ABSORPTION
- Unionized drug is absorbed and ionized drug is excreted.
- Acidic drug is absorbed in stomach and basic drug is absorbed in intestine.

Factors influencing absorption:
- **Physical state:** Liquid formulation (solution, syrup) is quickly absorbed than solid formulation (tablet, capsule).
- Aqueous (water) solubility increases the rate of absorption.
- The rate of disintegration and dissolution of a drug influences its absorption.
- High concentration of a drug facilitates its absorption.
- A large surface area increases the extent of drug absorption.
- Rich blood supply favors absorption of a drug.

Pharmacokinetics

- Parenteral route of administration increases the extent of absorption than the oral route.
- Food delays absorption of drugs like rifampin.
- Tetracyclines form insoluble complex with contents of food that may interfere with its absorption.
- Fatty food increases absorption of drugs like griseofulvin.
- Vitamin C enhances the absorption of iron.
- Liquid paraffin reduces absorption of fat soluble vitamins.
- Delayed gastric emptying and hypermotility alters absorption.
- Enterohepatic circulation increases the duration of action of drugs.
- First pass metabolism reduces the systemic absorption.

Bioavailability
- It is the rate and extent of absorption of a drug into the systemic circulation.
- It depends on the rate of disintegration and dissolution, concentration, aqueous solubility, surface area, route of administration, type of formulation, presence of food and first pass metabolism.
- Bioavailability is 100% through intravenous route.
- Microionized formulation is absorbed quickly.
- **Bioequivalence:** Two formulations from same manufacturer or from different manufacturers may be chemically equivalent but may not be biologically equivalent.

Distribution
- Once absorbed, the drug enters into cells or is distributed extracellularly.
- Drugs are either highly protein bound or minimally bound to plasma proteins.
- Drugs bind reversibly to plasma proteins.
- Protein bound drug is clinically inactive.
- It does not enter into cells, not metabolized and not excreted.
- Protein binding serves as a temporary storage site and prolongs the duration of action of drugs.
- Once plasma concentration of the free drug declines, bound drug dissociates from proteins.
- Bound drug does not enter CNS and does not cross placenta.
- Acidic drug binds to albumin and basic drug binds to α_1 acid glycoprotein.

- Highly protein bound drugs compete with each other for protein binding, one drug displacing the other from its bound site.
- Highly lipid soluble drugs enter cells, accumulate in CSF and in fat.
- Lipid solubility and protein binding capacity of a drug influences its distribution.
- NSAIDs, phenytoin, sulfonamides and warfarin have high protein binding capacity.
- Lidocaine, beta blockers, verapamil and bupivacaine have low protein binding capacity.

TISSUE STORAGE
Drugs are stored in many tissues:
- **Liver:** Chloroquine
- **Brain:** Chlorpromazine
- **Kidney:** Chloroquine
- **Skeletal muscles:** Emetine
- **Heart:** Digoxin
- **Adipose tissue:** Thiopentone
- **Thyroid:** Iodine
- **Retina:** Chloroquine
- **Iris:** Ephedrine
- **Bone:** Tetracyclines
- **Teeth:** Tetracyclines.

BIOTRANSFORMATION (METABOLISM)
Prodrug
- It is an inactive form of a drug.
- Prodrug should be converted into active drug.
- Levodopa, enalapril, dipivefrin, prednisolone are prodrugs.

First Pass Metabolism
- Drugs administered orally enter portal circulation and reach liver.
- They undergo presystemic metabolism in liver before entering into systemic circulation.
- Such presystemic metabolism reduces bioavailability or plasma concentration of drugs.
- First pass metabolism or presystemic metabolism is minimal through parenteral route.
- Organs commonly involved in first pass metabolism are liver, lung and intestine.

- Drugs with high first pass metabolism should be either given through parenteral route or as a high oral dose.
- Lidocaine and testosterone require parenteral administration to avoid first pass metabolism.
- Propranolol, verapamil and morphine can be administered at a high oral dose to compensate the presystemic metabolism.
- Glyceryl trinitrate is given through sublingual route to avoid the first pass metabolism.
- Isoprenaline undergoes first pass metabolism in intestine while general anesthetics undergo presystemic metabolism in lung.

PHASES OF METABOLISM

They are phase I and phase II reactions. The drugs become inactive or less active after phase I and are conjugated and excreted after phase II metabolism.

Phase I
- Oxidation
- Reduction
- Hydrolysis

Phase II
Conjugation

Phase I Reaction
- Both microsomal and non-microsomal enzymes are involved in phase I reaction.
- Cytochrome P450, flavin monooxygenases and epoxide hydrolases are microsomal enzymes.
- Monoamine oxidase, xanthine oxidase, alcohol and aldehyde dehydrogenase are non-microsomal enzymes.
- Codeine, indomethacin and phenytoin undergo oxidation.
- Chloramphenicol, naloxone and prontosil undergo reduction.
- Local anesthetics such as lidocaine and procaine undergo hydrolysis.

Phase II Reaction
- Conjugation facilitates the excretion of drugs.
- Glucuronidation, acetylation, sulfation, methylation, glutathionylation are the types of conjugation.

- Glucuronidation is the major route of conjugation.
- Paracetamol and morphine are mainly excreted as glucuronides.

Enzyme Induction

- Certain drugs can cause enzyme induction by stimulating hepatic microsomal enzymes.
- They may promote metabolism of coadministered drugs or may increase their own metabolism.
- They either reduce the duration of action of coadministered drugs or increase the level of toxic metabolites.
- Few such drugs are phenytoin, phenobarbitone and rifampin.
- Phenobarbitone induced enzyme induction reduces bilirubin level in congenital nonhemolytic jaundice.
- Tolerance to a drug can occur due to enzyme induction.

Enzyme Inhibition

- Drugs can inhibit hepatic enzyme mediated metabolism and increase the concentration of coadministered drugs.
- An enzyme inhibitor can inhibit the metabolism of another enzyme inhibitor.
- Cimetidine, erythromycin and clarithromycin are few such drugs.

Factors influencing drug metabolism:
- In neonates and infants the metabolic capacity of microsomal enzymes is poor. So, metabolism of drugs is less in this age group.
- Liver disease influences metabolism of drugs as it is the major site of metabolism.
- Enzyme inducers and inhibitors alter drug metabolism.

EXCRETION

- Drugs are excreted through urine, saliva, milk, bile, skin and lung.
- Majority of drugs are excreted through kidney.
- Ionized and unbound drugs are excreted through kidney.
- Glomerular filtration is the major route of renal excretion.
- Drugs excreted through tubular secretion are penicillin, probenecid, sulfonamides and salicylates.
- Acidic drugs are eliminated quickly in alkaline urine.
- Alkaline drugs are eliminated quickly in acidic urine.
- Renal disease impairs excretion of drugs increasing their plasma concentration.
- Drugs concentrate in kidney and can cause drug induced nephrotoxicity.

Pharmacokinetics

- Fluoroquinolones, cotrimoxazole and metronidazole require dose reduction in severe renal failure.
- Few drugs that require dose reduction even in mild renal failure are amphotericin B, cephalexin and acyclovir.
- Drugs are also excreted through other routes:
  - **Lungs:** Volatile general anesthetics
  - **Bile:** These drugs undergo enterohepatic circulation. Few such drugs are rifampin and erythromycin.
  - **Feces:** Ampicillin
  - **Milk:** Tetracyclines
  - **Skin:** Arsenic
  - **Saliva:** Lead.

First Order Kinetics
Rate of elimination of a drug is proportional to its plasma concentration.

Zero Order Kinetics
- A constant fraction of drug is excreted irrespective of its plasma concentration.
- The elimination kinetics of some drugs switches from first order to zero order kinetics when it reaches the saturation limit.
- Phenytoin, warfarin and theophylline are few such drugs whose elimination switches from first to zero order kinetics.

Plasma Half-life
- The time taken for a drug to reach half (50%) of its original plasma concentration is the plasma half-life of that drug.
- It depends on its rate of distribution, extent of metabolism and its excretion.
- The near complete elimination of a drug occurs after 4 to 5 half-lives.
- Similarly, on repeated administration, a drug reaches its steady-state plasma concentration or plateau after 4 to 5 half-lives.
- Plasma half-life of a drug helps to determine its dose and frequency of administration.

Therapeutic Drug Monitoring
Monitoring of plasma concentration is required
  A. For drugs with narrow therapeutic index such as lithium, theophylline or digoxin.

B. In drug overdose.
C. In renal failure.
D. To monitor compliance in schizophrenia and HIV patients.
E. For drugs like propranolol and antidepressants with high interindividual variation.

Drug Action can be Prolonged
- By prolonging the absorption from its site of administration
- By increasing its binding with plasma proteins
- By reducing its metabolism
- By inhibiting its excretion.

CHAPTER 4

Pharmacodynamics

- Pharmacodynamics refers to the mechanism of action of a drug.
- The drugs act through various mechanisms.
- Generally, they either stimulate or inhibit function. Adrenaline stimulates heart rate. Acetylcholine inhibits heart rate.
- They can also be used as a replacement. Levodopa is used as a replacement in Parkinsonism.

PHYSICAL PROPERTY
- Activated charcoal acts through adsorption.
- Mannitol acts through its osmotic property.
- Dimercaprol causes chelation of heavy metals.

CHEMICAL PROPERTY
Antacids neutralize gastric acid in peptic ulcer.

ENZYME INHIBITION
- Acetazolamide inhibits carbonic anhydrase.
- Disulfiram inhibits aldehyde dehydrogenase.
- Sildenafil inhibits phosphodiesterase-5 enzyme.

Drugs can also act through ion channels, transporters and receptors.

Through Ion Channels
- Nifedipine blocks calcium channel.
- Phenytoin blocks sodium channel.

Reuptake Inhibitors
- Fluoxetine inhibits serotonin reuptake.
- Desipramine inhibits reuptake of noradrenaline.

Transport Inhibitors
- Furosemide inhibits $Na^+K^+2Cl^-$ cotransport.
- Hydrochlorothiazide inhibits Na^+Cl^- cotransport.

Through Receptors

Drugs act through G-protein coupled receptors, ion channel receptors, transmembrane enzyme-linked receptors, Janus Kinase-signal transducers and activators of transcription (JAK-STAT) binding receptors and receptors regulating gene transcription.

A. G-protein Coupled Receptors
They are guanosine triphosphate (GTP) activated protein receptors. They act through Gs, Gi and Gq receptors.
  (i) Gs or Stimulation of adenyl cyclase-cyclic adenosine monophosphate (AMP) pathway: Adenosine
  (ii) Gi or Inhibition of adenyl cyclase-cyclic AMP pathway: Acetylcholine
  (iii) Gq or Phospholipase pathway: Histamine

B. Ion Channel Receptors
  (i) Nicotinic cholinergic receptor: Acetylcholine
  (ii) Gamma-aminobutyric acid (GABA) receptor: Diazepam

C. Enzyme Linked Receptors
Insulin stimulates tyrosine kinase activity of the receptor.

D. JAK-STAT Receptors
Prolactin.

E. Receptors Regulating Gene Transcription
Drugs acting on nuclear receptors such as corticosteroids.

- The amount of drug required for a therapeutic response determines potency of the drug.
- The efficacy is the maximal response elicited by a drug.
- Therapeutic index is the ratio between the median lethal dose and median effective dose.
- The range between minimal therapeutic effect and maximum toxic effect is called therapeutic window.
- Selectivity of a drug indicates its predominant action over its other pharmacological actions.
- Salbutamol has more selective bronchodilator action than cardiac action.
- The drug specificity refers to the range of actions of a drug.

Synergism
- Facilitation of action of one drug by another drug is known as synergism.
- It can be either additive or supra-additive.

Pharmacodynamics

Additive
- The total effect of two drugs is equal to the sum of their individual effects.
- The analgesic action of aspirin and paracetamol combination is equal to the sum of their individual analgesic action.

Supra-additive
- The combined effect of two drugs is more than their individual effect.
- Sulfamethoxazole and trimethoprim combination produces greater blockade of para-aminobenzoic acid (PABA). It is known as sequential blockade and results in higher pharmacological response than their individual action.

Antagonism
Inhibition of action of one drug by another drug.

Physical Antagonism
Adsorption of alkaloids by charcoal is based on its physical property.

Chemical Antagonism
Tannin inactivates alkaloids due to its chemical property.

Physiological/functional Antagonism
Adrenaline antagonizes the physiological actions of histamine.

Receptor Antagonism
Competitive Antagonism
- The antagonism between acetylcholine and atropine.
- It is reversible depending upon the concentration of agonists or antagonists.

Noncompetitive Antagonism
- The concentration of agonists or antagonists does not determine the reversal of drug action.
- Diazepam and bicuculline cause noncompetitive antagonism.

Nonequilibrium Antagonism
- The binding between the antagonist and its receptor is very tight.
- The antagonist dissociates very slowly.
- The antagonism between phenoxybenzamine and adrenaline is of nonequilibrium type.

CHAPTER 5

Adverse Drug Reactions

SIDE EFFECTS
- They are usually mild.
- They are unavoidable.
- They can be prevented by reducing the dose of drug.
- They may occur due to extension of pharmacological action of the drug.
- Nitrates induced vasodilatation is useful in angina but can result in hypotension.
- Sometimes they can be utilized therapeutically.
- Atropine induced dryness of mouth is used for reducing sialorrhea in Parkinsonism.
- Similarly constipation induced by codeine can be utilized in traveler's diarrhea.
- Side effects may also be unrelated to pharmacological action of the drug.
- Nausea induced by estrogens is unrelated to its antiovulatory action.

SECONDARY EFFECTS
- Compared to side effects, the secondary effects are severe in intensity.
- They may even require discontinuation of the drug.
- Superinfection following tetracycline therapy necessitates its discontinuation.

TOXIC EFFECTS
- These are severe adverse effects after prolonged therapy of high dose of drugs.
- They are either predictable or unpredictable.
- They can also be due to extension of the drug effect.
- Morphine induced respiratory depression and coma is an extension of its action.
- Streptomycin induced ototoxicity is unrelated to its pharmacological action.

INTOLERANCE
- Onset of toxic effect following a therapeutic dose is called intolerance.
- Some individuals are highly sensitive even to the therapeutic dose of a drug.
- Chloroquine induced vomiting, aspirin induced hematemesis are few examples of intolerance.

IDIOSYNCRASY
- Abnormal uncharacteristic response, due to either genetic or unknown mechanism.
- Primaquine induced hemolytic anemia in glucose-6-phosphate dehydrogenase (G6PD) deficient individual is due to idiosyncrasy.

DRUG ALLERGY
- It always has an immunological basis.
- These reactions are totally unrelated to drug action.
- They occur after a latent period of 1 to 2 weeks following exposure to drug.
- Even small dose can induce drug allergy.
- Allergic response is seen in skin, gastrointestinal tract (GIT), nasal tract, mucosa and blood.
- Sulfonamides, fluoroquinolones, angiotensin-converting enzyme (ACE) inhibitors and tetracyclines cause drug allergy.

Mechanisms of Drug Allergy
Humoral Mechanism
Type I Anaphylactic Reaction
- It is a medical emergency.
- The symptoms are itching, urticaria, swelling of lips, difficulty in breathing, wheeze, fall in BP, angioedema, palpitation and syncope.
- It is due to release of histamine, platelet-activating factor (PAF), leukotrienes and prostaglandins.
- Supportive measures and IM injection of 0.5 mL of 1 in 1000 solution of adrenaline in adults or 0.3 mL of 1 in 1000 solution of adrenaline in children is life saving.
- Intravenous glucocorticoid and intramuscular antihistamine are also helpful.

- Penicillins and cephalosporins can cause anaphylactic reaction.
- It can be detected through intradermal injection of a small test dose.

Type II Cytolytic Reaction
- It is mediated by IgG and IgM antibodies.
- Anemia, thrombocytopenia, leukocytosis, agranulocytosis or aplastic anemia and other blood dyscrasias can occur due to cytolytic reaction.
- These reactions subside on discontinuation of the drug.
- Sulfonamide induced granulocytopenia is caused by cytolytic reaction.

Type III Arthrus Reaction
- Serum sickness characterized by urticaria, arthritis, fever, arthralgia and lymphadenopathy occurs due to type III reaction.
- Penicillins can induce serum sickness.

Cell Mediated Mechanism
Type IV Delayed Hypersensitivity Reaction
- It is a T cell mediated response.
- It is a delayed response and usually occurs after 12 hours.
- Photosensitization, fever and rash can occur.
- Contact dermatitis caused by poison ivy is due to delayed hypersensitivity reaction.

PHOTOSENSITIVITY REACTION
- Both phototoxic and photoallergic responses can occur.
- Phototoxic reaction is more common.
- Phototoxic reaction is due to drugs or their metabolites which accumulate in skin and undergo photochemical reaction when exposed to light causing tissue damage.
- Fluoroquinolones, tetracyclines, dapsone and sulfonamides cause phototoxic reaction.
- They cause sunburn, hyperpigmentation and desquamation.
- Photoallergy is due to type IV delayed cell mediated immunity.
- Griseofulvin, chloroquine and chlorpromazine cause photoallergy.
- These drugs cause papular or eczematous rash.

DRUG DEPENDENCE
- Drugs can result in psychological or physical dependence.
- The person feels emotionally stable only if the drug is taken.

- Opioids such as morphine and heroin can induce such drug seeking behavior.
- Physical dependence is an adaptation of a person's physiological system to the effects of a drug.
- The discontinuation of drug usually results in withdrawal (abstinence) syndrome.
- Alcohol and benzodiazepines can result in physical dependence.

Drug Abuse
- Self medication and repeated use of drug.
- The person uses the drug either continuously or rarely.
- While opioids cause continuous use pattern, amphetamine causes occasional use pattern.

Drug Addiction
- Compulsive use and frequent relapse after abstinence, characterize drug addiction.
- Lysergic acid diethylamide (LSD), cannabis and opioids cause drug addiction.
- They can result in compulsive drug use or drug craving.
- They may not result in physical dependence.

Drug Habituation
- These drugs produce only mild discomfort on discontinuation.
- Physical dependence is absent.
- Coffee and tea cause habituation.

DRUG WITHDRAWAL REACTION
- Adverse reactions occur on sudden discontinuation of some drugs.
- Acute adrenal insufficiency occurs on abrupt cessation of corticosteroid therapy.
- Dose of β blockers should be reduced gradually to prevent their withdrawal effect.

TERATOGENICITY
- Unless absolutely necessary, drugs should not be administered during pregnancy.
- Drugs can cause fetal abnormalities if administered in women during pregnancy.

- These drugs cross placenta and can cause embryotoxicity.
- If given in the first few days, they can cause abortion.
- They can interfere with organogenesis if given during first trimester.
- Therefore, they result in fetal deformities during this period.
- If given at later stage, they can cause developmental abnormalities.
- Hence, only those drugs that are safe during pregnancy should be administered.
- Thalidomide, sex hormones, sodium valproate, ACE inhibitors, phenytoin and lithium are highly teratogenic drugs.
- Drugs are classified into five 'risk category' during pregnancy. Category A is safe drugs, category B indicates no risk in human, category C indicates that risk cannot be ruled out, category D means benefit outweighs risks and category X drugs are absolutely contraindicated.

CARCINOGENICITY
- Drugs can induce DNA mutation and can cause cancer.
- Anticancer drugs and estrogens are few such carcinogenic drugs.

DRUG INDUCED DISEASES
- Peptic ulcer induced by salicylates.
- Osteoporosis induced by corticosteroids.
- Parkinsonism induced by chlorpromazine.
- Stevens-Johnson syndrome induced by sulfonamides.

Treatment of Drug Overdose
- Ipecac syrup which contains emetine and cephaeline, to induce vomiting.
- Emesis should not be induced in poisoning due to corrosive substances.
- Gastric lavage with saline should be done only in hospital set up and it should not be attempted in corrosive poisoning.
- Activated charcoal, the universal antidote adsorbs most drugs.
- Diuretics, with either acidification or alkalinization of urine depending upon the pH of drug, to enhance the excretion of drug.
- Whole bowel irrigation with polyethylene glycol (PEG) to promote excretion of drug through feces.
- Administration of a specific antidote.

- Supportive measures are maintenance of airway, intravenous fluids, plasma expanders and vasopressor to maintain BP, assisted mechanical ventilation, antibiotics to prevent infection and intravenous glucose to facilitate nutrition.

CUMULATIVE TOXICITY

Drugs can accumulate and cause toxicity. Chloroquine and digoxin cause cumulative toxicity.

Nursing Responsibilities
- Patient should be informed about the drugs they are allergic to.
- Patient should be advised to avoid self medication as it is the common cause of drug overdose.
- Care should be taken not to induce hypernatremia while giving salt and water in the management of drug overdose.
- Activated charcoal should not be given in cyanide, arsenic, lithium and iron overdose.
- Charcoal and emetics should not be coadministered.

Chapter 6

Factors Modifying Drug Action

- Dose of a drug can be calculated according to body size and body weight.
- Young's formula and Dilling's formula are used to calculate the dose of a drug according to age.
- Sex of the patient also determines the action of drugs. Women are more sensitive to digoxin than men.
- Racial differences can also alter the response to drugs. Indians tolerate thiacetazone better than whites.
- The drug response can be altered by genetic variability. Succinylcholine apnea occurs in persons with atypical pseudocholinesterase.
- The effect of a drug depends upon the route of administration.
- Environmental factors influence drug action. Insecticides induce drug metabolism. Hypnotics taken at night time are more effective.
- Pathological states such as GIT, liver, kidney and heart disease can decrease the effect of a drug.
- Psychological factor alters the efficacy of drugs. Anxious patients may require more general anesthetic.

TOLERANCE
Prolonged use of a drug resulting in higher dose requirement for the same therapeutic response is known as tolerance.

Types

Innate Tolerance
- It is genetically mediated.
- Natural tolerance to atropine is found in rabbits.
- Ethanol tolerance seen in certain individuals is due to innate tolerance.

Acquired Tolerance
- Pharmacokinetic, pharmacodynamic and learned tolerance.
- **Pharmacokinetic:** Occurs due to changes in distribution or metabolism, e.g. barbiturate.

- **Pharmacodynamic:** Occurs due to changes in receptor density or efficacy, e.g. barbiturate.
- **Learned tolerance:** Occurs due to compensatory mechanism, e.g. alcohol.
- Tolerance may develop to sedative effect of chlorpromazine but not to its antipsychotic action.

Conditioned Tolerance
It is a learned adaptation to drug due to environmental cues such as sight or smell.

Cross Tolerance
- Tolerance occurs among pharmacologically related drugs.
- Cross tolerance occurs between morphine and pethidine.

Acute Tolerance (Tachyphylaxis)
- It is a rapid development of tolerance.
- Ephedrine, amphetamine and tyramine cause tachyphylaxis due to depletion of catecholamine from storage sites.
- Other reasons for development of tachyphylaxis are desensitization of receptors, slow dissociation of a drug from its receptor and internalization of receptors.

CHAPTER 7

Legal Aspects in Nursing Practice

- The five major responsibilities of nursing personnel are to give the right drug at right dose through right route at right time to the right patient.
- The therapy should confer maximum benefit with minimal harm.
- Since the effect of a drug is difficult to reverse, medication error should be avoided before administration of a drug.
- To respond quickly in an emergency, the nursing personnel should always anticipate and should have adequate knowledge about the adverse effects of drugs.
- A proper knowledge about the contraindications of drugs is also necessary.
- Proper assessment of patient's base line data, high risk patients and their ability for self-care are necessary before administration of a drug.
- A drug dose may vary depending upon the clinical condition. The antiplatelet dose of aspirin is lower than its dose required for arthritis.
- The oral dose of morphine is higher than its parenteral dose. Inadvertent parenteral administration of oral dose can prove to be fatal.
- Special care should be taken to avoid extravasation of intravenously administered drugs.
- Intravenous infusion should be monitored closely to detect infusion related reaction.
- The nursing personnel should read the details of prescription before administering a drug.
- They should identify the patient's name, age, sex and also verify the drug, dose, formulation and route of administration before starting therapy.
- They should educate the patient about the drug and should provide necessary emotional support.
- In the event of adverse effect, the patient should be advised to report immediately and these symptoms should be swiftly notified to the attending physician.

- In accordance with law, drugs in Schedule II, III and IV should not be dispensed to persons other than patients to whom they are prescribed.

IMPORTANT DRUG LAWS

- **1878—The Opium Act:** Controls cultivation, manufacture, possession, sale, import and export of opium.
- **1919—The Poisons Act:** Controls possession, import and sale of poisonous substances.
- **1940—The Drugs and Cosmetics Act:** Deals with operation related to allopathic, ayurvedic, siddha, unani, homeopathic drugs as well as cosmetics.
- **1954—The Drugs and Magic Remedies Act:** Prevents misleading advertisements.
- **1985—The Narcotic and Psychotropic Substances Act:** Prohibits cultivation, manufacture, purchase, sale and distribution of all narcotic and psychotropic substances.
- **1995—The Price Control/Drug Order:** Deals with control of prices of bulk drugs and drug formulations.

SECTION II

Autonomic Nervous System

- ✦ Cholinergics
- ✦ Anticholinergics
- ✦ Adrenergic Agonists
- ✦ Alpha Blockers
- ✦ Beta Blockers
- ✦ Skeletal Muscle Relaxants
- ✦ Ganglionic Stimulants and Blockers
- ✦ Local Anesthetics

CHAPTER 8

Cholinergics

Cholinergics are broadly classified as:
- Choline esters
- Natural alkaloids
- Anticholinesterases

CHOLINE ESTERS
The choline esters are:
- Acetylcholine
- Methacholine
- Carbachol
- Bethanechol

Acetylcholine
- It is a parasympathetic neurotransmitter.
- It is not used therapeutically as it is hydrolyzed within seconds.

Actions
- It causes vasodilatation mediated by endothelial nitrous oxide.
- It is vagomimetic and causes direct inhibition of heart.
- It decreases heart rate and blood pressure.
- It reduces conduction velocity.
- It decreases the force of cardiac contraction.
- It causes bronchoconstriction and increases tracheobronchial secretion.
- It increases tone and amplitude of gastrointestinal smooth muscles.
- It increases gastric and intestinal secretion.
- It promotes contraction of detrusor muscles.
- It reduces bladder capacity and increases voiding pressure.

Methacholine
- It has longer duration of action.
- It is highly selective and acts predominantly on muscarinic receptors.

- It has very minimal nicotinic action.
- It is used to evaluate the bronchial hyperactivity, to rule out bronchial asthma.
- This provocative test should be performed only in the presence of supportive measures such as oxygen, bronchodilator and emergency resuscitation equipment.
- This test is contraindicated in patients with known asthma, recent myocardial infarction (MI), pregnancy and uncontrolled hypertension.

Carbachol
- It is completely resistant to hydrolysis by cholinesterases.
- It has substantial nicotinic activity.
- It is used topically as a miotic and in glaucoma.

Bethanechol
- It is an analog of carbachol.
- It is completely resistant to cholinesterases.
- Its actions are predominantly muscarinic in gastrointestinal tract (GIT) and urinary bladder.
- It results in minimal nicotinic action.
- It is used for postoperative urinary retention and postoperative paralytic ileus.
- It is also used to improve smooth muscle motility in patients with diabetic autonomic neuropathy.
- Further, it is effective in neurogenic and hypotonic bladder.

Nursing Responsibilities
- Bethanechol should be given on empty stomach either 1 hour before or 2 hours after a meal.
- Adequate fluid replacement should be ensured in patients with bethanechol induced vomiting.
- In postoperative paralytic ileus, following administration of bethanechol, flatus indicates recovery of intestinal motility.

NATURAL ALKALOIDS
Natural cholinergic alkaloids are:
- Pilocarpine
- Arecoline
- Muscarine

Pilocarpine
- It acts on muscarinic receptors.
- It increases salivary secretion and stimulates sweat glands.
- It can cross the blood-brain barrier (BBB).
- It is effective in relieving xerostomia in Sjögren's syndrome.
- It is also used to increase salivation after head and neck radiation therapy.
- It is available as 'ocusert' or ocular insert for the treatment of glaucoma.

Muscarine
- It acts on muscarinic receptors.
- Its oral absorption is poor.
- It is not used therapeutically.

Arecoline
- It stimulates both muscarinic and nicotinic receptors.
- It readily crosses BBB.
- It is not used therapeutically.

Cevimeline
- It selectively acts on M_3 receptors.
- It increases salivary and lacrimal secretion.
- It has long duration of action.
- It is used in Sjögren's syndrome.

Contraindications of Cholinergic Alkaloids
- Bronchial asthma
- Chronic obstructive pulmonary disease (COPD)
- Peptic ulcer
- Hypotension and shock
- Hyperthyroidism.

Adverse Effects of Cholinergic Alkaloids
Diaphoresis, sialorrhea, diarrhea, nausea, vomiting, abdominal cramp and hypotension.

ANTICHOLINESTERASES
Anticholinesterases (AChE) are classified as reversible and irreversible agents.

Reversible, Long Acting AChE
- Physostigmine
- Neostigmine
- Pyridostigmine
- Ambenonium
- Demecarium
- Tacrine
- Donepezil
- Galantamine

Reversible, Short Acting AChE
Edrophonium

Irreversible, Long Acting AChE
- Echothiophate
- Malathion
- Parathion
- Diazinon
- Sarin
- Soman
- Tabun

Reversible Anticholinesterases
- They stimulate both muscarinic and nicotinic receptors.
- They bind with peripheral 'anionic or acetyl' and central 'cationic or esteric' sites of cholinesterase enzyme.
- The acetylated esteratic site of cholinesterase enzyme is stable but is slowly hydrolyzed.
- Therefore, they cause only temporary inhibition of the enzyme.
- Hence, binding at esteratic site of cholinesterase enzyme is reversible.

Physostigmine
Actions
- It is an alkaloid and a carbamate ester.
- It is a tertiary amine, crosses BBB and penetrates cornea.
- Its duration of action is short.
- It acts on both central and peripheral cholinergic receptors.
- It causes conjunctival hyperemia.
- It results in miosis and 'near vision'.
- It reduces intraocular pressure.

Cholinergics 37

- It is absorbed from GIT, mucous membrane and subcutaneous tissue.
- It can enter into systemic circulation following conjunctival instillation.

Uses
- Glaucoma
- Atropine overdose with central symptoms
- To reverse central anticholinergic symptoms due to tricyclic antidepressants (TCA), phenothiazines and antihistamines.

Neostigmine

Actions
- It does not cross BBB and acts on only peripheral cholinergic receptors.
- Its nicotinic action is more prominent than its muscarinic action.
- It accumulates in motor end plates and stimulates nicotinic receptors directly.
- Since it causes persistent stimulation of the nicotinic receptors, it promotes twitching and fasciculation of skeletal muscles resulting in paralysis.
- It increases the tone and motility of intestine.
- It increases gastric secretion.
- It decreases blood pressure and heart rate.
- It causes bronchoconstriction.
- It is absorbed poorly from GIT.

Uses
- Myasthenia gravis
- Paralytic ileus
- Atony of urinary bladder
- Reversal of paralysis induced by competitive neuromuscular blockers
- Cobra bite
- Atropine overdose without central symptoms.

Nursing Responsibilities
- Neostigmine does not reverse skeletal muscle paralysis induced by succinylcholine.
- It should not be administered in the presence of organic obstruction of bladder or intestine.
- It should be avoided in peritonitis.

Pyridostigmine
- Since its GIT absorption is poor, higher dose is required for oral administration.
- It has long duration of action.
- It is available as sustained release preparation.
- It is used in myasthenia gravis.

Nursing Responsibilities
Pyridostigmine prophylaxis reduces the mortality associated with nerve gas soman poisoning.

Ambenonium
- Its duration of action is longer than neostigmine and physostigmine.
- It is effective in myasthenia gravis.

Demecarium
- Structurally, it contains two molecules of neostigmine.
- It has longer duration of action than neostigmine.

Edrophonium
- It is a quaternary ammonium compound.
- It is a reversible anticholinesterase.
- Its duration of action is short as it is excreted quickly.
- It is used in the diagnosis of myasthenia gravis.

Rivastigmine, Tacrine and Donepezil
- They are lipophilic reversible anticholinesterases.
- Hence, they have more central than peripheral action.
- They have long duration of action.
- They are used in Alzheimer's disease.

Myasthenia Gravis
- It is an autoimmune neuromuscular disease.
- The prominent symptoms are weakness and fatigue.
- Remissions and exacerbations are the characteristic features.
- It occurs due to improper synaptic transmission at motor end plates.
- Defective neuronal transmission is due to development of antibodies to postsynaptic cholinergic nicotinic receptors.

Cholinergics

Diagnostic Test
- A rapid intravenous administration of 2 mg edrophonium improves muscle strength.
- Additional 8 mg after 45 seconds is required whenever the first dose fails to evoke a response.

Nursing Responsibilities
Intravenous (IV) atropine should be administered immediately if symptoms worsen after edrophonium.

Treatment
- Neostigmine 7.5 to 15 mg improves muscle strength for 2 to 4 hours (or).
- Pyridostigmine 30 to 60 mg provides improvement for 3 to 6 hours (or).
- Pyridostigmine is also available as a sustained release (SR) formulation of 180 mg (or).
- Ambenonium 2.5 to 5 mg causes improvement for 3 to 8 hours.
- Tolerance can occur for the therapeutic benefit of anticholinesterases.
- Glucocorticoids and thymectomy are helpful if the condition does not improve with anticholinesterases therapy.

Sustained release (SR) preparation should not be chewed but should be swallowed as a whole formulation.

Uses of Reversible Anticholinesterases
- Primary, secondary and congenital glaucoma.
- Postoperative paralytic ileus.
- Postoperative urinary retention.
- Tonic pupil due to local denervation.
- Myasthenia gravis.
- Breaking adhesions between iris and ciliary body.
- Prophylaxis of nerve gas soman poisoning.
- Alzheimer's disease.

Irreversible Anticholinesterases
- These agents bind mainly to centrally placed esteratic site of the enzyme and phosphorylate it.
- Such phosphorylated site undergoes minimal hydrolysis so, is highly stable for many hours.

- Further, aging or loss of an alkyl group enhances the stability of the phosphorylated enzyme.
- Hence these agents cause permanent inhibition of the cholinesterase enzyme.
- However, echothiophate binds to both anionic and cationic site.

Organophosphorus Compound Poisoning
- Symptoms are miosis, eye pain, vision impairment, redness, brow ache, hypotension, increased salivary and respiratory secretion, bronchospasm, nausea, vomiting, diarrhea, abdominal cramp, urination, fasciculation, convulsion, ataxia, slurred speech, respiratory paralysis and coma.

Treatment
- **Specific treatment: atropine and oximes.**
  - **Atropine** 2 mg IV every 5 to 10 minutes till dryness of mouth or till pupils dilate
  - **Oximes:** pralidoxime, obidoxime

Supportive Measures
- Protection of patient from further exposure by removing contaminated clothing.
- Maintenance of airway.
- Administration of oxygen.
- Artificial respiration, if necessary.
- IV Diazepam 5 to 10 mg if convulsions occur

Oximes
- They reactivate acetylcholinesterase enzyme.
- Organophosphates, except echothiophate bind to the esteratic site of the acetylcholinesterase enzyme.
- Oximes bind to the unoccupied anionic site of the acetylcholinesterase enzyme, phosphorylating the organophosphates attached to the esteric site, detaching them to reactivate the enzyme.
- They are effective only if given before 'aging' of the phosphorylated enzyme.
- Aging occurs due to loss of alkyl group resulting in a more stable acetylcholinesterase.

CHAPTER 9

Anticholinergics

Anticholinergics are broadly classified as:
- Natural alkaloids
- Semisynthetic derivatives
- Synthetic derivatives

NATURAL ALKALOIDS
They are atropine and scopolamine.

Atropine

Actions
- It increases the heart rate.
- It does not alter blood pressure and cardiac output.
- It causes cutaneous vasodilatation and 'atropine flush' at toxic doses.
- It reduces airway resistance and causes bronchodilatation.
- It reduces salivary and tracheobronchial secretion.
- It causes mydriasis and cycloplegia.
- This results in photophobia and blurred vision.
- It reduces gastrointestinal tract (GIT) motility, tone, amplitude of intestinal smooth muscles.
- It reduces intestinal secretion and promotes constipation.
- It reduces voiding pressure, promoting urinary retention.
- It is an antispasmodic and relaxes bile duct and ureters.
- It inhibits activity of sweat glands and skin becomes dry and hot.
- It is well absorbed orally.
- At toxic doses, it causes central nervous system (CNS) excitation.

Adverse Effects
- Blurring of vision, cycloplegia, urinary retention, dry mouth, hot flushed skin, fever, constipation, mydriasis, restlessness, disorientation, irritability and delirium.

Scopolamine

Actions
- It is also known as hyoscine.
- It penetrates cornea and crosses blood brain barrier (BBB).
- Unlike atropine, it is a CNS depressant at therapeutic dose.
- It causes fatigue, amnesia and drowsiness.
- Its duration of action is short.
- It inhibits the neural pathways from vestibular apparatus to vomiting center.
- So it is effective in motion sickness.
- It is effective only as a prophylactic, if given before undertaking a journey.
- It is available as transdermal patch for this purpose.
- It was formerly used as an anesthetic adjunct due to its ability to cause amnesia.

SEMISYNTHETIC DERIVATIVES OF ATROPINE
The drugs are:
- Homatropine
- Ipratropium bromide
- Tiotropium bromide

Homatropine
- It causes mydriasis and minimal cycloplegia.
- It is more potent than atropine
- It has short duration of action
- It is used for fundoscopy.

Ipratropium and Tiotropium
- They have selective action on respiratory system.
- They cause bronchodilatation and reduce respiratory and salivary secretion.
- They are given through inhalational route.
- Hence they are used in the treatment of respiratory conditions.
- Tiotropium is more effective than ipratropium.
- While ipratropium is available as aerosol or solution, tiotropium is available as dry powder which delays its onset of action.
- The effect of ipratropium persists only for 4 to 6 hours but tiotropium acts for 24 hours and can be administered once a day.

Anticholinergics 43

- They are very effective in chronic obstructive pulmonary disease (COPD) and in rhinorrhea of common cold.
- They are less effective in bronchial asthma.

SYNTHETIC DERIVATIVES OF ATROPINE
The drugs are:
- Cyclopentolate
- Tropicamide
- Glycopyrrolate
- Dicyclomine
- Pirenzepine
- Telenzepine
- Oxybutynin
- Solifenacin
- Darifenacin
- Tolterodine
- Trospium chloride
- Fesoterodine
- Trihexyphenidyl
- Biperiden

Cyclopentolate
- It causes mydriasis and cycloplegia rapidly
- It has short duration of action
- It is used for testing refractory error
- It is also used in iridocyclitis and keratitis.

Tropicamide
- Its onset of action is quick
- Its termination of effect is rapid
- It causes mydriasis and insufficient cycloplegia
- It is used for fundoscopy.

Glycopyrrolate
- It reduces bronchial and salivary secretion
- It does not cause central effects when given as anesthetic adjuvant
- It is used as anaesthetic adjuvant.

Dicyclomine
- It is a weak anticholinergic agent
- It has more selective action on smooth muscles

- It is a direct smooth muscle relaxant
- Hence, it is used as an antispasmodic agent
- It is used in dysmenorrhea, abdominal colic, motion sickness and morning sickness.

Pirenzepine, Telenzepine
- It is a selective M_1 blocker
- Telenzepine, its analog is highly potent
- It can be used in peptic ulcer
- It has minimal side effects.

Oxybutynin
- It is useful in overactive bladder
- It causes xerostomia
- It is available as transdermal patch, topical gel and oral extended release formulation
- Transdermal application minimizes its side effects.

Tolterodine
- It has greater bladder selectivity
- Fesoterodine, its prodrug is converted to its active metabolite tolterodine.

Trospium
- It is a quaternary amine
- It is effective in overactive bladder
- It is excreted mainly through kidneys.

Solifenacin, Darifenacin
- It is a selective M_3 blocker
- It is used in overactive bladder.

Trihexyphenidyl, Biperiden
- They are centrally acting atropine substitutes
- They are effective in 'drug induced Parkinsonism'
- They are also used as adjuvant to levodopa in Parkinsonism.

Uses of Anticholinergics
- Organophosphorus compound poisoning
- Intestinal, biliary and ureteric colic
- Fundoscopy examination

- For testing refractory error
- Keratitis, iridocyclitis
- Motion sickness
- Anesthetic adjuvant
- Overactive bladder
- Atrioventricular (AV) block
- Parkinsonism.

Atropine Overdose

- It can be either accidental or suicidal.
- Overdose of H_1 antihistamines, tricyclic antidepressants (TCA) and phenothiazines can also cause anticholinergic side effects.
- Dryness of mouth, restlessness, delirium, headache, palpitation, depression and circulatory collapse can occur.
- Intravenous administration of physostigmine is confirmatory if it does not elicit salivation, sweating, bradycardia, urination or defecation.

Treatment
- Gastric lavage
- IV physostigmine 2 mg. To be repeated if necessary.

Nursing Responsibilities
- Patient suffering from dryness of mouth induced by anticholinergics can benefit by chewing gum.
- In case of photophobia, patient is advised to wear dark glasses.
- To prevent toxicity due to high blood level, extended release preparation should not be crushed or chewed.

Adrenergic Agonists

Adrenergic agonists are broadly classified into:
- Directly acting adrenergic drugs
- Indirectly acting adrenergic drugs
- Mixed acting adrenergic drugs

DIRECTLY ACTING ADRENERGIC DRUGS
The drugs are:
  A. **Selective**
   Phenylephrine
   Clonidine
   Dobutamine
   Terbutaline
  B. **Nonselective**
   Adrenaline
   Noradrenaline
   Oxymetazoline
   Isoprenaline

INDIRECTLY ACTING ADRENERGIC DRUGS
- Amphetamine
- Tyramine
- Cocaine
- Selegiline
- Entacapone

MIXED ACTING ADRENERGIC AGONISTS
Ephedrine

Adrenaline/epinephrine
Actions
- It acts on both α and β receptors.
- It is a powerful cardiac stimulant.

- It increases heart rate, cardiac contractility, cardiac output and cardiac workload.
- It increases BP but decreases peripheral resistance.
- At small dose, it reduces blood pressure.
- It increases cerebral, muscular and splanchnic blood flow.
- It reduces cutaneous and renal blood flow.
- It increases the automaticity of sinoartial (SA) node and shortens the refractory period of atrioventicular node (AV) node.
- It decreases the tone and amplitude of intestinal contraction.
- It reduces the contraction of pregnant uterus at term.
- It relaxes detrusor muscle and causes retention of urine.
- It is a potent bronchodilator and inhibits the release of inflammatory mediators from mast cells.
- It increases blood glucose and free fatty acid levels.
- It inhibits insulin release and promotes glucagon release.
- It increases the number of circulating polymorphonuclear leucocytes.
- It causes mydriasis and reduces intraocular pressure.
- By increasing potassium uptake by skeletal muscles, it causes hypokalemia.
- It facilitates neuromuscular transmission.
- It is not effective orally.
- The absorption is slow through subcutaneous administration but rapid through intramuscular route.
- It can be also administered through intravenous and inhalational route.
- It is metabolised by catechol-o-methyl transferase (COMT) and monoamine oxidase (MAO).

Adverse Effects
- Throbbing headache, restlessness, tremor, palpitation, cardiac arrhythmia, cerebral hemorrhage.

Contraindications
- Hypertension
- Angina
- Hyperthyroidism
- In patients receiving monoamine oxidase inhibitors (MAOI) or tricyclic antidepressants (TCA).

Uses
- Anaphylaxis
- To prolong the action of local anesthetics
- Cardiac arrest or complete heart block
- Topical hemostatic agent for bleeding peptic ulcer during endoscopy
- Infectious croup.

Nursing Responsibilities
- Adrenaline should not be given through oral route
- Blood pressure should be monitored before topical application
- Heart rate to be monitored even when it is applied locally
- Adrenaline is a life saving drug in anaphylaxis.

Noradrenaline/norepinephrine

Actions
- It stimulates α receptors more than β_2 receptors.
- It increases systolic, diastolic and pulse pressure.
- It increases peripheral resistance.
- It does not alter cardiac output.
- It reduces renal, splanchnic and hepatic blood flow.
- It increases coronary blood flow.
- It is not effective orally.
- It is poorly absorbed after subcutaneous administration as it causes severe vasoconstriction.

Adverse Effects
- Hypertension
- Sloughing and necrosis at the infusion site in case of extravasation.

Contraindications
- Hypertension
- Angina
- In patients receiving MAOI or TCA.

Uses
- As vasopressor in shock.

Nursing Responsibilities
- BP should be monitored constantly during infusion of noradrenaline to prevent drug induced hypertension
- Renal output should also be monitored regularly in patients on IV infusion of noradrenaline as it reduces renal blood flow

- It should not be administered into normal saline infusion
- It should be given only with 5% dextrose solution.

Dopamine
Actions
- It is a precursor of noradrenaline and adrenaline.
- It is also a central neurotransmitter.
- It acts on dopamine, α_1 and β_1 adrenergic receptors.
- At low dose, dopamine dilates renal, mesenteric and coronary blood vessels.
- Moderate dose increases heart rate.
- High dose increases blood pressure.

Contraindications
In patients receiving MAOI or TCA.

Adverse Effects
Nausea, vomiting, angina, arrhythmia and headache.

Uses
- Cardiogenic shock
- Septic shock
- Congestive heart failure with oliguria.

Nursing Responsibilities
- Infusion of IV fluids or whole blood is necessary before infusion of dopamine in shock
- An antiemetic drug should be kept ready during infusion of dopamine
- Dopamine infusion should be given through calibrated infusion pump into larger veins
- During dopamine infusion, it is important to monitor heart rate.

Fenoldopam
Actions
- It is a dopamine agonist and acts on dopamine receptors.
- It has rapid onset of action.
- It has minimal oral bioavailability as it undergoes extensive first pass metabolism.
- It dilates coronary, renal and mesenteric arteries.
- It is used in hypertensive emergency.

Adverse Effects
Flushing, dizziness, headache and tachycardia.

Nursing Responsibilities
It should be administered only through calibrated infusion pump.

Dopexamine
- It is a synthetic analog of dopamine.
- It acts on dopamine and β_2 receptors.
- It inhibits reuptake of catecholamines.
- It is effective in severe congestive heart failure, shock and sepsis.

NONSELECTIVE BETA RECEPTOR AGONISTS
Isoprenaline
Actions
- It acts on β_1, β_2 and β_3 adrenergic receptors.
- It increases the rate and force of contraction of heart.
- It increases cardiac output.
- It can cause palpitation and arrhythmia.
- It decreases the diastolic pressure as it reduces peripheral resistance.
- It relaxes intestinal and bronchial smooth muscles.
- It reduces histamine release from mast cells.
- Its absorption is adequate when given as aerosol formulation.

Adverse Effects
Palpitation, flushing, headache, arrhythmia.

Uses
To increase heart rate in heart block.

Nursing Responsibilities
Even through inhalational route, it should not be given to patients with bronchial asthma.

Dobutamine
Actions
- It acts on α_1 and β_1 receptors.
- It increases force of contraction of heart.
- It increases cardiac output.
- It has a very short half-life of 2 minutes.
- Tolerance develops to its pharmacological action.
- It is administered as intravenous infusion.

Adrenergic Agonists

Adverse Effects
Tachycardia, hypertension.

Uses
Cardiogenic shock.

Nursing Responsibilities
- It should be administered through calibrated infusion pump.
- Heart rate and BP should be monitored during its infusion.

SELECTIVE SHORT ACTING β_2 ADRENERGIC RECEPTORS
Metaproterenol/Orciprenaline
Actions
- It acts on β_2 adrenergic receptors.
- In addition to dilatation of bronchial muscles it can also stimulate heart.
- On oral administration, the onset of action is slow and its duration is short.
- Through inhalational route, its onset of action is quick and the duration of action is long.

Uses
- Chronic obstructive pulmonary disease (COPD)
- Bronchial asthma
- Treatment of acute bronchospasm.

Nursing Responsibilities
It should be given only as inhalation in acute bronchial spasm.

Albuterol
Actions
- It is a selective β_2 receptor agonist and causes significant bronchodilatation.
- It is available as metered dose inhaler.
- It can be administered orally as well as through inhalational route.
- The action starts within 15 minutes through inhalational route.
- It is administered orally to prevent preterm labor.
- It is the drug of choice in acute asthma.

Levalbuterol
- It is an albuterol enantiomer.
- It causes bronchodilatation.

- It is available as a solution for nebulizer and as metered dose inhaler.

Pirbuterol
- It is a bronchodilator.
- It is available only as metered dose inhaler.

TERBUTALINE
Actions
- It is a bronchodilator and acts on β_2 receptors.
- It can be administered through oral, subcutaneous or inhalational route.
- It is used for long-term therapy.

Uses
- Bronchial asthma
- Status asthmaticus
- Chronic obstructive pulmonary disease

SELECTIVE LONG ACTING β_2 AGONISTS
Salmeterol
Actions
- It is a selective β_2 agonist.
- It has slow onset of action but prolonged duration of action.
- So, it is not suitable for acute exacerbations of bronchial asthma.
- It provides symptomatic relief and improves lung function in COPD.
- It is given with ipratropium or theophylline in COPD.
- It is very effective in nocturnal asthma.

Adverse Effects
- It is usually well tolerated.
- It can result in tremor, hypokalemia and can increase plasma glucose level.

Uses
- Bronchial asthma
- Chronic obstructive pulmonary disease

Nursing Responsibilities
It should not be administered more than two times a day.

Formoterol

Actions
- It has a long duration of action and its effect persists upto 12 hours.
- When administered through inhalational route the onset of action is very quick.
- It is very effective in nocturnal asthma.

Uses
- Nocturnal asthma
- Chronic obstructive pulmonary disease
- Prophylactic agent in exercise induced asthma.

Nursing Responsibilities
For patients suffering from nocturnal asthma, formoterol and salmeterol are suitable.

Arformoterol

Actions
- Arformoterol is twice as potent as formoterol.
- It inhibits histamine and leukotrienes release.
- It is approved for long-term therapy in COPD.

Adverse Effects
- Tremor, insomnia, tachycardia, cramps, hypokalemia, hyperglycemia.

Uses
- Chronic obstructive pulmonary disease
- Emphysema
- Chronic bronchitis.

Carmoterol
- It has five times more selective action on β_2 receptors.
- It has rapid onset and long duration of action.
- Hence, it is suitable for once daily administration.
- It is used in COPD and in bronchial asthma.

Indacaterol
- It has quick onset of action.
- Its duration of action is longer than salmeterol and formoterol.
- It is effective in COPD and bronchial asthma as once daily administration.

- Unlike salmeterol, it does not antagonize the action of short acting β_2 agonists.
- Minimal development of tachyphylaxis occurs on continuous use.

Ritodrine
- It is used as uterine relaxant to arrest premature labor.
- Its oral absorption is quick but incomplete.
- Hence, it is administered intravenously in premature labor.
- It causes relaxation of uterine muscle by stimulating β_2 receptors.

Adverse Effects of Selective β_2 Agonists
- Tremor is the common side effect.
- Tolerance, tachycardia, hypokalemia, hyperglycemia and increased lactate level can also occur.

Nursing Responsibilities for Selective β_2 Agonists
Blood sugar should be monitored periodically during administration of selective β_2 agonists especially in diabetics.

SELECTIVE α_1 ADRENERGIC AGONISTS

Phenylephrine

Actions
- It is a selective α_1 agonist.
- It causes marked vasoconstriction.
- It is administered through intravenous and intranasal route.
- It causes mydriasis and is also available as eye drops.

Uses
- Nasal decongestant
- As mydriatic for fundoscopy.

Nursing Responsibilities
It is preferred to atropine substitutes as mydriatic in elders for fundoscopy where cycloplegia is not required.

Mephentermine

Actions
- It acts both directly and indirectly.
- It is administered through intramuscular route.
- It has quick onset of action and the effect persists for a long period.
- It increases blood pressure and cardiac contraction.

Adrenergic Agonists

Adverse Effects
Hypertension, arrhythmia
Uses
Hypotension during spinal anesthesia.

Metaraminol
- It acts both directly and indirectly.
- It has direct vascular action.
- It releases noradrenaline indirectly.

Uses
- Hypotension.
  - **Off label use:** Paroxysmal atrial tachycardia

Midodrine
- It is a prodrug and the action is due to its active metabolite.
- It stimulates α_1 receptors and causes contraction of arterial and venous smooth muscles.

Uses
Postural hypotension in patients with autonomic neuropathy.

Nursing Responsibilities
Dose is titrated by frequent monitoring of blood pressure.

SELECTIVE α_2 ADRENERGIC AGONISTS

Clonidine
See Section VI, Chapter 31

Apraclonidine
- Unlike clonidine, it does not cross BBB.
- It reduces intraocular pressure by reducing production of aqueous humor.
- It is used as short-term adjunctive in therapy of glaucoma.

Brimonidine
- It crosses blood brain barrier (BBB) resulting in sedation and hypotension.
- It reduces intraocular pressure by reducing aqueous humor production and by increasing its outflow.
- It is used in open angle glaucoma and in patients with ocular hypertension.
- It should be used cautiously in cardiac patients.

Guanfacine
Actions
- It has more selective action at α_2 receptors and lowers blood pressure.
- Its efficacy is similar to clonidine.
- It is available as sustained release preparation.
- It can cause mild withdrawal syndrome on sudden discontinuation.

Adverse Effects
Dry mouth, sedation

Uses
Attention deficit hyperactivity disorder (ADHD) in children.

Guanabenz
Similar to guanfacine but undergoes high first pass metabolism.

Alpha Methyl Dopa
See Section VI, Chapter 31

Tizanidine
- It is a α_2 receptor agonist and a muscle relaxant.
- It is used in spasticity associated with cerebral and spinal lesions.

MISCELLANEOUS DRUGS
Amphetamine
Actions
- It increases both systolic and diastolic blood pressure.
- It causes reflex bradycardia but can cause cardiac arrhythmias at high doses.
- It does not alter cerebral blood flow.
- It increases bladder capacity and contracts external sphincter.
- It is a powerful CNS stimulant and stimulates cortical as well as reticular activating system.
- It increases alertness, ability to concentrate and reduces fatigue.
- It improves self-confidence and causes euphoria.
- It postpones the need for sleep and stimulates wakefulness.
- It improves physical and mental performance.
- It also reduces appetite.
- Prolonged use can result in fatigue and depression.
- It stimulates medullary respiratory center, increasing rate and depth of respiration.

Adrenergic Agonists

Adverse Effects
- Headache, dizziness, panic, aggressiveness, confusion, insomnia, suicidal and homicidal tendency
- Dry mouth, metallic taste, nausea, vomiting, diarrhea
- Restlessness, talkativeness, palpitation, arrhythmia
- Tolerance, dependence

Uses
- Approved by FDA in narcolepsy, ADHD, nocturnal enuresis.
- Off label use in obesity.

Nursing Responsibilities
- Acidification of urine facilitates excretion of amphetamine in drug overdose.
- The drug should be administered only under medical supervision.

Methamphetamine
- It releases dopamine and other catecholamine in brain.
- Low dose results in predominant central action while high dose causes sustained increase of blood pressure and cardiac output.
- It is a recreational drug with abuse potential listed under schedule II controlled substances.
- It is a controlled substance under federal regulations.

Methylphenidate
- It is a mild central nervous system (CNS) stimulant.
- Its cerabrospinal fluid (CSF) concentration exceeds its plasma concentration.
- It is a drug with abuse potential and listed under schedule II controlled substances.
- It is used for narcolepsy and ADHD.
- It is contraindicated in glaucoma.

Dexmethylphenidate
- It is also listed under schedule II of controlled substances.
- It is indicated in ADHD.

Premoline
- It has more CNS and minimal cardiac action.
- It has prolonged duration of action.
- So, it can be administered once daily.
- It is not available now as it can cause hepatotoxicity.
- It is indicated in ADHD.

Ephedrine

Actions
- It acts on both α and β receptors.
- It increases heart rate, cardiac output and peripheral resistance.
- It is a CNS stimulant and a powerful bronchodilator.
- Its action is prolonged and persists for several hours.
- It also causes urinary retention.

Adverse Effects
Hypertension, insomnia

Uses
- Narcolepsy
- Spinal shock during spinal anesthesia.
- Urinary incontinence in men with benign prostatic hypertrophy (BPH).
- Strokes-Adams attack with complete heart block.

Nursing Responsibilities
Due to variability in ephedrine content of ephedrine containing dietary preparations, patients should be advised not to use them to avoid overdose of the drug.

Therapeutic uses of adrenergic agonists (sympathomimetics)
- Shock
- Hypotension
- Hypertension
- Cardiac arrest
- Local hemostatic agent
- To prolong the duration of action of local anesthetics
- Nasal decongestion
- Bronchial asthma
- Anaphylaxis
- Glaucoma
- Narcolepsy
- Obesity
- ADHD

CHAPTER 11

Alpha Blockers

Alpha blockers are classified as:
- Nonselective α blockers
- Selective $α_1$ blockers
- Selective $α_2$ blockers

SELECTIVE $α_1$ BLOCKERS

The drugs are:
- Prazosin
- Terazosin
- Tamsulosin
- Silodosin
- Alfuzosin
- Bunazosin
- Indoramin
- Urapidil

Common Adverse Effects of $α_1$ Blockers
- First dose effect – hypotension following initial dose.
- Orthostatic hypotension
- Syncope
- Asthenia
- Headache, dizziness.

Prazosin

Actions
- It has greater $α_1$ receptor selectivity and blocks all $α_1$ receptor subtypes.
- It causes peripheral vasodilatation and reduces the venous return.
- This in turn reduces cardiac preload.
- It reduces blood pressure but does not cause reflex tachycardia.
- Oral absorption is good and it is extensively metabolized in liver.

Adverse Effects
See common adverse effects of $α_1$ blockers.

Uses
Hypertension.

Off Label Use
Benign prostatic hypertrophy (BPH)

Terazosin

Actions
- Although less potent, it is highly selective to α_1 receptors.
- It is well absorbed orally with 90% bioavailability.
- It has long duration of action and can be administered once daily.
- It is very effective in BPH as it induces apoptosis of prostatic smooth muscle cells.

Adverse Effects
See common adverse effects of α_1 blockers.

Uses
- Benign prostatic hypertrophy
- Hypertension

Doxazosin

Actions
- It causes a more selective blockade of α_1 receptors.
- It has long duration of action and can be administered once daily.
- It induces apoptosis of prostatic smooth muscle cells.
- It is effective in long-term management of BPH.

Adverse Effects
See common adverse effects of α_1 blockers.

Uses
- Benign prostatic hypertrophy
- Hypertension.

Alfuzosin

Actions
- It has high affinity for α_1 receptors.
- It is extensively used in BPH.
- It induces apoptosis of prostatic cells.
- It is not approved in the treatment of hypertension.

- It is available as extended release preparation.
- Extended release preparation of alfuzosin should be administered after meal at same time everyday.

Adverse Effects
See common adverse effects of α_1 blockers.

Contraindications
It should not be administered to patients on enzyme inducers and those with prolonged QT syndrome.

Tamsulosin

Actions
- It selectively blocks α_{1A} subtype receptors present in prostate.
- Hence, tamsulosin is suitable for therapy of BPH.
- It is not approved for the treatment of hypertension.

Adverse Effects
Abnormal ejaculation

Other Adverse Effects
See common adverse effects of α_1 blockers.

Silodosin

Actions
- It causes more selective blockade of α_{1A} receptors.
- It is approved for the treatment of BPH.
- It is not very effective in the treatment of hypertension.

Adverse Effects
Retrograde ejaculation

Other Adverse Effects
See common adverse effects of α_1 blockers.

Nursing Responsibilities of α_1 Blockers
- Patient should be advised to take the first dose during night time to prevent 'first dose effect'.
- Patient should be given reassurance that this 'first dose effect' disappears on continuation of therapy.
- Patient should be warned not to increase the dose suddenly without physician's advice otherwise, they can suffer from syncope.

SELECTIVE α_2 BLOCKERS
Yohimbine is a selective α_2 blocker.

Yohimbine
Actions
- It is a competitive antagonist of α_2 receptors.
- It readily crosses BBB.
- It increases heart rate and blood pressure.

Adverse Effects
Tremor

Uses
- Erectile dysfunction
- Diabetic neuropathy
- Postural hypotension.

NONSELECTIVE α BLOCKERS
The drugs are:
- Phenoxybenzamine
- Phentolamine.

Phenoxybenzamine
Actions
- Phenoxybenzamine is a nonselective, classical antagonist of α receptors.
- It is an irreversible antagonist.
- It reduces blood pressure by causing peripheral vasodilatation.
- It causes reflex tachycardia.

Adverse Effects
- Postural hypotension
- Cardiac arrhythmia.

Uses
- Inoperable malignant pheochromocytoma
- It is given 1 to 3 weeks prior to surgery in pheochromocytoma.

Phentolamine
Actions
- Phentolamine is a nonselective, competitive antagonist of α receptor.

- It is a reversible α receptor blocker.
- It reduces blood pressure by causing peripheral vasodilatation.
- It causes reflex tachycardia.

Adverse Effects
- Postural hypotension
- Cardiac arrhythmia.

Uses
- Short-term control of blood pressure in pheochromocytoma.
- Pseudo bowel obstruction in patients with pheochromocytoma.
- Hypertensive crisis following abrupt discontinuation of clonidine.
- Prevention of dermal necrosis.

Ergot Alkaloids
See Section III, Chapter 17

Indoramin
Actions
- It is a selective, competitive α_1 receptor blocker.
- It also blocks the histamine and serotonin receptors.
- It undergoes high first pass metabolism.

Adverse Effects
- Dry mouth, sedation
- Failure of ejaculation

Uses
- Prophylaxis of migraine
- Hypertension
- Benign prostatic hypertrophy
- Raynaud's phenomenon.

Beta Blockers

Beta blockers are classified as:
- Nonselective β blockers
- Selective $β_1$ blockers
- Selective $β_1$ third generation blockers

NONSELECTIVE β BLOCKERS

The drugs are:
- Propranolol
- Nadolol
- Penbutolol
- Pindolol
- Timolol

Common Properties of Nonselective β Blockers
- They block both $β_1$ and $β_2$ adrenergic receptors.
- They reduce the heart rate, cardiac contractility, cardiac output and conduction velocity.
- They increase the refractory period.
- They cause bronchoconstriction in patients with COPD.
- They reduce plasma free fatty acid and high density lipoprotein chlorestrol (HDLC) levels.
- They increase low density lipoprotein chlorestrol (LDLC) and triglyceride levels.
- They blunt the hypokalemic action of adrenaline.

Adverse Effects of Nonselective β Blockers
- Bradycardia and bradyarrhythmia
- Bronchoconstriction
- Fatigue
- Insomnia, nightmare, sexual dysfunction
- In diabetic patients on insulin, they delay the recovery from hypoglycemia.

Uses of Nonselective β Blockers
- Angina
- Myocardial infarction
- Hypertension
- Cardiac arrhythmia
- Pheochromocytoma
- Glaucoma
- Hyperthyroidism
- Prophylaxis of migraine
- Variceal bleeding in portal hypertension
- Hypertrophic obstructive cardiomyopathy
- Acute panic symptoms

Nursing Responsibilities
- Patients should be informed not to discontinue β blockers abruptly.
- Patients should be advised not to miss even a single dose of β blocker.
- Monitoring the ECG and BP is absolutely essential during therapy.

Propranolol
Actions
- It has membrane stabilizing effect (MSA).
- It does not have intrinsic sympathomimetic activity (ISA).
- It blocks both $β_1$ and $β_2$ adrenergic receptors.
- It is completely absorbed orally, highly lipophilic and undergoes high first pass metabolism.
- Inter-individual differences determine its plasma concentration.
- Repeated increase in dose is required to attain maximum therapeutic benefit.
- It has short half-life but prolonged antihypertensive effect.
- Food increases its absorption on prolonged therapy.
- Sustained release formulation of propranolol is available.
- It can be administered IV in life-threatening arrhythmia.

Adverse Effects
See common adverse effects of nonselective β blockers.

Uses
- Hypertension
- Angina
- Myocardial infarction
- Ventricular arrhythmia

- Supraventricular tachycardia
- Pheochromocytoma
- Essential tremor
- Prophylaxis of migraine

Off Label Uses
- Parkinsonian tremor
- Akathisia
- Generalized anxiety disorder
- Variceal bleeding

Nadolol

Actions
- It is a long acting drug and blocks both β_1 and β_2 receptors.
- It neither has ISA nor MSA.
- It is incompletely absorbed and has minimal inter-individual differences.

Adverse Effects
See common adverse effects of nonselective β blockers.

Uses
- Hypertension
- Angina

Off Label Uses
- Parkinsonian tremor
- Migraine prophylaxis
- Variceal bleeding

Timolol

Actions
- It does not have either MSA or ISA.
- It is a nonselective blocker and blocks both β_1 and β_2 adrenergic receptors.
- On topical administration, it reduces intraocular pressure.
- It is available as eye drops for use in glaucoma.
- Systemic absorption can occur after topical application in eye.
- This can cause bronchoconstriction in patients with bronchial asthma.

Adverse Effects
See common adverse effects of nonselective β blockers.

Uses
- Open angle glaucoma
- Intraocular hypertension
- Hypertension
- Migraine prophylaxis

Pindolol
Actions
- It is a nonselective β blocker.
- It has high ISA and low MSA.
- It has low lipid solubility.
- It is well absorbed so it causes minimal inter-individual differences.
- It reduces exercise-induced increase in cardiac output and tachycardia.

Adverse Effects
See common adverse effects of nonselective β blockers.

Uses
- Angina
- Hypertension

SELECTIVE β_1 BLOCKERS
The drugs are:
- Atenolol
- Acebutolol
- Esmolol
- Metoprolol
- Bisoprolol

Metoprolol
Actions
- It is a selective β_1 blocker.
- It has no ISA and MSA.
- Although completely absorbed, it has low oral bioavailability as it undergoes high first pass metabolism.
- It is generally administered two times a day.
- Extended release preparation of metoprolol is available for once daily administration.

Adverse Effects
Bradycardia, dizziness, fatigue, hypotension.

Uses
- Angina
- Secondary prevention after myocardial infarction
- Vasovagal syncope
- Congestive heart failure (CHF)
- Migraine prophylaxis

Nursing Responsibilities
Twenty four hours BP and heart rate should be monitored to assess its therapeutic response.

Atenolol

Actions
- It is a selective β_1 blocker.
- It does not have either ISA or MSA.
- It is incompletely absorbed.
- Since it is hydrophilic, its central nervous system (CNS) concentration is low.
- Hence, the incidence of CNS side effects such as depression and nightmare are minimal.
- It can cause inter-individual difference in plasma concentration.

Adverse Effects
Hypotension, fatigue, dizziness

Uses
- Hypertension
- Angina
- Arrhythmia
- Coronary artery disease

Esmolol

Actions
- It has a very short duration of action.
- It is a selective β_1 blocker.
- It has no ISA or MSA.
- It is given as slow intravenous administration in arrhythmia.

Adverse Effects
Bradycardia, dizziness, fatigue, hypotension

Uses
- Supraventricular tachycardia
- Perioperative hypertension.

Nursing Responsibilities
Esmolol infusion should not be given in persons with normal BP or to those on β blockers.

Acebutolol
Actions
- It is a selective β_1 receptor antagonist.
- It has both ISA and MSA.
- It is well absorbed orally and it undergoes high first pass metabolism.
- It is lipophilic and attains high concentration in CNS.

Adverse Effects
Bradycardia, dizziness, fatigue, hypotension

Uses
- Hypertension
- Myocardial infarction
- Ventricular and atrial arrhythmias

Bisoprolol
Actions
- It has high selectivity to β_1 receptors.
- It has neither ISA nor MSA.
- It is well absorbed and attains adequate plasma concentration.

Adverse Effects
Bradycardia, dizziness, fatigue, hypotension

Uses
- Hypertension
- Stable CHF
- Ischemic heart disease
- Arrhythmia

IIIrd GENERATION β_1 BLOCKERS
They have additional cardiovascular effects. The drugs are:
- Betaxolol
- Labetalol

- Carvedilol
- Bucindolol
- Celiprolol
- Nebivolol
- Carteolol

Betaxolol

Actions
- It does not have ISA but has minimal MSA.
- It has high oral bioavailability.
- It causes minimal adverse effects.

Uses
- Hypertension
- Glaucoma
- Angina.

Labetalol

Actions
- It blocks α_1, β_1 and β_2 receptors.
- It has both MSA and ISA.
- It causes vasodilatation and reduces blood pressure.
- It maintains renal, coronary and cerebral blood flow.
- It does not reduce peripheral blood flow.
- It is completely absorbed.
- It undergoes extensive first pass metabolism.
- Still it is available as oral preparation for long-term therapy of chronic hypertension.
- It is also available as intravenous formulation in hypertensive emergency.

Uses
- Hypertensive emergency
- Hypertension
- Pheochromocytoma

Carvedilol

Actions
- It blocks α_1, β_1 and β_2 receptors.
- It has both antioxidant and anti-inflammatory property.
- It reduces synthesis of reactive oxygen species (ROS) and inhibits ROS mediated apoptosis.

- It blocks calcium channel at high doses.
- It has MSA but no ISA.
- It is rapidly absorbed and is highly lipophilic.

Uses
- Hypertension
- Left ventricular dysfunction following myocardial infarction (MI)
- Congestive heart failure

Bucindolol
Actions
- It is a strong β_1 and β_2 blocker but weak blocker of α_1 receptors.
- It reduces afterload as it causes peripheral vasodilatation.
- It is well absorbed and extensively bound to plasma proteins.
- It increases HDLC but does not affect triglycerides.

Celiprolol
Actions
- It blocks β_1 receptors but is an agonist at β_2 receptors.
- It has no MSA but has ISA.
- It reduces heart rate and blood pressure.
- It has low lipid solubility so has minimal CNS action.
- It does not undergo high first pass metabolism.
- It is a weak bronchodilator.
- It increases vascular nitric oxide production and reduces oxidative stress.

Uses
- Hypertension
- Angina

Nebivolol
Actions
- It is a IIIrd generation selective β_1 blocker.
- It reduces BP and preserves cardiac output.
- It induces endothelial nitric oxide release.
- It has antioxidant property.
- It maintains splanchnic blood flow.
- It increases insulin sensitivity and does not alter lipid profile.
- It does not have MSA or ISA.
- Less fatigue and minimal sexual dysfunction are its advantage.

Uses
Hypertension

GLAUCOMA
- Increased intraocular pressure causing progressive degeneration of optic nerves.
- The normal intraocular pressure (IOP) is 21 mm of Hg.
- Drugs that reduce IOP are effective in the therapy of glaucoma.
- They either reduce the production of aqueous humor or increase its drainage.

I. Prostaglandins
The $PGF_{2\alpha}$ agonists are effective at low concentration in therapy of glaucoma. They increase aqueous humor drainage. The drugs used are:
- Latanoprost
- Bimatoprost
- Travoprost

II. Beta blockers
They reduce aqueous humor production. The drugs used are:
- Timolol
- Betaxolol
- Carteolol
- Metipranolol
- Levobunolol

III. Adrenergics

A. Nonselective Adrenergic Agonists
They reduce aqueous humor production and also facilitate its drainage. The drugs are:
- Adrenaline
- Dipivefrine

B. Selective α_2 Agonists:
They facilitate drainage of aqueous humor. The drugs are:
- Apraclonidine
- Brimonidine

IV. Carbonic Anhydrase Inhibitors

They reduce aqueous humor formation. The drugs used are:
- Acetazolamide
- Dorzolamide

V. Cholinergics

They increase drainage of aqueous humor. They are rarely used now. They are:
- Pilocarpine
- Physostigmine

Drugs Used in Open Angle Glaucoma

β blockers, adrenergic agonists, prostaglandins, carbonic anhydrase inhibitors and cholinergics.

Narrow Angle or Acute Congestive Glaucoma
- It is a medical emergency.
    It is treated by:
- IV hypertonic mannitol
- IV acetazolamide
- Topical timolol
- Topical apraclonidine.

Chapter 13: Skeletal Muscle Relaxants

Skeletal muscle relaxants are broadly classified as:
  A. Centrally acting muscle relaxants
  B. Peripherally acting muscle relaxants which is sub classified as:
     I. Neuromuscular or nondepolarizing competitive blockers
     II. Depolarizing blockers
     III. Directly acting skeletal muscle relaxants

NEUROMUSCULAR BLOCKERS
The drugs are:

A. Long Acting
- D-Tubocurarine
- Doxacurium
- Pancuronium
- Pipecuronium
- Metocurine

B. Intermediate Acting
- Atracurium
- Cisatracurium
- Rocuronium
- Vecuronium

C. Short Acting
- Mivacurium

D. Ultrashort Acting
- Gantacurium

Actions
- They block the binding of acetylcholine at nicotinic cholinergic receptors in motor end plate.
- They cause motor weakness that progress to flaccid paralysis.
- The rapidly moving muscles are paralyzed first.

- Order of paralysis is from eye, jaw, laryngeal muscles and progress to limb and trunk muscles.
- Finally they result in paralysis of diaphragm.
- Recovery occurs in the reverse order.
- Oral absorption is minimal and they do not cross BBB.
- They are effective only through IM or IV route.
- They cause histamine release from mast cells.
- Histamine release is minimal with pancuronium bromide, pipecuronium bromide, vecuronium bromide and rocuronium bromide.
- They also potentiate the curarimimetic action of aminoglycosides.
- Rocuronium bromide has rapid onset of action.
- Hence, it is used in 'rapid induction anesthesia' for relaxation of jaw and laryngeal muscles to facilitate endotracheal intubation.
- Hence they have good cardiovascular stability, do not result in hypotension and do not cause bronchospasm.
- Atracurium besylate and cisatracurium besylate are preferred in patients with renal dysfunction.
- Both atracurium besylate and cisatracurium besylate undergo spontaneous elimination by plasma esterase.
- This process of elimination is known as 'Hoffman elimination'.
- Gantacurium chloride is an ultrashort acting drug.

Drug Interaction

Tetracycline, aminoglycoside, clindamycin, lincomycin, polymyxin B and colistin potentiate the neuromuscular blockade of competitive blockers.

Adverse Effects

- Bronchospasm, apnea
- Hypotension

Uses

- Adjuvant during surgery to facilitate muscular relaxation.
- During laryngoscopy, bronchoscopy and esophagoscopy.
- During electroconvulsive therapy (ECT).

Nursing Responsibilities

Either atropine or glycopyrrolate and a vasoconstrictor should be kept ready during neostigmine administration for reversal of skeletal muscle relaxants to counteract bronchospasm and to stabilize the blood pressure.

DEPOLARIZING MUSCLE RELAXANTS
Actions
- Succinylcholine is a depolarizing skeletal muscle relaxant.
- It acts by 'dual mechanism'.
- It causes fasciculation followed by neuromuscular blockade and respiratory paralysis.
- The order of paralysis starts from chest, abdomen and then proceeds to other muscles.
- It undergoes hydrolysis by plasma and hepatic butyrylcholinesterase.
- Hence it is extremely short acting with very rapid onset of action and quick termination of effect.
- Continuous IV administration is required to prolong its effect.
- It causes succinylcholine apnea in patients with atypical pseudocholinesterase.
- Muscle soreness is common after its use.
- It causes minimal histamine release, but life-threatening hyperkalemia.

Contraindications
- Rhabdomyolysis
- Hyperkalemia
- Children <8 years
- Paraplegia, hemiplegia, spinal cord injury, muscular dystrophy
- Should not be given in patients receiving digoxin and potassium sparing diuretics.

Uses
- Adjuvant to anesthetics during surgery.
- During laryngoscopy, bronchoscopy and esophagoscopy.
- During ECT.

Nursing Responsibilities
- Patient will have muscle soreness after succinylcholine administration.
- It should be avoided with drugs causing hyperkalemia.

Sugammadex
Actions
- It is a reversal agent for competitive neuromuscular agents.
- It chelates these agents and forms insoluble complex, promoting their excretion.

- It has high affinity for vecuronium bromide and rocuronium bromide.

Adverse Effects
Dysgeusia, hypersensitivity.

Nursing Responsibilities
Sugammadex induced hypersensitivity reaction is often self-limiting.

DIRECTLY ACTING SKELETAL MUSCLE RELAXANT
Actions
- Dantrolene is a directly acting skeletal muscle relaxant.
- It blocks the release of calcium from sarcoplasmic reticulum of skeletal muscles.
- It is given IV in the treatment of malignant hyperthermia.

Adverse Effects
Fatigue, hepatotoxicity

Uses
- Malignant hyperthermia
- Neuroleptic malignant syndrome
- Spasticity
- Hyperreflexia

Malignant Hyperthermia
- Susceptibility is due to autosomal dominant genetic trait.
- It is a life-threatening medical emergency.
- It is common when succinylcholine is combined with halogenated anesthetics such as halothane, sevoflurane or isoflurane.
- Body temperature increases by 1°C in every 5 minutes.
- Uncontrolled release of calcium from sarcoplasmic reticulum causes rigidity, hyperthermia, tachycardia and metabolic acidosis.

Treatment
IV dantrolene

Nursing Responsibilities
- In malignant hyperthermia, rapid cooling is essential to reduce body temperature immediately.
- 100% oxygen should be administered.
- Acidosis should be managed.

Centrally Acting Muscle Relaxants

The drugs are:
- Mephenesin
- Carisoprodol
- Chlorzoxazone
- Methocarbamol
- Benzodiazepines
- Baclofen
- Tizanidine

Actions
- They decrease spinal and supraspinal reflexes.
- Therefore they reduce rigidity and spasticity.
- By inhibiting reticular activating system, they reduce wakefulness and cause sedation.
- Eventhough they reduce the muscle tone, they do not inhibit the voluntary movements.

Uses
- Paraplegia
- Hemiplegia
- Cerebral palsy

CHAPTER 14

Ganglionic Stimulants and Blockers

GANGLIONIC STIMULANTS

Actions
- Nicotine stimulates the autonomic ganglia.
- It can cause stimulation as well as desensitization of receptors.
- It can stimulate and inhibit both sympathetic and parasympathetic ganglia.
- It is a weak analgesic at low doses but causes tremor at high doses.
- It stimulates vomiting through both central and peripheral actions.
- It causes tachycardia and increases blood pressure.
- It increases the tone and motility of intestine.
- Initially, it increases salivary and bronchial secretions but later it reduces them.
- It is well absorbed from respiratory tract, buccal mucosa and skin.
- It has limited absorption from the intestine.

Nursing Responsibilities
Since the absorption of nicotine from nicotine gum is slow from the intestine, it prolongs the effect of nicotine and preferred in de-addiction.

GANGLION BLOCKERS
The drugs are:
- Trimethaphan
- Mecamylamine
- Hexamethonium

Actions
- They reduce BP in patients in erect posture than in those in recumbent posture.
- They reduce cardiac output in those with normal cardiac function but increase it in cardiac failure patients.

- They reduce the intestinal motility, cause mydriasis, cycloplegia, xerostomia, and urinary retention.
- They have unpredictable oral absorption.

Adverse Effects

Postural hypotension, visual disturbances, dry mouth, urinary retention, constipation or diarrhea.

Uses:
- Hypertensive crisis
- Controlled hypertension.

CHAPTER 15

Local Anesthetics

The drugs are:
- Lidocaine/lignocaine
- Cocaine
- Bupivacaine
- Ropivacaine
- Procaine
- Chloroprocaine
- Articaine
- Mepivacaine
- Prilocaine
- Tetracaine
- Benzocaine
- Proparacaine
- Dyclonine
- Pramoxine

Actions
- They inhibit generation and conduction of nerve impulses.
- They abolish pain first, followed later by sensation of temperature, touch, deep pressure and motor function.
- Their duration of action can be prolonged by adrenaline which causes vasoconstriction delaying their absorption from the site of injection.
- They stimulate CNS causing restlessness, tremor and convulsion.
- Central nervous system (CNS) stimulation is followed by depression resulting in drowsiness.
- Except cocaine, all other local anesthetics inhibit heart rate and force of cardiac contraction.
- They relax bronchial and vascular smooth muscles.

LIDOCAINE
Actions
- Its onset of action is quick and duration of action is long.
- On oral administration, it undergoes high first pass metabolism.

- It is available as topical, mucosal and ophthalmic formulation.
- It is also available as transdermal patch and oral patch.
- It can be given through intramuscular route.
- It is administered into cerebrospinal fluid (CSF) in lumbar space for spinal anesthesia.
- It is administered into epidural space for epidural anesthesia.
- In order to delay its absorption and to prolong its duration, it is usually combined with a vasoconstrictor, adrenaline.

Adverse Effects

Tinnitus, dizziness, drowsiness, seizures, respiratory depression, dysgeusia

Uses

- Suitable local anesthetic for procedures requiring intermediate duration of anesthesia such as dental procedures, venipuncture and skin grafting.
- Arrhythmia

COCAINE

Actions

- Unlike other local anesthetics, it increases blood pressure.
- It causes mydriasis.
- It is a sympathomimetic drug with both direct and indirect action.
- On topical application in respiratory tract, in addition to its anesthetic action, it shrinks the mucosa.
- It causes euphoria and has high potential for abuse.
- It is a controlled substance under Schedule II drugs.

Uses

Topical application for upper respiratory tract for anesthetic and mucosal shrinking action.

BUPIVACAINE

Actions

- It has long-duration of action and results in prolonged anesthesia.
- It causes more sensory than motor blockade.
- It dissociates very slowly from cardiac sodium channels causing cardiotoxicity.
- Hence, bupivacaine induced ventricular arrhythmia is difficult to treat.

Adverse Effects
Ventricular arrhythmia

Uses
Obstetric anesthetic

Articaine
It has rapid onset and intermediate duration of action.

CHLOROPROCAINE
Actions
- The onset of action is quick and the termination of effect is rapid.
- It causes prolonged sensory as well as motor blockade.
- It can be administered through epidural and spinal route.
- Earlier preparation containing sodium metabisulfite was neurotoxic and is no more used.
- Current preparation containing calcium ethylenediaminetetra-acetic acid (EDTA) as preservative is safe and not neurotoxic but causes tetany of paraspinous muscle and results in back pain following epidural anesthesia.
- This is due to binding of muscular calcium to the preservative EDTA.

MEPIVACAINE
Actions
- It is an intermediate acting local anesthetic.
- It is not effective as topical anesthetic.
- Its duration of action is longer than lidocaine.
- It is much safer than lidocaine and has high therapeutic index.
- It accumulates in acidic pH of neonatal blood.
- Hence it is toxic to neonates and not preferred as obstetric anesthetic.

PRILOCAINE
Actions
- It is an intermediate acting local anesthetic.
- It is a mild vasodilator and does not require the vasoconstrictor, adrenaline.

- It causes minimal CNS toxicity.
- It is suitable for IV regional block.
- It is not used as obstetric anesthetic as it causes neonatal methemoglobinemia.

ROPIVACAINE

Actions

- It is a long-acting local anesthetic.
- Its actions are similar to bupivacaine but it is less cardiotoxic.
- It is more motor sparing than bupivacaine.
- It is suitable for epidural and regional anesthesia.

PROCAINE

Actions

- It is a low potency infiltration anesthetic.
- It has slow onset of action and short duration of action.
- It is occasionally used for diagnostic nerve blocks.
- It inhibits the action of sulfonamides.

TETRACAINE

Actions

- It is more potent but has slow onset of action.
- It has long duration of action.
- It is slowly metabolized resulting in systemic toxicity.
- It is given as spinal anesthetic when prolonged anesthesia is required.

DYCLONINE

Actions

- The onset of action is quick but the duration of action is short.
- It is also absorbed through skin and mucous membrane.
- It is a component of 'over-the-counter' sore throat, lozenges.
- It is used for topical anesthesia during endoscopy.
- It is used topically for pain due to oral mucositis and pain following cancer chemotherapy or radiation therapy.

PRAMOXINE
Actions
- It is a surface anesthetic and can be applied on skin and mucous membrane.
- It is available as lotion, cream, foam, wipes, gel, spray and as ear drops.
- It should not be used as local anesthetic in eyes as it causes irritation.
- It can be used safely in patients allergic to other local anesthetics.

Benzocaine
It results in sustained action but can cause methemoglobinemia.

PROPARACAINE
Actions
- It causes minimal irritation to eyes as it is less antigenic.
- It can be applied topically on cornea and conjunctiva.
- It can be used for patients allergic to other local anesthetics.

Nursing Responsibilities
- Care should be taken not to apply local anesthetics on abraded skin or mucous membrane as it can be absorbed.
- Excess application in infants for reducing pain and itching in napkin rash can result in systemic absorption.
- Injection of local anaesthetic containing adrenaline should be avoided in fingers, toes, nose and ears to reduce risk of gangrene.
- Care should be taken not to inflate the tourniquet for more than 2 hours during IV regional block anesthesia to avoid nerve damage.
- The tourniquet should remain inflated for a minimum period of 15 to 20 minutes.
- Oxygen, IV fluids, and vasopressor are necessary if BP falls below 30% of its resting value during spinal anesthesia.
- Local anesthetics should be instilled as single drop at a time in the eye. Subsequent drops should be instilled only if the anesthetic action is inadequate.
- Patients should be advised against self-medication of local anesthetic in eyes as it can cause pitting or sloughing of corneal epithelium.

SECTION III

Autacoids

- Antihistamines
- Serotonin Agonists and Antagonists
- Lipid Derived Autacoids

CHAPTER 16

Antihistamines

Antihistamines are broadly classified as:
- H_1 antihistamines
- H_2 antihistamines: **See Section IX, Chapter 50**

H_1 ANTIHISTAMINES

These drugs act by blocking H_1 receptors. The drugs are further subclassified as:
  A. Highly sedative, first generation H_1 antihistamines
  B. Nonsedative, second generation H_1 antihistamines

First Generation H_1 Antihistamines
- Diphenhydramine
- Dimenhydrinate
- Hydoxyzine
- Promethazine
- Meclizine
- Cinnarizine
- Cyproheptadine
- Chlorpheniramine

Actions
- They inhibit histamine mediated bronchoconstriction.
- They block H_1 receptor mediated vasodilatation but not H_2 receptor mediated vasodilatation.
- They inhibit edema, itch, pain and allergy mediated by histamine.
- These agents have strong anticholinergic property.
- They are well absorbed orally and enter the central nervous system (CNS).
- Hence they cause sedation.
- They inhibit the release of leukotrienes and platelet activating factor.
- They do not cause psychomotor impairment.

- Promethazine, cyclizine and meclizine are used in motion sickness and vertigo.
- Dimenhydrinate and meclizine are used in Meniere's disease.
- Promethazine has additional local anesthetic property.
- Hydoxyzine concentrates in skin.

Second Generation H_1 Antihistamines
- Cetirizine
- Fexofenadine
- Loratadine
- Levocetirizine
- Azelastine
- Rupatadine
- Ketotifen
- Ebastine

Actions
- These compounds are highly selective in action.
- They attain minimal CNS concentration.
- So, they cause minimal sedation.
- They do not have anticholinergic property.
- Rupatadine inhibits platelet activating factor (PAF) receptor that contributes to its anti-inflammatory activity.

Cetirizine
- It is a metabolite of hydroxyzine and acts on peripheral H_1 histamine receptors.
- Although it crosses blood-brain barrier (BBB) poorly, it can cause somnolence at higher doses.
- It concentrates in skin and has superior efficacy in urticaria and atopic dermatitis.
- It can be safely administered during pregnancy.

Fexofenadine
- It is a metabolite of terfenadine but does not cause cardiotoxicity.
- It does not cause sedation or psychomotor impairment.
- It is not safe in pregnancy as it causes teratogenicity.

Azelastine
- It has good topical action and available as intranasal preparation.
- It is teratogenic and should not be used during pregnancy.
- It is administered intranasally for seasonal allergic rhinitis.
- It can cause stinging sensation through this route.

Common Adverse Effects of H_1 Antihistamines
- Sedation, hangover, dizziness, tinnitus, fatigue, incoordination, blurred vision, diplopia, euphoria
- Epigastric distress, constipation, dry mouth, urinary retention
- Drug fever, photosensitization
- Leukopenia, agranulocytosis, hemolytic anemia

Uses of H_1 Antihistamines
- Allergy
- Limited efficacy in bronchial asthma, anaphylaxis and angioedema
- Seasonal rhinitis
- Allergic conjunctivitis
- Urticaria
- Pruritus
- Atopic dermatitis
- Contact dermatitis
- Symptomatic in rhinorrhea of common cold
- Motion sickness
- Vertigo

Nursing Responsibilities
- Patients on H_1 antihistamines should be told to avoid driving vehicles.
- Elders above 65 years can tolerate only low dose second generation H_1 antihistamines.

Chapter 17: Serotonin Agonists and Antagonists

SEROTONIN ANTAGONISTS
- Methysergide
- Risperidone
- Cyproheptadine
- Katanserin
- Ondansetron
- Granisetron

Methysergide

Actions
- It is an ergot derivative.
- It is neither a selective serotonin agonist nor a selective serotonin antagonist.
- It is not effective in acute migraine.
- It can cause inflammatory fibrosis.
- Hence it is rarely used.

Adverse Effects
Pleuropulmonary fibrosis, retroperitoneal fibrosis, endocardial and coronary fibrosis.

Uses
- Migraine prophylaxis.
- Other vascular headache.

Nursing Responsibilities
Patients should be informed not to take methysergide continuously for prophylaxis of migraine.

Cyproheptadine

Actions
- It blocks both histamine and serotonin receptors.
- It has an additional weak anticholinergic property.
- It causes CNS depression.

Adverse Effects
Increased appetite, weight gain, sedation, dry mouth.

Uses
- Allergy
- Pruritus
- Appetite stimulant

Off Label Uses
- Carcinoid syndrome
- Post-gastrectomy dumping syndrome
- Migraine prophylaxis

Katanserin

Actions
- It is a serotonin antagonist.
- It also blocks α adrenergic and histamine receptors.
- It inhibits platelet aggregation mediated by serotonin.
- It dilates both arteries and veins.
- It lowers BP in hypertensive persons.

Uses
Schizophrenia, migraine, depression

Atypical Antipsychotics
The atypical antipsychotics clozapine and risperidone have serotonin blocking property.

SEROTONIN AGONISTS
- Sumatriptan
- Naratriptan
- Rizatriptan
- Almotriptan
- Eletriptan
- Zolmitriptan
- Cisapride
- Buspirone, ipsapirone, gepirone

Triptans

Actions
- They cause selective vasoconstriction of cranial vessels.
- They also inhibit release of proinflammatory neuropeptides.

- They can be given orally, intranasally and subcutaneously.
- Zolmitriptan has higher oral bioavailability than sumatriptan.
- The bioavailability of naratriptan is 70%.
- Rizatriptan is available as orally dissolving formulation.

Adverse Effects
- Transient myocardial infarction (MI) and coronary artery vasospasm in patients with coronary artery disease (CAD).
- Sumatriptan causes pain and stinging at the site of injection.
- Sumatriptan nasal spray causes bitter taste.
- Oral administration of triptans causes fatigue, paresthesia, flushing, drowsiness and tightness of chest.

Contraindications
- Coronary artery disease
- Cerebrovascular disease
- Peripheral vascular disease
- Uncontrolled hypertension

Uses
Acute migraine

Nursing Responsibilities
- Subcutaneous route is preferred in migraine patients with nausea and vomiting.
- The relief of pain is quicker with sumatriptan nasal spray.
- A 24 hours gap should be maintained between administration of triptans and ergot alkaloids.
- Patients should be warned not to take triptans more than thrice within 1 month.

Ergot Alkaloids

Actions
- They block serotonin, dopamine and adrenergic receptors.
- They have low oral bioavailability due to high first pass metabolism.
- Rectal suppository increases their plasma concentration.
- Although they have short half-life, their action persists for 24 hours.
- They cause vasoconstriction of cerebral vessels.
- They are not suitable for prophylaxis of migraine.

- Ergotamine and dihydroergotamine are used in migraine.
- Ergometrine is used in postpartum hemorrhage.

Adverse Effects
Nausea, vomiting, weakness of limbs, numbness, tingling, local edema, itching.

Uses
- Moderate frequent migraine
- Severe infrequent migraine
- Postpartum hemorrhage

Nursing Responsibilities
Incidence of nausea and vomiting is two times higher after oral than after parenteral administration.

Buspirone
- It is a serotonin agonist.
- Gepirone and ipsapirone are other drugs.
- It is effective in treatment of anxiety.

Migraine
- It is characterized by unilateral throbbing headache.
- The two forms of migraine are 'common migraine without aura' or 'classic migraine with aura'.
- One episode of migraine lasts from few hours to many days.
- Photophobia, hyperacusis and mood disturbance are common symptoms.

Therapy of Acute Migraine
- **Mild:** Analgesics such as Nonsteroidal anti-inflammatory drugs (NSAIDs)
- **Moderate:** NSAIDs alongwith triptans/ergot alkaloids
- **Severe:** Triptans/ergot alkaloids.

Prophylaxis
- **Beta blocker:** Propranolol
- **Calcium channel blocker:** Flunarizine
- **Antiepileptics:** Gabapentin
- **Tricyclic antidepressants (TCA):** Amitriptyline

CHAPTER 18
Lipid Derived Autacoids

USES OF PROSTAGLANDINS
Abortion
- Prostagladins E (PGE_2) (dinoprostone) and PGE_1 (misoprostol) are used.
- They are effective during first trimester.
- Dinoprostone can induce abortion during second trimester of pregnancy.
- They can be administered as intravaginal pessary.
- They can be combined with mifepristone.
- They are contraindicated in ectopic pregnancy.
- They can cause nausea, vomiting, bleeding, uterine hyperactivity.
- They are indicated in missed abortion, molar gestation and midterm abortion.

Cervical Priming, Induction and Augmentation of Labor
- Low dose of PGE_2 (dinoprostone) and PGE_1 (misoprostol) applied intravaginally are effective.
- Intracervical gel or vaginal insert of dinoprostone can be used.
- Dinoprostone should be removed after 12 hours or at the onset of labor.
- A maximum of only 3 doses within a period of 24 hours can be used.
- Vaginal misoprostol should be repeated every 4 to 6 hours.

Peptic Ulcer
- PGE_1 (misoprostol) is used.
- It is effective in NSAID induced gastritis.

Glaucoma
- $PGF_{2\alpha}$ analogs latanoprost and travoprost is used.

Maintenance of Patency of PDA
- PGE_1 analog alprostadil is used.

Pulmonary Hypertension
- PGI_2 (epoprostenol) is used.

Erectile Dysfunction
- PGE_1 (alprostadil) is used.

Leukotriene Antagonist
See Section X, Chapter 53

SECTION IV

Central Nervous System

- Ethyl Alcohol
- General Anesthetics
- Sedatives and Hypnotics
- Antiepileptic Drugs
- Drugs used in Neurodegenerative Disorders
- Opioid Analgesics

CHAPTER 19

Ethyl Alcohol

ACTIONS

- It acts as a counterirritant and rubifacient when applied topically.
- At low concentration, it stimulates appetite and increases gastric secretion.
- At higher concentration, it reduces the gastric secretion.
- It causes chronic diarrhea and malabsorption.
- It causes chronic pancreatitis.
- It is a central nervous system (CNS) depressant.
- It promotes the inhibitory activity of gamma-aminobutyric acid (GABA) and inhibits the excitatory action mediated through N-Methyl-D-aspartate (NMDA) receptors.
- Its euphoric effect and alcohol craving are mediated through dopaminergic system.
- These effects diminish in chronic users.
- If stopped suddenly, it causes withdrawal syndrome.
- It interferes with mental coordination and causes apathy.
- It causes slurred speech and unsteady gait.
- Although it is a mild vasodilator, on chronic use it increases blood pressure.
- It may precipitate arrhythmia and cardiomyopathy.
- It dilates skin vessels and causes feeling of warmth.
- It causes dose related hepatotoxicity resulting in cirrhosis, hepatitis or fatty degeneration of liver.
- Chronic intake of alcohol reduces muscle strength and promotes atrophy.
- It promotes diuresis by inhibiting the release of vasopressin.
- It is teratogenic and causes fetal alcohol syndrome.
- It is metabolized by alcohol dehydrogenase and aldehyde dehydrogenase.
- On chronic use, it acts as an enzyme inducer and induces metabolism of coadministered drugs.
- It follows first order kinetics of excretion initially but switches over to zero order kinetics when it reaches saturation level.

ADVERSE EFFECTS
- Osteoporosis
- Megaloblastic anemia
- Microcytic anemia
- Pancreatitis
- Esophageal cancer
- Hepatotoxicity
- Diarrhea
- Nutritional deficiency
- Vitamin B deficiency resulting in peripheral neuropathy, Korsakoff's psychosis and Wernicke's encephalopathy.

USES
- Antiseptic
- Appetizer
- Topical application in fever
- Trigeminal neuralgia
- Methyl alcohol poisoning

NURSING RESPONSIBILITIES
- Ethyl alcohol can be used for sponging in patients with high fever.
- It can also be used to prevent bed sores.
- It is a household remedy for fainting attack.
- Patients with ethanol induced hepatotoxicity should be advised to take vitamin E.
- Diarrhea and pruritus ani are common in chronic alcoholics.

TREATMENT OF ALCOHOL ADDICTION
Disulfiram
- It is an antabuse and used for de-addiction of alcohol.
- It inhibits aldehyde dehydrogenase and inhibits alcohol metabolism.
- Thereby it increases the plasma level of acetaldehyde.
- Ingestion of alcohol in patients treated with disulfiram causes dizziness, headache, flushing, palpitation, nausea, vomiting and hypotension.
- It does not prolong the abstinence or reduce alcohol craving.

Ethyl Alcohol

Adverse Effects
- Headache
- Urticaria
- Tremor
- Fatigue
- Metallic or garlic taste
- Acne.

Nursing Responsibilities
- De-addiction should be initiated only in 'hospital set-up'.
- In patient's willing for de-addiction, it is important to rule out alcohol consumption for atleast 12 hours prior to administration of disulfiram.

Naltrexone
- It is an opioid antagonist and given daily for maintenance of abstinence.
- It blocks the dopaminergic pathway involved in alcohol craving and euphoria.
- It prolongs the abstinence period and reduces craving for alcohol.
- It has higher oral bioavailability than naloxone.
- It has longer duration of action.
- It can cause nausea, more frequently in women.
- Naltrexone can also cause hepatotoxicity.
- Nalmefene has better bioavailability and longer duration of action.
- Nalmefene does not cause hepatotoxicity.

Acamprosate
- It is a GABA agonist and NMDA antagonist.
- It reduces alcohol craving.
- It prolongs abstinence.
- It can cause diarrhea and headache.

TREATMENT OF METHYL ALCOHOL POISONING
- Gastric lavage
- Sodium bicarbonate to correct acidosis.
- Correction of hypokalemia and hypoglycemia, if present.
- Ethyl alcohol is life saving and recommended as it competes with methanol for aldehyde dehydrogenase.

- Fomepizole to inhibit alcohol dehydrogenase.
- Alkalinization of urine to promote excretion.

Fomepizole
- It inhibits alcohol dehydrogenase and inhibits the metabolism of methyl alcohol.
- It is very effective but costly.
- It can cause headache and dizziness.
- It can also be used to treat ethylene glycol poisoning.

CHAPTER 20

General Anesthetics

These agents cause reversible loss of consciousness. They are:
I. **Inhalational anesthetics**
   - **Volatile liquids:** Diethyl ether, halothane, enflurane, isoflurane, desflurane, sevoflurane
   - **Gas:** Nitrous oxide, xenon.
II. **Intravenous anesthetics**
   - **Barbiturates:** Thiopentone sodium, methohexital
   - Propofol
   - **Dissociative anesthetic:** Ketamine
   - α_2 **agonists:** Dexmedetomidine
   - **Miscellaneous:** Etomidate

DIETHYL ETHER

Advantages
- It is a good analgesic.
- It does not need a special apparatus.
- It is a good skeletal muscle relaxant and bronchodilator.
- It does not require preanesthetic medication.
- It does not precipitate cardiac arrhythmia.
- Incidence of hepatotoxicity and nephrotoxicity is minimal.

Disadvantages
- It is an irritant and increases salivary secretion.
- Both induction of anesthesia and emergence from anesthesia are slow.
- It is inflammable so cautery should not be used.
- It is a central nervous system (CNS) stimulant and may cause convulsion.

ETHYL CHLORIDE
- It is inflammable.
- It is nonirritant.
- It has local anesthetic action.
- So it is used for incision and drainage.

TRICHLOROETHYLENE
- It is noninflammable.
- It is nonirritant.
- It is a potent analgesic.
- The onset of action is quick.
- It causes inadequate muscle relaxation.
- It is not used now.

HALOTHANE
Advantages
- It is a volatile liquid.
- It is a low cost, noninflammable and nonirritant anesthetic.
- The induction of anesthesia is slow.
- Emergence from anesthesia depends upon the duration of anesthesia.
- It is a good maintenance agent.
- It is a bronchodilator.
- It inhibits pharyngeal and laryngeal reflexes, facilitating smooth tracheal intubation.
- It causes minimal postoperative vomiting.
- It is used as inducing agent in children as it causes minimal side effects in this age group.

Disadvantages
- It is a poor muscle relaxant and a poor analgesic.
- It has low safety margin.
- A special apparatus is necessary for induction of halothane anesthesia.
- It inhibits the centrally mediated ventilatory response to hypercapnea.
- It causes cerebral vasodilatation and increases intracranial pressure.
- It sensitizes the heart to catecholamines and can cause cardiac arrhythmia.
- It causes hypotension which disappears on continuous administration.
- It potentiates the risk of malignant hyperthermia when coadministered with succinylcholine.
- It can cause hepatotoxicity due to its toxic metabolite, trifluoroacetyl chloride

Nursing Responsibilities
- It is necessary to check if halothane container is sealed tightly as it is highly volatile at room temperature and prone for evaporation.
- The amber bottle of halothane should not be exposed to direct sun light as it can undergo spontaneous breakdown in the presence of light.
- It is not a suitable obstetric anesthetic.
- In uncooperative children, for whom preoperative IV line is difficult to start, halothane can be used as an inducing agent.

ENFLURANE
Advantages
- It is noninflammable and is used as maintenance agent.
- It has better muscle relaxant property.
- It is a bronchodilator.
- It does not increase the respiratory rate.

Disadvantages
- Since it has a relatively slow induction and recovery, it is not suitable as an inducing agent.
- It causes hypotension.
- It has low safety margin.
- It can cause malignant hyperthermia when given with succinylcholine.
- It stimulates CNS and can precipitate seizure.
- It increases intracranial pressure.
- It inhibits the ventilatory response to hypoxia and hypercapnia.

Nursing Responsibilities
- Although a bronchodilator, it causes a rapid and shallow breathing during anesthesia.
- Although the seizure induced by enflurane is self-limiting, it cannot be used as anesthetic in epileptic patients.
- The urine output falls during anesthesia but improves as the effect of enflurane wanes.

ISOFLURANE
Advantages
- It is a good skeletal muscle relaxant and a bronchodilator.
- It is a coronary vasodilator and maintains the cardiac output.

- The depth of anesthesia is achieved quickly.
- The emergence from anesthesia is also quick.
- It is safe in patients with ischemic heart disease.
- It does not cause hepatotoxicity.
- It is a preferred maintenance agent for neurosurgical procedures.

Disadvantages
- Since it is an airway irritant, it stimulates cough and laryngospasm.
- It has a modest risk for increased intracranial pressure.
- It can cause malignant hyperthermia when combined with succinylcholine.
- It has a low safety margin.
- Its odor is pungent. So it is not suitable as an inducing agent.

Nursing Responsibilities
Since it potentiates the action of skeletal muscle relaxants, concurrent administration of these drugs should be avoided.

DESFLURANE

Advantages
- The induction of anesthesia is very rapid.
- The emergence from anesthesia is also rapid.
- It can be used for maintenance of anesthesia.
- It can also be used for outpatient surgery due to rapid onset and recovery.
- It is a bronchodilator.
- It maintains the cardiac output.
- It maintains the blood flow to kidney, brain and heart.
- It does not cause nephrotoxicity.

Disadvantages
- It needs a special vapourizer.
- It causes rapid fluctuation in depth of anesthesia.
- It is an airway irritant, induces cough, bronchospasm and increases salivary secretion.
- It is not a suitable inducing agent due to its irritant nature.
- It can cause malignant hyperthermia when combined with succinylcholine.
- It has low safety margin.
- It increases intracranial pressure.

Nursing Responsibilities
- Always check if desflurane bottle is sealed tightly as it is highly volatile.
- Change of color in the apparatus should be watched for and carbon dioxide absorbers should be refilled as soon as the color changes to prevent airway burns and injury due to exothermic reaction.

SEVOFLURANE
Advantages
- The induction of anesthesia and the emergence from anesthesia are rapid.
- It is suitable as outpatient anesthetic due to its rapid recovery.
- It is preferred as inducing agent in children.
- It is suitable for patient's prone for myocardial ischemia as it does not increase the heart rate.
- It is a potent bronchodilator and it does not induce hepatotoxicity.

Disadvantages
- Compound A, a metabolite of sevoflurane causes nephrotoxicity.
- It can cause malignant hyperthermia when combined with succinylcholine.
- It has low safety margin.

Nursing Responsibilities
- It is necessary to store sevoflurane in the sealed containers.
- It should be administered with fresh gas flow of 2L/minute to wash out compound A.

NITROUS OXIDE
Advantages
- It is a potent analgesic.
- It is a nonirritant and noninflammable anesthetic.
- The onset of anesthesia and emergence from anesthesia are rapid.
- It does not potentiate the curarimimetic action of skeletal muscle relaxants.
- Hence it does not cause malignant hyperthermia.
- It is also used as anesthetic for minor procedures such as tooth extraction.

- It facilitates the uptake of coadministered anesthetic (second gas effect).

Disadvantages
- It requires a special apparatus for administration.
- It should be combined with another anesthetic adjunct as it is not effective if given alone.
- It is a poor skeletal muscle relaxant.
- It increases the intracranial pressure.
- It causes diffusional hypoxia during emergence from anesthesia.
- It can cause spontaneous abortion among female medical professional and female nursing staff exposed to nitrous oxide frequently.
- It causes violent delirium and hallucination.

Contraindications
- Pneumothorax
- Obstructed middle ear
- Pulmonary bulla
- Obstructed bowel loop

Nursing Responsibilities
- To prevent diffusional hypoxia, always ensure that 100% oxygen is administered during recovery of nitrous oxide.
- Since it can cause vitamin B_{12} deficiency, peripheral blood smear should be done to rule out megaloblastic anemia.
- Whenever an opioid analgesic is given as preanesthetic medication, blood pressure should be monitored to prevent hypotension.

XENON

Advantages
- The induction of anesthesia and the emergence from anesthesia is rapid.
- It is a potent analgesic.
- It has minimal cardiorespiratory side effects.
- It does not increase intracranial pressure.
- It does not cause hepatotoxicity or nephrotoxicity.

General Anesthetics

Disadvantages
- It is a rare gas.
- It cannot be manufactured easily.
- It is very expensive.
- It should be administered either with oxygen or with propofol.

THIOPENTONE SODIUM

Advantages
- It is an ultra-short acting anesthetic. So, it has quick onset and rapid recovery.
- The induction of anesthesia is smooth.
- It reduces the intraocular and intracranial pressure.
- It does not cause cardiac arrhythmia
- It can be used as an inducing agent.
- It can also be used as an anesthetic agent for minor procedures.
- It does not cause malignant hyperthermia.

Disadvantages
- It is a respiratory depressant and a myocardial depressant.
- It is a poor analgesic and a poor muscle relaxant.
- It promotes release of histamine and causes bronchospasm and laryngospasm.
- It crosses placenta.
- It can precipitate acute porphyria.

Nursing Responsibilities
- Never mix thiopentone and other drugs in the same syringe during induction, otherwise it can precipitate.
- Wait till thiopental is totally cleared from IV line before administering other drugs through the same IV line.
- Never administer thiopentone to patients in sitting posture to prevent fainting due to hypotension.
- Patient should not be discharged immediately after emergence from thiopentone anesthesia as they may be disoriented.
- It should be noted that the recovery from anesthesia is always delayed during subsequent administration of thiopentone.
- Even inadvertent injection of thiopentone into arteries should be avoided as it causes necrosis.
- Methohexital causes pain at site of injection more frequently than thiopentone.

PROPOFOL

Advantages
- It is the most frequently used intravenous anesthetic.
- It is available as fospropofol, its prodrug.
- It causes rapid induction and quick emergence even after multiple administration.
- Rapid shift to alert stage helps in discharging patients from the recovery room quickly.
- It decreases cerebral blood flow.
- It decreases intracranial and intraocular pressure.
- It causes minimal bronchospasm so is safe for asthmatics.
- It can be used both for induction and for maintenance.
- Lower doses can be infused continuously for long-term maintenance of anesthesia.
- It has antiemetic property.
- It is safe during pregnancy.
- It does not trigger malignant hyperthermia.

Disadvantages
- Even low maintenance dose, it can cause apnea in some individuals.
- It can result in opisthotonus and choreiform movements.
- It can cause hypotension and can also induce sedation.
- It can induce propofol infusion syndrome (PRIS).

Nursing Responsibilities
- Wait for longer recovery period in neonates although children recover quickly.
- Always check and avoid the propofol formulation containing sodium metabisulfite as it does not have the benefit of the bronchodilator property of propofol.
- Soon after the recovery from anesthesia, the patients can be discharged and need not be monitored for 24 hours.
- During induction, signs of PRIS should be watched for.

ETOMIDATE

Advantages
- The onset of anesthesia is quick and the duration of anesthesia is short.

- It has relative cardiovascular stability.
- So, it is mainly used in patients with a risk of hemodynamic instability.
- It does not potentiate the action of coadministered skeletal muscle relaxants.
- It decreases the intraocular and intracranial pressure.
- It does not cause histamine release.

Disadvantages
- It has no analgesic action and can cause pain at the site of injection.
- It can cause myoclonic movements during induction.
- It induces nausea, vomiting and hiccups.
- It suppresses the synthesis of cortisol.

Nursing Responsibilities
- The anesthetic adjuvants suitable for suppressing myoclonic movement occurring during induction of etomidate are benzodiazepines or opioids.
- Monitor the patient for seizures during etomidate anesthesia.
- Pain at injection site can be reduced by using the local anesthetic lignocaine.

KETAMINE

It is a phencyclidine derivative. It is both lipophilic and water soluble.

Advantages
- It causes dissociative anesthesia resulting in amnesia and profound analgesia.
- It is safe in asthmatics as it is a potent bronchodilator.
- It increases blood pressure.
- So, it is preferred in patients with risk of hypotension.
- It has quick onset of action and prolonged duration of action.
- It can be used both as inducing and maintenance agent.
- It is safe in children.

Disadvantages
- It can induce nystagmus and catalepsy.
- It increases intracranial pressure.
- It also increases intraocular pressure.

- Emergence delirium during recovery can occur.
- It increases myocardial oxygen consumption.
- So it should be avoided in patients with risk of myocardial ischemia.

Contraindication
- Hypertension
- Cerebral ischemia

Nursing Responsibilities
- Patient should be kept under observation for about 24 hours after recovery and should not be discharged immediately as ketamine can cause emergence delirium.
- Patient will have unpleasant dreams, delusion or hallucination during the first hour of ketamine recovery.
- To prevent ketamine induced emergence delirium, benzodiazepines can be used as preanesthetic medication.

ANESTHETIC ADJUVANTS
- They are used to reduce the dose of anesthetics.
- They also promote specific component of anesthesia.
- They are benzodiazepines, α_2 agonists, skeletal muscle relaxants and analgesics.

BENZODIAZEPINES
Actions
- They cause amnesia, sedation and reduce anxiety.
- Midazolam is often preferred as anesthetic adjuvant as it has rapid onset and short duration of action.
- Hence it is given as infusion for prolonged sedation or maintenance of anesthesia.
- It can be given through oral, IM, IV or rectal route.
- Midazolam is particularly useful in young children.
- It causes minimal venous irritation during administration.
- Occasionally it causes apnea.
- Lorazepam and diazepam can also be used.

Nursing Responsibilities
Diazepam and lorazepam are not preferred due to the solvent propylene glycol found in these formulations which causes high venous irritation.

DEXMEDETOMIDINE

Actions
- It is a α_2 agonist approved by FDA as an anesthetic adjuvant.
- It causes sedation, analgesia but not anesthesia.
- It causes minimal respiratory depression.
- The sedation induced by dexmedetomidine resembles normal sleep.
- The patient on dexmedetomidine is easily arousable.
- Hence it is preferred for sedating patients on mechanical ventilation with endotracheal intubation.
- It can cause hypotension, bradycardia, nausea and dry mouth.

Nursing Responsibilities
- Complaint of nausea and dry mouth is frequent when dexmedetomidine is given as anesthetic adjuvant.
- If it is available as aqueous solution of hydrochloride salt, it is necessary to dilute it in normal saline before administration.
- Always administer dexmedetomidine through intravenous route.
- Never administer it intrathecally or through any other routes.

ANALGESICS
- They help in reducing the dose of general anesthetics to minimize the 'pain induced' hemodynamic changes.
- The opioid analgesics, morphine, pethidine, fentanyl, sufentanil, alfentanil and remifentanil are useful as anesthetic adjuvants.
- Remifentanil is ultra-short acting and more suited for procedures that do not require analgesia during postoperative period.

Nursing Responsibilities
Nausea, vomiting and pruritus are common during the postoperative period, if opioids are used as anesthetic adjuvants.

MUSCLE RELAXANTS
- Succinylcholine, vecuronium bromide are the commonly used agents.
- They are administered during induction of anesthesia to facilitate muscle relaxation for endotracheal intubation and laryngoscopy.
- Succinylcholine can potentiate malignant hyperthermia if combined with halogenated anesthetics such as halothane.

CHAPTER 21

Sedatives and Hypnotics

These drugs have calming effect and result in sedation. They are effective in the treatment of insomnia.

The drugs are:
- Benzodiazepines
- Novel benzodiazepine receptor agonists (Z compounds)
- Barbiturates
- Melatonin agonists

BENZODIAZEPINES

Ultra Short Acting
Midazolam

Short Acting
Triazolam

Intermediate Acting
- Estazolam
- Temazepam
- Alprazolam
- Lorazepam
- Nitrazepam
- Oxazepam

Long Acting
- Chlordiazepoxide
- Clonazepam
- Diazepam
- Flurazepam
- Chlorazepate

Actions
- They act on gamma-aminobutyric acid ($GABA_A$) receptors and facilitate GABA induced inhibition.

- They cause sedation, hypnosis and reduce anxiety.
- They promote muscle relaxation and cause anterograde amnesia.
- They also have anticonvulsant property.
- They reduce the time required for falling asleep.
- They also reduce the number of awakenings during sleep.
- They induce apnea if combined with opioids.
- They reduce the muscle tone.
- Hence they should be avoided in patients with obstructive sleep apnea.
- They reduce blood pressure and increase heart rate.
- They reduce the nocturnal gastric secretion markedly.

Adverse Effects
- Lightheadedness
- Blurred vision
- Vertigo
- Nausea
- Increased reaction time
- Motor incoordination
- Confusion
- Anterograde amnesia
- Residual day time sedation (hangover)
- Dependence
- Drug abuse.

Uses
- Insomnia
- Anxiety
- Status epilepticus
- Anesthetic adjuvant

Nursing Responsibilities
- Sedative hypnotics should always be administered just before bedtime to prevent accidental fall.
- Never mix benzodiazepines with other drugs in the same syringe as it may precipitate.
- Intramuscular injection of diazepam should be given deeply to reduce pain.
- They should be infused slowly into larger veins.
- Patients on benzodiazepines should be warned not to drive.

- Patients on flurazepam complain of nightmares during 1st week of therapy.
- Flunitrazepam is the 'date rape drug'. It is banned in many countries.
- Taper benzodiazepines slowly before discontinuation after chronic use.

NOVEL BENZODIAZEPINE RECEPTOR AGONISTS

They are structurally unrelated to benzodiazepines. Being GABA agonist, they cause sedation and hypnosis. They are used in sleep onset insomnia. They do not cause rebound insomnia even after abrupt discontinuation. They are:
- Zaleplon
- Zolpidem
- Eszopiclone

Zaleplon
- It reduces the time required for falling asleep.
- Its duration of action is short.
- Hence, it can be administered even 4 hours before anticipated waking time.

Zolpidem
- It induces overnight sleep and should be given at bedtime.
- It is not suitable for late night administration.
- If given late, it causes morning sedation and delayed reaction time.
- Its effect may persist for about a week after discontinuation.
- Tolerance and physical dependence occur rarely.
- It is useful for short-term treatment of chronic insomnia.

Eszopiclone
- It is used for treatment of transient and chronic insomnia.
- It is preferred for patients who have difficulty in falling asleep.
- It is also useful in patients who have difficulty in staying asleep.
- Tolerance does not occur even after 12 months of therapy.
- Adverse effects are abnormal dreams, nausea and anxiety.

Nursing Responsibilities

Patients should be informed that eszopiclone is bitter in taste.

Flumazenil
- It is a benzodiazepine receptor antagonist.
- It is used for the treatment of benzodiazepines overdose.
- It is also used for reversal of sedative effect of benzodiazepines.
- It should be administered only through intravenous route.

Nursing Responsibilities
- Flumazenil should be administered intravenously as series of small injections instead of a bolus dose.
- It should not be given with barbiturates and tricyclic antidepressants.

MELATONIN CONGENER
Ramelteon
Actions
- It is an analog of melatonin and induces sleep.
- It reduces the time taken for falling asleep.
- Taken half an hour before bedtime, it induces sleep.
- In spite of its ability to undergo high first pass metabolism, it is given orally.
- It is effective in both transient and chronic insomnia.
- It does not impair cognitive function the next morning.
- It does not cause rebound insomnia.
- It does not result in tolerance even after 6 months of use.
- It does cause withdrawal effects on discontinuation.

BARBITURATES
- Phenobarbitone
- Pentobarbitone
- Secobarbitone
- Mephobarbitone
- Butabarbitone
- Methohexitone

Actions
- They facilitate central nervous system (CNS) depression by promoting $GABA_A$ mediated inhibition.
- They inhibit cortical pyramidal cells and have anticonvulsant property.
- They increase total sleep time but alter all stages of sleep.

- They reduce the time taken for falling asleep and also reduce night time awakening.
- Tolerance develops to their sedative effect within a few days.
- Tolerance develops through both pharmacokinetic and pharmacodynamic mechanism.
- Abrupt discontinuation results in rebound increase in sleep.
- They also develop cross tolerance to other CNS depressants.
- They cause drug dependence.
- They cause respiratory depression.
- They result in cough, hiccup and sneezing.
- Barbiturates are enzyme inducers.
- They stimulate the metabolism of coadministered drugs.
- They also stimulate the metabolism of vitamin K and vitamin D.
- They cause day time sedation and 'after effect'.
- They reduce intestinal absorption of calcium and interfere with bone mineralization.

Adverse Effects
- Respiratory depression
- Impaired bone mineralization
- Hypersensitivity reaction
- Paradoxical excitement and delirium
- Exfoliative dermatitis.

Nursing Responsibilities
- Intravenous administration of barbiturates should always be slow to prevent sudden fall in BP.
- Apnea, cough and laryngospasm can occur even during slow IV administration.
- Barbiturates may increase perception to pain in elders.
- Patients on barbiturates should be advised against driving.

Therapy of Barbiturate Poisoning
- IV fluids for correction of hypovolemia.
- Forced diuresis with furosemide after correction of hypovolemia.
- Alkalinization of urine.
- Mechanical ventilation.
- Hemodialysis if renal function is compromised.

CHAPTER 22

Antiepileptic Drugs

Antiepileptic drugs are given as monotherapy to minimize adverse effects. However, failure to control seizure with a single drug necessitates substitution with another drug. More drugs are required in patients with more than one type of seizure. The drugs used in the treatment of epilepsy are:

Sodium channel modulators:
- Phenytoin
- Carbamazepine
- Topiramate

Inhibition of T type calcium current:
- Ethosuximide

Gamma-aminobutyric acid (GABA) mediated inhibition:
- Phenobarbitone
- Benzodiazepines

GABA modulators:
- Gabapentin
- Tiagabine
- Vigabatrin

N-methyl-D-aspartate (NMDA) antagonism (Inhibition of excitatory neurotransmitter):
- Felbamate

Sodium channel modulator and T type calcium current inhibitor:
- Sodium valproate
- Lamotrigine

Miscellaneous:
- Zonisamide
- Levetiracetam
- Acetazolamide

PHENYTOIN

Actions
- It inhibits seizure but does not cause central nervous system (CNS) depression.

- It abolishes tonic phase but not the clonic phase of tonic clonic seizure.
- It modulates sodium channel and blocks the propagation of neuronal impulses.
- It is available as rapid release and extended release formulation.
- It is an enzyme inducer and induces metabolism of coadministered drugs.
- It is teratogenic.
- Its rate of excretion shifts from first order to zero order kinetics depending upon its plasma concentration.
- It has low water solubility and is not preferred for intravenous administration.
- Fosphenytoin, its prodrug is highly water soluble and preferred for intravenous administration.

Adverse Effects
- Gingival hyperplasia
- Osteomalacia
- Megaloblastic anemia
- Hirsutism
- Drug allergy
- Hyperglycemia
- Hypersensitivity reaction
- Stevens-Johnson syndrome
- Neutropenia, leukopenia, agranulocytosis
- Lymphadenopathy resembling Hodgkin's disease and malignant melanoma
- Fatal hepatic necrosis

Uses
- Generalized tonic clonic seizure
- Partial seizure
- Cardiac arrhythmia

Nursing Responsibilities
- Epileptics on phenytoin should be advised not to take oral contraceptive pills (OCPs) for avoiding unplanned pregnancy and to follow other methods of contraception as phenytoin induces contraceptive failure.
- Patient should be advised to always use the same formulation from the same manufacturer for better control of seizure.

- Periodic monitoring of plasma concentration of phenytoin is necessary.
- Patients having gingival hyperplasia should be advised to maintain proper oral hygiene.
- Since hirsutism in women necessitates dosage adjustment, it should be reported to the attending physician.
- Monitor blood count and blood glucose in patients taking phenytoin.

BARBITURATES
Actions
- Phenobarbitone has anti-seizure activity even at low doses.
- It potentiates the synaptic inhibition mediated through stimulation of $GABA_A$ receptors.
- It is an enzyme inducer and increases the metabolism of coadministered drugs.

Adverse Effects
- Sedation
- Nystagmus
- Ataxia
- Irritability in children
- Agitation in elderly
- Drug allergy
- Megaloblastic anemia
- Osteomalacia

Uses
- Partial seizure
- Generalized tonic-clonic seizure

Nursing Responsibilities
Neonates of mothers treated with barbiturates during pregnancy will suffer from bleeding due to hypoprothrombinemia.

CARBAMAZEPINE
Actions
- It is a sodium channel modulator and inhibits transmission of nerve impulses.

- It is converted to its active epoxide metabolite which is further metabolized to inactive compounds.
- It is also an enzyme inducer.
- It is teratogenic.

Adverse Effects
- Ataxia, vertigo, diplopia, blurred vision
- Drowsiness
- Agranulocytosis, aplastic anemia
- Hypersensitivity reaction
- Elevation of aspartate aminotransferase (AST) and alanine aminotransferase (ALT).

Uses
- Generalized tonic-clonic seizure
- Simple and complex partial seizure
- Trigeminal neuralgia.

Nursing Responsibilities
- Monitor the patient for severe skin reaction during therapy of carbamazepine.
- Serum AST and ALT to be monitored to detect hepatotoxicity.
- Complete blood count should be done to rule out leukopenia and thrombocytopenia.

OXCARBAZEPINE
Actions
- It is a prodrug and is converted to its active metabolite.
- It modulates sodium channel and inhibits transmission of nerve impulses.
- It is a less potent enzyme inducer than carbamazepine.
- It is given as monotherapy for partial seizure in adults.

ETHOSUXIMIDE
Actions
- It inhibits T type (transient type) calcium current in thalamic neurons.
- On chronic administration, its cerebrospinal fluid (CSF) concentration equals its plasma concentration.
- Its half-life is long, around 50 hours in adults and 30 hours in children.

Adverse Effects
- Nausea, vomiting, anorexia, hiccup
- Dizziness, headache
- Agitation, restlessness, aggressiveness
- Urticaria
- Lethargy
- Aplastic anemia, leukopenia, thrombocytopenia, pancytopenia
- Stevens-Johnson syndrome

Uses
Absence seizure

Nursing Responsibilities
- Splitting the dose will reduce the incidence of nausea, vomiting and sedation.
- It aggravates restlessness and agitation in patient's with a prior history of psychiatric disturbance.
- Complete blood count should be done to rule out bone marrow depression.

SODIUM VALPROATE
Sodium valproate was a 'chance discovery' (serendipity). It is a broad spectrum antiepileptic drug.

Actions
- It modulates sodium channel and inhibits T type calcium current.
- It increases GABA by promoting its synthesis and inhibiting its metabolism.
- Its CSF concentration is equal to its plasma concentration.
- It is an enzyme inhibitor.

Adverse Effects
- Nausea, vomiting, anorexia
- Tremor, ataxia, sedation
- Acute pancreatitis
- Increase in AST and ALT level, hyperammonemia
- Alopecia, weight gain and rash

Uses
- Partial seizure
- Generalized tonic-clonic seizure

- Absence seizure
- Myoclonic seizure

Nursing Responsibilities

- It should never be combined with clonazepam. Such a combination increases the risk of absence seizures.
- Administration of sodium valproate after meals or as enteric coated formulation delays its peak plasma concentration.
- Serum AST and ALT levels should be monitored as it is hepatotoxic.
- Serum amylase should be monitored as it can cause pancreatitis.

BENZODIAZEPINES

- Clonazepam and chlorazepate are useful for long-term management of seizure.
- Midazolam is preferred for intermittent bouts of refractory seizure.
- Diazepam and lorazepam are effective in status epilepticus.
- Benzodiazepines result in GABA mediated synaptic inhibition.
- They cause drowsiness, lethargy, dizziness, hypotonia, aggression, hyperactivity and irritability.

Diazepam

- The onset of action is immediate on intravenous administration.
- Its half-life is 1 to 2 days.
- It is redistributed immediately.
- So its duration of action is short.
- Hence it is not suitable for treatment of status epilepticus.
- Its metabolite desmethyl diazepam is less active with a long half-life of about 60 hours.

Clonazepam

- Tolerance develops to its antiepileptic action within 6 months.
- Intranasal spray is available for recurrent seizures.
- Its half-life is around 23 hours.
- It is effective in absence seizure and myoclonic seizure in children.

Lorazepam

- It has long duration of action with intermediate half-life.
- Hence, it is more suited for management of status epilepticus.

Antiepileptic Drugs

Nursing Responsibilities
- Rectal administration of diazepam reduces the high-risk febrile seizure in children.
- Since prolonged therapy of benzodiazepines can result in behavioral disturbances in children, parents should be informed about the same.
- Since sudden discontinuation of benzodiazepine can result in status epilepticus, patients should be warned not to stop it abruptly.

GABAPENTIN AND PREGABALIN

Actions
- They are GABA agonists but they do not mimic GABA action.
- Their antiepileptic activity is mediated through the cortical membrane protein.
- They are not metabolized and are excreted as such.

Adverse Effects
Gabapentin is usually well tolerated but can cause fatigue, somnolence, dizziness and ataxia.

Uses
- Partial seizure.
- It is also used in the treatment of newly diagnosed partial or generalized seizure, migraine, chronic neuropathic pain and bipolar disorder.

Nursing Responsibilities
Patient on gabapentin should be warned not to drive.

VIGABATRIN

Actions
- It is a GABA analog and inhibits GABA transaminase irreversibly.
- Thereby it increases the concentration of GABA in brain.
- It acts by facilitating GABA mediated neuronal inhibition.
- It is useful in infantile spasm in children less than 2 years.
- It is also used as an adjunct in refractory complex partial seizures.
- It is a reserve drug as it causes progressive and permanent bilateral loss of vision.

Nursing Responsibilities

Patient should be advised to inform the attending physician about any alteration or difficulty in vision as soon as it occurs to prevent permanent loss of vision.

LAMOTRIGINE

Actions

- It modulates sodium channel and inhibits transmission of nerve impulses.
- It also inhibits glutamate release.
- Sodium valproate increases its plasma concentration.
- It potentiates the toxicity of carbamazepine.
- It is used as monotherapy as well as combination therapy with other antiepileptic drugs.

Adverse Effects

- Double vision, dizziness, ataxia
- Nausea, vomiting
- Rash.

Uses

- Partial seizure
- Secondarily generalized tonic-clonic seizure in adults
- Lennox-Gastaut syndrome in children and in adults.

Nursing Responsibilities

Children suffer more frequently with rash than the adults.

LEVETIRACETAM

Actions

- The antiepileptic action is mediated through synaptic vesicle protein.
- It is used as an adjunct.
- It is rapidly and completely absorbed.
- It is not bound to plasma proteins.

Adverse Effects

Dizziness, asthenia and somnolence.

Uses
It is used as an adjunct in:
- Refractory generalized myoclonic seizure
- Refractory partial seizure
- Generalized tonic-clonic seizure

Nursing Responsibilities
Patient on levetiracetam should be warned against driving.

TIAGABINE
Actions
- It acts by reducing the neuronal reuptake of GABA.
- It is used as an adjunctive with other anti epileptic drugs.
- It is rapidly absorbed and is extensively bound to plasma proteins.

Adverse Effects
- Somnolence
- Dizziness
- Tremor

Uses
Refractory partial seizure

Contraindication
Absence seizure

Nursing Responsibilities
Patient should be advised against driving.

TOPIRAMATE
Actions
- It is effective as monotherapy and as add on therapy.
- It has broad spectrum antiepileptic action.
- It modulates sodium channel and inhibits neuronal transmission.
- It inhibits excitatory neurotransmission mediated by glutamate.
- It enhances GABA mediated synaptic inhibition.
- It facilitates potassium current induced hyperpolarization.
- It is a weak carbonic anhydrase inhibitor.
- It is rapidly absorbed and is minimally bound to plasma proteins.

Adverse Effects
- Somnolence, weight loss, fatigue
- Renal calculi
- Cognitive impairment

Uses
- Refractory partial seizure
- Refractory generalized tonic-clonic seizure
- To reduce drop attack in Lennox-Gastaut syndrome
- Prophylaxis of migraine

Nursing Responsibilities
Patient should be warned about driving as it can cause somnolence.

FELBAMATE

Actions
- It is approved for partial seizure.
- It has dual action.
- It potentiates GABA action.
- It also inhibits NMDA mediated excitatory neurotransmission.
- It can cause aplastic anemia.

Adverse Effects
Hepatotoxicity

Uses
- Resistant partial and secondarily generalized seizures
- Lennox-Gastaut syndrome

Nursing Responsibilities
- Periodic monitoring of complete blood count is absolutely necessary.
- Liver enzymes should be monitored as it can cause hepatotoxicity.

ZONISAMIDE

Actions
- It inhibits T type calcium current.
- By modulating sodium channel it inhibits propagation of neuronal impulses.

Antiepileptic Drugs 131

- It inhibits carbonic anhydrase enzyme.
- It is well absorbed orally.
- It has a very long half-life.
- It is used as an adjunct.
- Lamotrigine increases the plasma concentration of zonisamide.

Adverse Effects
- Somnolence
- Ataxia
- Nervousness
- Anorexia
- Fatigue

Uses
Refractory partial seizure

Nursing Responsibilities
- Patient should be warned about the potential of zonisamide to cause somnolence.
- Painful urination in patients on zonisamide indicates the possibility of renal calculi.

LACOSAMIDE
- It modulates the sodium channel and inhibits the transmission of neuronal impulses.
- It is used as an adjunct.
- It is effective for refractory partial seizure.

Nursing Responsibilities
It can be administered as an injection for short-term use when oral administration is not possible.

RUFINAMIDE
- It modulates sodium channel and inhibits repetitive firing of neurons.
- It can be given in children above 4 years and in adults.
- It is used as adjunct for treatment of seizure associated with Lennox-Gastaut syndrome.

STATUS EPILEPTICUS
- It is a medical emergency requiring immediate treatment.
- The seizure occurs rapidly and continuously for a period of 15 minutes.
- Drugs should be administered only through IV route and not by intramuscular (IM) route.
- IV lorazepam 4 to 8 mg given over 1 to 2 minutes is the first line drug.
- It should be repeated if the seizure is not controlled within 5 minutes.
- Diazepam is an alternative when lorazepam is not available.
- The dose of diazepam is 10 mg and should be administered intravenously.
- In children, it can be administered rectally.
- Midazolam is ultra-short acting drug and a substitute for diazepam.
- Following lorazepam, IV fosphenytoin 20 mg should be administered.
- BP and other vital parameters should be monitored.
- Oral therapy with antiepileptic drugs should be started immediately after the seizure is controlled.

Nursing Responsibilities in Therapy of Epilepsy
- Monotherapy in epilepsy is ideal as it causes minimal side effects.
- The minimum period of therapy should extend upto 2 years.
- Cessation of therapy is possible only if the patient is seizure free for atleast 2 years.
- The therapeutic dose of all antiepileptic drugs should be tapered before stopping them completely.
- Patient should be closely monitored during the first 4 months after complete discontinuation of antiepileptic drug.
- Patients prone for recurrent seizures should be warned about driving vehicles.
- Enzyme inducing antiepileptic drugs nullify the benefit of oral contraceptive pills.
- Neonates of mothers treated with enzyme inducing antiepileptic drugs suffer from intracerebral hemorrhage.
- Hypoventilation can be anticipated during an episode of status epilepticus, respiratory assistance should be provided.
- Diazepam should never be given IM in status epilepticus. It should always be given through IV route.

CHAPTER 23

Drugs in Neurodegenerative Disorders

THERAPY OF PARKINSONISM
Parkinsonism is characterized by bradykinesia, muscular rigidity and resting tremor. The loss of dopaminergic neurons in substantia nigra causes dopamine deficiency. Therapy is mainly aimed at restoring function through replacement of dopamine. The drugs are:
- Levodopa/carbidopa
- Catechol-O-methyl transferase (COMT) inhibitors
- Dopamine agonists
- Monoamine oxidase (MAO) inhibitors
- Others

Levodopa

Actions
- It is a prodrug and the metabolic precursor of dopamine.
- It is inactive as such and decarboxylated into dopamine
- It is more effective when combined with carbidopa.
- Carbidopa is a peripheral dopa decarboxylase inhibitor and does not cross blood-brain barrier.
- It prevents the peripheral conversion of levodopa to dopamine.
- Therefore, it facilitates the entry of levodopa into brain.
- It also inhibits the peripheral side effects of dopamine such as nausea, vomiting and tachycardia.
- 100 mg of levodopa is combined with 25 mg of carbidopa and given twice or thrice daily.

Adverse Effects
- Nausea
- 'Wearing off' phenomenon on long-term use.
- Dyskinesia when the dose and frequency of administration is increased to reduce the 'wearing off' phenomenon.
- 'On/off' phenomenon (**on**-severe dyskinetic reactions, **off**-no beneficial effects)
- Hallucination and confusion
- Orthostatic hypotension

- Neuroleptic malignant syndrome causing rigidity, hyperthermia and confusion.

Nursing Responsibilities
- Levodopa should not be administered with high protein meals as this impairs its absorption.
- Severe nausea indicates that the dose of carbidopa may be inadequate.
- Sustained release preparation of levodopa will have unpredictable oral absorption.
- The dose of levodopa should not be increased without the approval of the attending physician failing which dyskinesia will occur.
- Patient's should be warned against abrupt withdrawal of levodopa as it can precipitate 'neuroleptic malignant syndrome'.

Dopamine Receptor Agonists
- Apomorphine
- Bromocriptine
- Pramipexole
- Ropinirole

Ropinirole and Pramipexole
Actions
- They have longer duration of action.
- They are very effective in 'on-off' phenomenon in controlling motor fluctuation.
- They are well absorbed and well tolerated.
- Ropinirole is available as sustained release preparation and can be administered once daily.

Adverse Effects
- Confusion, hallucination
- Orthostatic hypotension
- Fatigue, somnolence
- Nausea.

Nursing Responsibilities
- Somnolence can be very severe and can cause accidents. Hence, patient's on these drugs should be warned against driving.
- Patient should be advised not to get up quickly from sitting or lying down position to avoid orthostatic hypotension.

Apomorphine
- It is administered through subcutaneous route of administration.
- It is useful as 'rescue therapy' for intermittent and fluctuating 'off' episode.
- An antiemetic drug should be given before and after administration of apomorphine as it is a powerful emetic.
- It can cause QT prolongation and injection site reaction.

Nursing Responsibilities
- It is ideal to give one test dose of apomorphine before starting therapy to check patient's tolerability as it is an emetic.
- Sudden increase in the dose of apomorphine causes hallucination and can result in drug abuse.
- Ondansetron and other $5HT_3$ agonists should not be used as antiemetics during apomorphine therapy.
- Bromocriptine: See Section VIII, Chapter 41

Catechol-O-methyl Transferase (COMT) Inhibitors
They are:
- Tolcapone
- Entacapone

Actions
- They inhibit the peripheral conversion of levodopa to dopa.
- Therefore, they facilitate the entry of levodopa into CNS.
- They inhibit the metabolism of both levodopa and dopamine.
- Tolcapone has long-duration of action.
- Entacapone has short-duration of action.

Adverse Effects
- Nausea, confusion, vivid dreams, hallucination
- Orthostatic hypotension.

Nursing Responsibilities
- Periodic monitoring of liver function is necessary for tolcapone but not for entacapone.
- Patient on COMT inhibitors should be advised to avoid sudden positional change to prevent dizziness.
- Patient should be informed about the capacity of these drugs to cause vivid dreams.

Selective MAO-B Inhibitors
They are
- Rasagiline
- Selegiline
- Selegiline and rasagiline are selective MAO-B inhibitors
- They cause irreversible inhibition of MAO-B and inhibit the metabolism of dopamine.
- They are neuroprotective and delay the rate of neurodegeneration in Parkinson disease.
- They do not cause 'cheese reaction'.

Selegiline
- It potentiates levodopa induced motor cognitive impairment.
- It is available as mouth dissolving tablet or as transdermal patch.

Rasagiline
- As monotherapy, it is effective in early Parkinson disease.
- It is used as adjunct to reduce 'off' phenomenon in advanced Parkinsonism.

Other Drugs in Parkinsonism
They are:
- Trihexyphenidyl
- Amantadine

Anticholinergics
- Trihexyphenidyl and benztropine are effective.
- They have moderate efficacy in Parkinsonism.
- Sedation, mental confusion, blurred vision, constipation and urinary retention are some adverse effects.

Amantadine
- It is an antiviral agent.
- It alters striatal dopamine release.
- It also has anticholinergic property.
- It has modest efficacy in Parkinsonism.
- It is usually well tolerated.
- It is effective in dopamine induced dyskinesia.
- It causes lethargy, nausea, vomiting, sleep disturbance or dizziness.

Drugs in Neurodegenerative Disorders

Nursing Responsibilities
Patient should be informed that the adverse effects of amantadine are often reversible.

THERAPY OF ALZHEIMER'S DISEASE
Alzheimer's disease is characterized by neuronal dysfunction and neuronal degeneration in temporal lobe causing memory loss.

Anticholinesterases
- They are first line drugs in the treatment of Alzheimer's disease.
- Rivastigmine, donepezil and galantamine are the anticholinesterases used.
- They are reversible anticholinesterases.
- They improve the cognitive function.
- They cause abnormal dreams, gastrointestinal tract (GIT) distress and muscle cramps.

Nursing Responsibilities
They should be used cautiously in patient with history of syncope.

Memantine
- It is an antagonist of NMDA glutamate receptors.
- It is an alternative to anticholinesterases.
- It reduces the rate of progression of the condition.
- Headache and dizziness can occur.
- Behavioral and psychological symptoms of dementia (BPSD) in Alzheimer's disease.
- Atypical antipsychotics risperidone, quetiapine and olanzapine reduce the agitation and psychosis in Alzheimer's disease but they can cause high side effects.
- Hence, selective serotonin reputake inhibitors (SSRIs) are preferred in this condition.

THERAPY OF HUNTINGTON'S DISEASE
The symptoms are motor incoordination and cognition impairment. It starts in midlife and progresses to involuntary movements such as dysphagia and dysarthria. Later, memory impairment and loss of balance occurs.

Tetrabenazine
- Tetrabenazine is effective in controlling the symptoms.
- It causes depletion of catecholamines.
- It has short-duration of action.
- It can cause suicidal tendency and hypotension.

THERAPY OF AMYOTROPHIC LATERAL SCLEROSIS (ALS)
It is characterized by rapidly progressing muscle atrophy. Riluzole is used in this condition.

Riluzole
- It is well absorbed orally and is highly protein bound.
- It inhibits sodium channel.
- It also inhibits the release of excitatory neurotransmitter, glutamate.
- Further, it blocks NMDA receptors.
- Other agents used to reduce the spasticity in ALS are the centrally acting muscle relaxants baclofen and tizanidine.

CHAPTER 24

Opioid Analgesics

Analgesics are classified as opioid and non-opioid analgesics. Opioid analgesics are:
Natural opioids:
Morphine
Semisynthetic opioids:
- Codeine
- Heroin

SYNTHETIC OPIOIDS

A. Morphine Analogs
- Pethidine (meperidine)
- Fentanyl
- Sufentanil
- Alfentanil
- Remifentanil
- Methadone
- Etorphine

B. Agonists-antagonists
- Pentazocine
- Buprenorphine
- Butorphanol
- Nalbuphine

C. Opioid with Other Actions
- Tramadol

D. Opioids Lacking Analgesic Action
- Loperamide
- Noscapine
- Diphenoxylate
- Dextromethorphan

E. Opioid antagonists:
- Nalorphine
- Naltrexone
- Naloxone

MORPHINE
It acts on μ, κ, σ and nociceptin/orphanin (N/OFQ) receptors.

Actions
Central Nervous System (CNS)
- It inhibits pain perception and increases the ability to tolerate pain.
- It causes analgesia, euphoria, drowsiness, cognitive impairment, and difficulty in concentration.
- In pain free individuals, it can result in unpleasant sensation.
- It does not impair consciousness.
- Unlike alcohol, it does not cause motor incoordination.
- It reduces continuous dull pain better than sharp intermittent pain.
- Euphoria and physical dependence is mediated through mesocorticolimbic dopamine system.

Respiration
- It causes respiratory depression and irregular breathing.
- It reduces rate, tidal exchange and minute volume.
- It inhibits the response of respiratory center to hypercapnia.
- It also reduces the response of respiratory center to hypoxic drive.
- It causes sleep apnea and respiratory depression in newborn.

Neuroendocrine Function
- It reduces the level of cortisol, testosterone, estrogen and progesterone.
- It increases prolactin level.

Other CNS Actions
- It causes bilateral pinpoint pupil.
- It reduces intraocular pressure.
- It can cause seizure.
- By stimulating chemoreceptor trigger zone (CTZ) and vestibular apparatus, it causes nausea.

Cardiovascular System (CVS)
- It causes peripheral vasodilatation due to histamine release.
- This results in orthostatic hypotension.
- It reduces preload and cardiac workload.
- It increases intracranial pressure.

Gastrointestinal tract (GIT) and Genitourinary Tract
- It prolongs gastric emptying time.
- It inhibits intestinal transit time.
- It inhibits gastric, intestinal and pancreatic secretion.
- It increases the tone and amplitude of circular muscles.
- It causes contraction of anal sphincter and promotes constipation.
- It increases intrabiliary pressure.
- It causes urinary retention.

Skin
- It causes vasodilatation, flushing of face, neck and upper thorax.
- It also causes urticaria and pruritus.
- These effects are due to morphine induced histamine release.

Other Actions
- It causes immunosuppression.
- It causes minimal reduction in body temperature.

Absorption and Metabolism
- Morphine can be administered through oral, rectal, subcutaneous, intravenous, intraspinal and epidural routes.
- It undergoes significant first pass metabolism and enterohepatic circulation.
- Both morphine and its conjugate morphine-6-glucuronide are active.

Precautions and Contraindications
- Bronchial asthma
- Chronic obstructive pulmonary disease (COPD)
- Cor pulmonale
- Kyphoscoliosis
- Emphysema
- Head injury
- Acute abdomen
- Hypovolemic shock.

Adverse Effects
- Respiratory depression
- Dysphoria, dizziness
- Nausea and vomiting
- Pruritus
- Constipation
- Urinary retention
- Hypotension.

Uses
- Myocardial infarction pain
- Cancer pain
- Fracture pain
- Postoperative pain.

Opioid Poisoning
It is characterized by pin point pupil, respiratory depression and coma.

Treatment
- Maintenance of vital functions.
- 0.4 to 0.8 mg of IV naloxone reverses the effects of morphine and increases the respiratory rate within 1 to 2 minutes.

PETHIDINE (MEPERIDINE)
- It is ten times less potent than morphine.
- It causes miosis at therapeutic dose but causes mydriasis at toxic doses.
- It causes minimal constipation.
- Urinary retention is less common.
- It is not used in the treatment of diarrhea or cough.
- Its metabolite norpethidine can cause convulsion.
- Hence, it is not used in chronic pain.
- It has a minimal tendency to cause nausea and vomiting.
- It does not delay labor.
- It has local anesthetic property.
- It suppresses respiration.
- It causes vasodilatation.
- It delays gastric emptying.
- It increases intracranial pressure.

HEROIN
- It is three times more lipophilic than morphine.
- Hence, it enters CNS faster than morphine.
- It has rapid onset and has high addiction liability.

CODEINE
- It is methyl morphine.
- It has low affinity to opioid receptors.
- Demethylation to morphine causes analgesia.
- It suppresses cough and used in the treatment of dry cough.
- It causes minimal dependence.

PROPOXYPHENE
- It is used in mild to moderate pain.
- It is less potent than codeine.
- Its actions are similar to morphine.

TRAMADOL
- It is an analog of codeine.
- In addition to its action on μ receptors, it also inhibits reuptake of noradrenaline and serotonin.
- It is used in moderate pain and in labor pain.

DIPHENOXYLATE
- It is a pethidine congener.
- It is used in diarrhea.
- At high doses, it causes euphoria.
- Chronic administration of diphenoxylate causes euphoria and physical dependence.

LOPERAMIDE
- It reduces GIT motility.
- It acts on both circular and longitudinal muscles of GIT.
- It reduces gastrointestinal secretion.
- It is used in diarrhea.
- It causes abdominal cramps.

FENTANYL
- It is 100 times more potent than morphine.
- It has rapid onset of action.

- Its duration of action is very short.
- It does not cause histamine release.
- Hence, it has good cardiovascular stability.
- It is highly lipid soluble.
- It is used as an anesthetic adjuvant to local anesthetics through epidural route.
- It can be administered through intravenous, intrathecal or epidural route.
- It is given for acute postoperative and chronic pain.
- It is also available as transdermal patch and lollipop oral preparation.
- It can cause muscle rigidity, itching, respiratory depression, nausea and vomiting.

SUFENTANIL, ALFENTANIL AND REMIFENTANIL
- They are more potent than fentanyl.
- Sufentanil is 1000 times as potent as morphine.
- Alfentanil and remifentanil are more potent than sufentanil.
- They have quick onset and short duration of action.
- They have good cardiovascular stability.
- They are also useful as anesthetic adjuvants.
- The onset and duration of action of remifentanil is much more rapid.
- Hence, it is used in short procedures requiring intense analgesia.
- Remifentanil can also be used for long neurosurgical procedures.
- It should not be given through intraspinal route.
- Alfentanil can be administered through intraspinal route.

METHADONE
- It acts similar to morphine but with lower intensity.
- It causes analgesia, mild euphoria, miosis and respiratory depression.
- It is extensively bound to plasma proteins and accumulates in brain.
- It is released slowly from bound sites after discontinuation.
- Therefore, it has extended duration of action.
- So it is used for suppressing withdrawal symptoms of morphine.
- The development of tolerance is very slow.
- It is used in chronic pain and in opioid abstinence syndrome.
- It should not be used in labor.
- It prolongs QT interval.

AGONISTS-ANTAGONISTS

Pentazocine, buprenorphine, nalbuphine and butorphanol are partial agonist-antagonist of opioid receptors.

Pentazocine
- It causes analgesia.
- It also causes sedation and respiratory depression.
- At higher dose, instead of euphoria, it causes dysphoria.
- Unlike other opioid agonists, it increases blood pressure.
- So it should not be given in patients with coronary artery disease.
- It has lower dependence liability than morphine.
- It is used in moderate to severe pain.
- In morphine dependent individuals, it can precipitate withdrawal syndrome.

Nalbuphine
- It is equipotent to morphine.
- Its onset and duration of action is similar to morphine.
- It does not alter blood pressure even in patient with myocardial infarction.
- It causes abstinence syndrome in morphine addicts.
- Physical dependence occurs on prolonged administration.
- Abrupt discontinuation causes withdrawal syndrome.
- It causes headache and sweating.
- It is used as an analgesic agent.

Butorphanol
- It is more potent than morphine
- It is used in acute pain.
- It increases cardiac workload.
- So it is not suited for myocardial infarction pain.
- Nasal formulation of butorphanol is effective in migraine pain.
- Physical dependence can develop to its actions.
- It causes nausea, drowsiness and a feeling of floating.

Buprenorphine
- It is more potent than morphine.
- It is slowly released from its binding sites.
- Therefore, it can be used to induce abstinence in opioid dependent patient.
- Withdrawal symptoms can occur on sudden discontinuation.

OPIOID ANTAGONISTS

Nalorphine
- Nalorphine is not a complete antagonist.
- So it is not effective in the treatment of opioid poisoning.

NALOXONE

Actions
- It antagonizes all subtypes of morphine receptors.
- Hence, it is a complete antagonist and reverses all the actions of morphine.
- It stimulates respiration and increases the blood pressure.
- It does not cause tolerance or physical dependence.
- It can be administered through subcutaneous (SC), intramuscular (IM) or intravenous (IV) route.
- A single dose can precipitate withdrawal symptoms in opioid dependent patients.

Uses
- Opioid poisoning
- Reversal of hypotension due to shock, stroke and spinal cord injury.

NALTREXONE

Actions
- Naltrexone is more potent than naloxone.
- It has higher oral bioavailability.
- The duration of action is longer than naloxone.
- It blocks the euphoria induced by opioids.
- It is used in de-addiction of opioids and alcohol.

Nursing Responsibilities in Opioid Therapy
- Although an opioid analgesic, pentazocine should never be given as analgesic in myocardial infarction.
- Patient should be monitored for atleast 2 weeks for symptoms of physical dependence after discontinuation of buprenorphine.
- Morphine is unsuitable as obstetric analgesic as it can cause neonatal respiratory depression.

- Inspite of its ability to cause addiction, morphine should be continued in terminally ill cancer patients.
- The patient should be rested in bed before administering intravenous opioids to prevent them from fainting.
- Do not apply fentanyl transdermal patch on abraded skin.
- Informed consent should be obtained from patient after explaining the risks and benefits of chronic opioid therapy.
- Documentation of opioid therapy should be done.
- It is necessary to monitor the respiratory rate in patients on opioids.

SECTION V

Psychopharmacology

- Pharmacotherapy of Depression and Anxiety
- Pharmacotherapy of Psychosis and Mania
- Drug Addiction

CHAPTER 25
Pharmacotherapy of Depression and Anxiety

Antidepressant drugs are classified as:
- Selective serotonin reuptake inhibitors (SSRIs)
- Selective noradrenaline reuptake inhibitors (SNRIs)
- Tricyclic antidepressants (TCAs)
- Monoamine oxidase inhibitors (MAOIs)
- Miscellaneous agents.

The challenges faced during therapy with antidepressant drugs are:
- Therapeutic lag due to early onset of side effects
- Switch over from depressive to manic episode
- A risk of suicidal tendency.

SELECTIVE SEROTONIN REUPTAKE INHIBITORS (SSRIs)

The drugs are citalopram, escitalopram, fluvoxamine, paroxetine, sertraline, fluoxetine.

Actions
- They are safer than TCAs.
- They inhibit the reuptake of serotonin at the presynaptic terminals.
- Thereby, they facilitate serotonergic neurotransmission.
- They are well-tolerated and administered once daily.
- Fluoxetine is available as once weekly formulation.
- They inhibit hepatic enzymes and increase the plasma concentration of TCAs, warfarin, paclitaxel, and tamoxifen.
- They cause withdrawal syndrome on sudden discontinuation.
- They do not cause anticholinergic and cardiovascular side effects.
- They do not cause sedation as they do not block histamine or α-adrenergic receptors.

Adverse Effects
- Anxiety, irritability, insomnia
- Vomiting, diarrhea
- Erectile dysfunction, delayed ejaculation occur more commonly with paroxetine

- Withdrawal syndrome characterized by headache, insomnia, dizziness, and nausea
- Paroxetine increases the risk of congenital cardiac malformations
- Venlafaxine increases the risk of perinatal complications.

Uses
- Obsessive compulsive disorder (OBC)
- Panic disorder
- Social anxiety
- Generalized anxiety disorder (GAD)
- Posttraumatic stress disorder (PTSD)
- Premenstrual dysphoric syndrome
- Postmenopausal vasovagal symptoms.

Drug Interactions
With MAOIs, they cause serotonin syndrome resulting in hyperthermia, tremor, muscular rigidity, irritability, confusion.

Nursing Responsibilities
Withdrawal effect is very severe with paroxetine and venlafaxine on discontinuation but does not occur with fluoxetine.

SEROTONIN NORADRENALINE REUPTAKE INHIBITORS (SNRIs)
The drugs are duloxetine, venlafaxine, milnacipran.

Actions
- They inhibit reuptake of both serotonin and noradrenaline.
- Thereby, they facilitate the neurotransmission of serotonin and noradrenaline.
- They are available as extended release and immediate release formulation.
- Duloxetine should not be given in patients with hepatic and renal dysfunction.

Adverse Effects
- Insomnia, headache
- Nausea, constipation
- Sexual dysfunction.

Uses
- Depression
- Pain
- Anxiety disorders
- Fibromyalgia.

Off-label Uses
- Hot flushes
- Autism
- PTSD
- Binge eating disorder
- Venlafaxine in posttraumatic disorder
- Off-label use of duloxetine in stress urinary incontinence.

Nursing Responsibilities
BP should be monitored in patients on immediate release preparation venlafaxine as it can cause diastolic hypertension.

ATYPICAL ANTIDEPRESSANTS (MISCELLANEOUS AGENTS)
The drugs are atomoxetine, reboxetine, mirtazapine, nefazodone, trazodone, mianserin.

Actions
- They block serotonin and α- adrenergic receptors.
- Mirtazapine and mianserin block H_1 histamine receptors and cause sedation.

Adverse Effects
- Mirtazapine causes somnolence, weight gain, rarely agranulocytosis
- Trazodone rarely causes priapism.
- Nefazodone causes liver failure.

Uses
- Depression
- Trazodone in insomnia along with SSRI or SNRI.

Nursing Responsibilities
- Complete blood count should necessarily be monitored in patients on mirtazapine.

- Fever or sore throat in patients on mirtazapine requires further investigation as it can be due to agranulocytosis.
- Priapism should be watched for in patients on trazodone and it requires surgical treatment.

Bupropion
- It acts through multiple mechanisms.
- It facilitates neurotransmission of both noradrenergic and dopaminergic neurons.
- It also increases the presynaptic release of noradrenaline and dopamine.

Adverse Effect
Seizure.

Uses
- Depression
- Smoking cessation
- Seasonal depressive disorder
- Attention deficit hyperactive disorder (ADHD).

Nursing Responsibilities
Extended release preparation of bupropion reduces the risk of seizure, its main side effect.

TRICYCLIC ANTIDEPRESSANTS (TCAs)
The drugs are amitriptyline, clomipramine, doxepin, imipramine, trimipramine, amoxapine, desipramine.

Actions
- They are not used as first-line drugs as they are highly toxic.
- They inhibit noradrenaline and serotonin neurotransmission.
- They also block histamine, α- adrenergic and muscarinic receptors.
- They lower the seizure threshold.

Adverse Effects
- Seizures.
- Anticholinergic side effects such as dry mouth, blurred vision, cycloplegia, constipation, urinary retention, tachycardia.
- Orthostatic hypotension, sedation, weight gain.

Uses
- Major depression
- Neuropathic pain
- Insomnia at low dose.

Nursing Responsibilities
- Patients on TCA should be monitored for abnormal muscular movements.
- To reduce dizziness and fainting attacks, the patients on TCA should be advised not to change their posture suddenly.

MONOAMINE OXIDASE INHIBITORS (MAOIs)
The drugs are phenelzine, tranylcypromine, selegiline, isocarboxazid.

Actions
- Their efficacy is comparable to TCA yet, they are rarely used due to their higher toxicity profile.
- Selegiline is reversible selective MAO-B inhibitor.
- All others are irreversible, nonselective 'suicide' inhibitors.

Adverse Effect
Hypertensive crisis with food containing tyramine.

Use
Depression.

Drug Interactions
They undergo many drug interactions. They should not be coadministered with SSRIs, SNRIs, TCAs, bupropion, opioids, anesthetics, and alcohol to prevent serotonin syndrome.

Nursing Responsibilities
- Patients should be encouraged to use transdermal patch of selegiline instead of its oral formulation as this minimizes the incidence of hypertensive crisis.
- Patients on irreversible, nonselective MAOI should be advised to avoid cheese, red wine and fava beans in their diet.
- Liver enzymes should be monitored in patients on MAOI.

Atypical Antipsychotics in Depression
- Quetiapine, aripiprazole and olanzapine are used.
- Aripiprazole and SSRIs/SNRIs combination or olanzapine and SSRIs are approved by FDA for the treatment of resistant major depression.

Anxiolytics
The anxiolytics are benzodiazepines, SSRIs, SNRIs, azapirone, buspirone and β-blockers.

Benzodiazepines
The drugs used are alprazolam, chlordiazepoxide, clonazepam, diazepam, lorazepam, clorazepate and oxazepam.

Actions
They facilitate GABA mediated inhibition of neurotransmission.

Adverse Effects
Sedation, slow reaction time, short-term amnesia, frequent fall, habituation, abuse, and dependence.

Uses
Acute and chronic management of:
- Panic disorder
- Generalized anxiety disorder (GAD).

Nursing Responsibilities
Elders taking benzodiazepines should be warned against the possibility of loss of balance.

SSRIs, SNRIs and Buspirone
- SSRIs and SNRIs venlafaxine are the first-line drugs in the treatment of anxiety disorders.
- Fluvoxamine is used in obsessive compulsive disorder (OCD).
- Venlafaxine is well-tolerated and used in anxiety.
- Buspirone is effective in chronic management of generalized anxiety disorder.
- Long-term therapy of buspirone is required in the management of GAD.

Nursing Responsibilities
The dose of SSRIs and SNRIs should be decreased gradually before discontinuation.

CHAPTER 26

Pharmacotherapy of Psychosis and Mania

ANTIPSYCHOTIC DRUGS
They are classified as:
- Typical antipsychotic agents
- Atypical antipsychotic drugs.

Common uses of antipsychotic drugs
- Posttraumatic stress disorder
- Obsessive compulsive disorder
- Tourette's disorder
- Autism
- Huntington's disease
- Generalized anxiety disorder (GAD)
- As antiemetic.

TYPICAL ANTIPSYCHOTIC DRUGS
They are:
- Chlorpromazine
- Perphenazine
- Fluphenazine
- Trifluoperazine
- Haloperidol
- Loxapine
- Molindone
- Thioridazine.

Actions
- They alter the dopaminergic pathway.
- Typical antipsychotics mainly block dopamine D_2 receptors.
- They also block histamine, muscarine and α_1-adrenergic receptors.
- Blockade of cholinergic receptors result in anticholinergic side effects and histamine receptor blockade causes sedation.
- Tolerance develops to anticholinergic and antihistaminic side effects.

- Adrenergic α_1-receptor blockade causes orthostatic hypotension.
- These agents are highly lipophilic and accumulate in brain.
- They are extensively bound to plasma proteins.
- They cross placenta and are secreted in milk.
- Therapeutic benefit occurs on once daily administration.
- They are well-absorbed orally.
- Long-acting injectable formulations are available for IM injection.

Adverse Effects
- Tardive dyskinesia—painless repetitive involuntary tic-like movements
- Akathisia or restlessness
- Extrapyramidal symptoms
- Acute dystonia
- Neuroleptic malignant syndrome—autonomic instability characterized by fluctuations in BP, pulse and respiratory rate, other features are pyrexia, myoglobinemia and nephrotoxicity. Antipsychotics should be discontinued immediately
- Orthostatic hypotension
- Sedation
- Anticholinergic side effects
- Hyperprolactinemia
- Weight gain.

CHLORPROMAZINE
Actions
- It quietens the aggressive patient.
- Patient becomes indifferent to his/her surroundings.
- It causes psychomotor slowing and emotional quietening.
- It is a neuroleptic and causes catatonia and catalepsy.
- It induces sleep and impairs concentration.
- It does not affect cognition or memory.
- It has antiemetic property.
- It is well-absorbed and undergoes enterohepatic circulation.
- It causes tolerance on continuous administration.

Adverse Effects
- Orthostatic hypotension, hyperprolactinemia, seizure.
- Photosensitivity with yellow discoloration due to melanin deposition.

- Visual disturbance due to pigment deposition in retina.
- Extrapyramidal symptoms, tardive dyskinesia.
- Anticholinergic side effects like blurring of vision, dry mouth, urinary retention, etc.
- Galactorrhea, impotence, gynecomastia.
- Weight gain, loss of diabetes control.
- Neuroleptic malignant syndrome.

Uses
- Maniac depressive psychosis
- Schizophrenia
- Huntington's disease
- Senile psychosis
- Alcoholic psychosis
- Emesis.

Haloperidol
- It is more effective in patients with aggressive behavior.
- It is a mild sedative and results in minimal orthostatic hypotension.
- It causes extrapyramidal symptoms similar to parkinsonism.

ATYPICAL ANTIPSYCHOTICS
They are:
- Ziprasidone
- Sertindole
- Olanzapine
- Clozapine
- Quetiapine
- Sulpiride
- Aripiprazole
- Risperidone
- Paliperidone
- Iloperidone
- Asenapine
- In addition to D_2-blockade, they also block serotonin receptors
- Risperidone blocks α_2-receptors also
- Except risperidone and paliperidone, they do not cause hyperprolactinemia
- They result in minimal extrapyramidal side effects
- The incidence of tardive dyskinesia is low

- They cause minimal anticholinergic side effects
- The frequency of orthostatic hypotension is also low.

Clozapine

- It blocks dopaminergic, serotonergic and adrenergic receptors.
- It controls both positive and negative symptoms of schizophrenia.
- It does not cause hyperprolactinemia.
- It results in very minimal extrapyramidal side effects.
- It reduces the seizure threshold.
- It is also available as 'oral dissolving tablet' (ODT).

Adverse Effects

- Sedation, orthostatic hypotension, weight gain
- Agranulocytosis, seizure
- Anticholinergic side effects
- Hyperglycemia, hypertriglyceridemia.

Uses

Refractory schizophrenia.

Olanzapine

- It blocks dopamine and serotonin receptors.
- It is not safe in children.
- It controls negative symptoms of schizophrenia.
- It decreases seizure threshold.
- It does not cause extrapyramidal side effects.
- It does not increase prolactin level. So, it does not result in amenorrhea, impotence and galactorrhea.
- It is available as 'oral dissolving tablet' (ODT).
- It increases the incidence of stroke in elderly.

Adverse Effects

- Nausea, constipation
- Sedation, weight gain
- Hyperglycemia, hypertriglyceridemia.

Uses

- Schizophrenia
- SSRI resistant PTSD
- Acute mania of bipolar disorder.

Quetiapine
- Its actions are similar to olanzapine but it should be administered twice daily.
- Unlike olanzapine, it causes only minimal weight gain.
- The incidence of extrapyramidal symptoms and hypertriglyceridemia is minimal.
- It causes moderate hyperglycemia.
- It does not control the negative symptoms of schizophrenia.

Adverse Effects
- Sedation
- Orthostatic hypotension
- Weight gain
- Akathisia
- Urinary retention
- QT prolongation.

Uses
- Schizophrenia
- SSRI resistant, post-traumatic stress disorder (PTSD)
- Manic episode of bipolar disorder.

Risperidone

Actions
- It blocks dopamine, serotonin, histamine and adrenergic receptors.
- It is safe in children but not safe in elders.
- It is effective in calming aggressive patients.
- The effect of long-acting formulation of risperidone takes 4 weeks for the onset of action and extends upto 6 weeks after its discontinuation.
- It is available as 'oral dissolving tablet' (ODT).
- It can be safely administered during pregnancy.
- The incidence of hyperglycemia and hypertriglyceridemia is minimal.

Adverse Effects
- Hyperprolactinemia
- Insomnia
- Orthostatic hypotension
- Dizziness.

Uses
- SSRI resistant schizophrenia
- PTSD
- OCD
- GAD
- Acute mania of bipolar disorder of children and adults.
- Autism.

Ziprasidone
- It blocks dopamine and $5HT_2$ receptors but facilitates the action of $5HT_1$ receptors.
- It does not cause hyperglycemia.
- It can be safely used in children.

Uses
- Schizophrenia in adults and children
- Manic episode of bipolar disorder in adults and children.

Paliperidone
- It causes minimal drug interactions but can cause hyperprolactinemia.
- Long-acting injectable formulation is also available for use.

Iloperidone
- It causes minimal weight gain but it prolongs QT interval.
- It does not cause hyperglycemia or hypertriglyceridemia.

Aripiprazole
- It blocks dopamine and $5HT_2$ receptors but facilitates the action of $5HT_1$ receptors.
- It does not cause hyperglycemia, hypertriglyceridemia or hyperprolactinemia.
- Hence, it is suited for long-term therapy of schizophrenia.
- It is also available as 'oral dissolving tablet' (ODT).

Adverse Effect
Akathisia.

Uses
- Schizophrenia
- Acute mania in bipolar disorder.

Schizophrenia
- Schizophrenia is characterized by split mind with disturbance in perception, thinking and behavior.
- Patients suffer from delusion, hallucination and illusion.
- It commonly occurs at younger age group.
- Patient may suffer from paranoid delusion.
- Symptoms can be positive with agitation, aggressiveness, irritability, hallucination and delusion or negative with social withdrawal.
- Antipsychotics afford symptomatic relief and are not curative.
- The drugs should be continued lifelong even after therapeutic benefit is obtained.
- Typical antipsychotic agents such as chlorpromazine are cheap but result in extrapyramidal symptoms, sedation and other side effects.
- Atypical antipsychotic drugs are costly and are reserve drugs.
- Clozapine controls both positive and negative symptoms but can cause agranulocytosis.
- Clozapine is preferred in refractory schizophrenia.
- The duration of therapy in schizophrenia is long. So, those atypical antipsychotic drugs prone for causing weight gain and metabolic disturbance should be avoided.
- Aripiprazole and ziprasidone are preferred in treatment of schizophrenia.

Nursing Responsibilities in Antipsychotic Agents
- Patients should be motivated to take the drug daily for better clinical outcome.
- Family members should also be given counseling to offer adequate emotional support to the patient.
- Liquid oral formulations should be dispensed in dark bottles as they are light sensitive and the patient taking them should be warned about the possibility of oral candidiasis.
- Deep IM injections are preferred and subcutaneous route should be avoided as it causes tissue irritation.
- Patients on clozapine should be advised to take stool softeners regularly to prevent constipation. The nursing personnel should enquire periodically about their bowel habits to prevent constipation mediated bowel obstruction.

- Hence fluid intake, renal output and bowel distention should also be monitored.
- Serum triglycerides and blood glucose should be monitored regularly in patients on clozapine and olanzapine.
- Serum total cholesterol should be monitored in patients taking clozapine, quetiapine and olanzapine.
- Patients on clozapine should be warned against driving and operating dangerous machinery as it can induce seizure.
- Periodic monitoring of complete blood count is necessary for patients on clozapine as it causes agranulocytosis.
- Since chlorpromazine, clozapine, quetiapine and risperidone can cause orthostatic hypotension, patients on these drugs should be warned against sudden postural change.
- The rate of oral absorption is similar for both mouth dissolving and liquid formulation of chlorpromazine.
- Contact dermatitis can occur due to contact of chlorpromazine on skin.
- Dystonia causing oculogyric crisis involving extraocular muscles following therapy with typical antipsychotic drugs can be frightening to patients. Hence, patients should be warned about the same.

Drugs in Bipolar Disorder

- Bipolar disorder is a lifelong condition with high recurrence rate in patients with manic episodes.
- Lithium is the drug of choice as it is a mood stabilizer.
- The drugs effective in acute mania are sodium valproate, divalproex, carbamazepine, olanzapine, risperidone, aripiprazole and ziprasidone.
- Lamotrigine is effective in bipolar maintenance for depressive episodes.
- Aripiprazole, olanzapine are effective for prophylaxis of manic episodes of bipolar disorder.
- Aripiprazole and risperidone are approved by FDA for acute mania in children and adults.

Lithium

Actions
- It inhibits the transmission of nerve impulses by replacing sodium ions.

- It reduces the release of noradrenaline and dopamine.
- It enhances the release of serotonin.
- It is a mood stabilizer.
- It reduces the turnover of arachidonic acid in brain.
- It is absorbed completely, concentrates initially in ECF and later on in other tissues.
- Once daily administration is effective in bipolar disorder.
- Since it is a drug with low therapeutic index, plasma concentration should be monitored.
- Its therapeutic action starts after 5 to 7 days.
- It is neuroprotective and effective in dementia of neurodegenerative Alzheimer's, Parkinson's and Huntington's disease.

Adverse effects
- Polyuria and nephrogenic diabetes insipidus.
- Fine hand tremor, cognitive impairment, seizure.
- Weight gain, hypothyroidism, dermatitis, folliculitis.

Uses
- Bipolar disorder
- Resistant major depression.

Nursing Responsibilities
- Plasma concentration should be monitored regularly as it is a drug of narrow therapeutic index.
- It is necessary to monitor renal function as it can cause nephrogenic diabetes insipidus.

# CHAPTER 27

Drug Addiction

Drugs causing addiction are alcohol, central nervous system (CNS) stimulants, cannabis, opioids, tobacco, cocaine, anti-anxiety drugs, psychedelics such as lysergic acid diethylamide (LSD).

- Chewing cocoa leaves causes slow absorption of cocaine from buccal mucosa.
- Children of alcoholic parents have higher tendency to develop alcohol addiction.
- Addiction can be psychological or physical.

TREATMENT

- **Ethanol:** Disulfiram, acamprosate, naltrexone
- **Nicotine:** Nicotine gum, nicotine patch, nicotine inhaler, nicotine nasal spray, bupropion, varenicline, rimonabant
- **Opioids:** Methadone, clonidine, lofexidine, naltrexone
- **Cocaine:** Topiramate, modafinil
- **Cannabinoid:** Rimonabant
- **LSD:** Acidification of urine enhances its excretion in drug overdose. LSD induced agitation is controlled by diazepam.

Nursing Responsibilities

Chlorpromazine should never be given in LSD induced agitation.

SECTION VI

Cardiovascular System

- ✦ Antianginal Drugs
- ✦ Diuretics
- ✦ Drugs in Heart Failure
- ✦ Antihypertensive Drugs
- ✦ Antiarrhythmic Agents

CHAPTER 28

Antianginal Drugs

Imbalance between myocardial blood supply and the requirement causes myocardial ischemia. Angina is the classical symptom of myocardial ischemia and occurs in two forms:
1. Typical stable exertional angina
2. Variant or Prinzmetal angina

Severe and frequent episodes of stable angina with pain occurring at rest is called unstable angina. Antianginal drugs are used either to treat or to prevent angina.

Drugs used in angina are:
- Nitrates
- Beta-blockers
- Calcium channel blockers
- Potassium channel openers
- Miscellaneous drugs.

NITRATES

The drugs are:
- Glyceryl trinitrate (GTN) or nitroglycerin
- Isosorbide dinitrate
- Isosorbide mononitrate.

Actions

- Nitrates are the 'first line drugs' in the treatment of angina.
- They are prodrugs and liberate nitric oxide.
- Nitric oxide stimulates cyclic guanosine monophosphate (GMP) resulting in vasodilatation.
- They relax the smooth muscles of major veins.
- This results in peripheral pooling of venous blood.
- Such peripheral venous pooling reduces the 'preload'.
- This in turn, reduces the end diastolic pressure of both left and right ventricles.
- Slight fall in peripheral resistance of arterioles promotes reduction of 'afterload'.
- These actions reduce the cardiac workload.

- They cause coronary vasodilatation.
- Nitrates also relax GIT, bronchial, gallbladder, biliary tract, ureteric and uterine smooth muscles.

Uses
- Exertional, variant and unstable angina.
- Congestive heart failure
- Non-ST segment elevated myocardial infarction (Non-STEMI)
- Acute MI
- Biliary colic
- Spasm of esophagus
- Cyanide poisoning.

Contraindications
Nitrates should not be administered in patients receiving phosphodiesterase 5 inhibitors such as sildenafil and tadalafil.

Adverse Effects
- Headache
- Flushing
- Tachycardia
- Dizziness, sweating
- Rash
- Tolerance.
- Methemoglobinemia.

Tolerance
- Tolerance frequently occurs with the use of long acting or sustained release preparations of nitrates.
- Higher doses of nitrates can also result in tolerance.
- It is due to the inability of smooth muscles to convert nitrates to nitric oxide, a vasodilator.
- Cross tolerance among nitrates is common.

Glyceryl Trinitrate
- It is administered through sublingual route to avoid first pass metabolism.
- It has quick onset and short duration of action.
- It terminates the anginal attack quickly.
- It is cheaper and very effective.
- So, it is preferred during acute attack.

- A sustained release oral preparation is used for chronic prophylaxis.
- Cutaneous transdermal application is also available for use.

Isosorbide Dinitrate
- It is short acting by sublingual route and long acting by oral route.
- It also undergoes significant first pass metabolism through oral route.
- The sustained release preparation prolongs the duration for 6 to 10 hours.

Isosorbide Mononitrate
- It is a metabolite of isosorbide dinitrate.
- It undergoes minimal first pass metabolism.
- It has good oral absorption and longer duration of action.
- It is also available as sustained release formulation.
- A gap of 7 hours is required when it is given twice daily.

Nursing Responsibilities
- Nitrate preparations should be kept in air tight glass containers to protect from light, heat and moisture.
- Since active tablets cause burning sensation when kept under the tongue, it should be asked for, especially in elderly patients.
- The nitrate tablet should always be kept in bedside table and within reach of the patient for immediate use during acute attack.
- If pain does not reduce after three tablets, the patient should be referred immediately to the physician.
- Transdermal applications should not be rubbed and should be applied on non hairy site, at the same time everyday.
- The site of transdermal application should be changed frequently.
- Transdermal patch should be removed at least 8 to 12 hours daily, to prevent the development of tolerance.
- Long acting nitrate preparation can result in tolerance.

CALCIUM CHANNEL BLOCKERS
The drugs are:
- **Phenylalkylamine:** Verapamil
- **Benzothiazepine:** Diltiazem
- **Dihydropyridines:**
  - Amlodipine
  - Nifedipine

- Nicardipine
- Felodipine
- Isradipine
- Nisoldipine
- Clevidipine.

Actions
- They are considered to be the third line drugs in MI.
- They block the L (long lasting) type of calcium channels.
- They prevent contraction of myocardial and vascular smooth muscle cells.
- Phenyl alkylamine has more cardiac actions.
- Dihydropyridines result in more vascular actions.
- Benzothiazepine result in equal cardiac and vascular actions.
- They cause systemic arterial vasodilatation and reduce the afterload.
- They also increase the coronary blood flow.
- They inhibit the SA node and reduce the heart rate.
- They also inhibit the AV conduction in heart.
- Amlodipine, diltiazem and verapamil are preferred in angina as they cause minimal reflex tachycardia.
- Nicardipine is also approved but not used widely.

Common Adverse Effects
- Dizziness, headache, flushing, tachycardia.
- Aggravation of gastroesophageal reflux disease (GERD), constipation.
- Peripheral edema
- Conduction defects
- Urinary retention
- Rash, elevated liver enzymes

Common Uses
- Classic or exertional angina
- Prinzmetal or variant angina
- Hypertension
- Arrhythmia
- Hypertrophic cardiomyopathy
- Prophylaxis of migraine

Verapamil
Actions
- It inhibits SA and AV node conduction.
- It has minimal vascular action.
- So, it causes minimal reflex tachycardia.
- It also causes coronary vasodilatation.

Adverse Effects
- Constipation, bradycardia
- Prolonged QT syndrome.

Contraindications
- SA and AV node conduction block
- Low BP
- Digitalis toxicity.

Uses
- Variant angina
- Exertional angina
- Paroxysmal supraventricular tachycardia (PSVT)
- Hypertension
- Hypertrophic cardiomyopathy.

Diltiazem
Actions
- It results in modest cardiac and vascular actions.
- It decreases heart rate and blood pressure.
- It causes minimal reflex tachycardia.

Adverse Effects
Dizziness, edema, headache

Contraindications
- Coadministration of digitalis
- Conduction defect
- Low BP

Uses
- Classic or exertional angina
- Variant angina
- Hypertension, arrhythmia
- Raynaud's disease

Dihydropyridine Calcium Channel Blockers

Most dihydropyridine calcium channel blockers share common pharmacological actions, side effects, contraindications and therapeutic uses. Incidence of reflex tachycardia is high except for amlodipine.

Amlodipine
Actions
- It reduces afterload.
- It also increases coronary blood flow.
- It has a long duration of action and can be given once daily.
- It causes minimal plasma fluctuation.
- Hence, it causes minimal reflex tachycardia.

Adverse Effects
- Peripheral edema, headache
- Palpitations, flushing.

Contraindications
- Digitalis toxicity
- Low BP

Uses
- Hypertension
- Classic or exertional angina
- Variant angina
- Heart failure
- Raynaud's disease

Nifedipine
- It is a potent vasodilator.
- So, it increases both coronary and peripheral blood flow.
- The incidence of reflex tachycardia is very high.
- It is less effective and may worsen the angina.

Adverse Effects
- Headache, flushing
- Dizziness, palpitation, peripheral edema

Contraindication
Low BP

Uses
- Hypertension
- Raynaud's disease
- Preterm labor

Antianginal Drugs

Nimodipine
- It has high lipid solubility.
- It inhibits cerebral vasospasm.
- It is indicated in patients with neurological defects associated with cerebral vasospasm after subarachnoid hemorrhage.

Nicardipine
It acts more selectively on coronary vessels to cause coronary vasodilatation.

Nisoldipine
It results in 1000 times more potent vascular than cardiac action.

Isradipine
Isradipine results in moderate cardiac depressant activity.

Felodipine
- It has long half-life, so, can be given as once daily dosage.
- It provides symptomatic relief in Raynaud's disease.

Other Calcium Channel Blockers

Clevidipine
- It is a novel dihydropyridine calcium channel blocker.
- It is available as intravenous preparation.
- It has quick onset and rapid termination of action.
- It selectively dilates arterial smooth muscles.

Use
Perioperative hypertension

Flunarizine
- Flunarizine acts by inhibiting the T (transient) type calcium channels found in thalamus.
- It is not used in angina.

Use
Prophylaxis of migraine

Nursing Responsibilities
- Extended release preparation should not be crushed and should be administered as full tablets.
- Cardiac status, liver enzymes, platelet count should be monitored periodically.

BETA BLOCKERS IN ANGINA
The drugs are:
- Propranolol
- Atenolol
- Timolol
- Metoprolol.

Actions
- The cardioselective beta blockers atenolol, timolol and metoprolol, block β_1 receptors.
- The nonselective β blocker propranolol blocks both β_1 and β_2 receptors.
- They reduce myocardial oxygen consumption.
- This reduces the workload of the heart.
- They limit cardiac workload, both at rest and during exercise or exertion.
- Hence, they reduce the severity and frequency of anginal attack.

Uses
- Unstable angina
- Exertional angina
- Post MI
- Other details: See Section II, Chapter 12

Nursing Responsibilities
- Beta blockers should not be stopped abruptly and the dose should be reduced gradually.
- Other details: See Section II, Chapter 12

Frequently used Drug Combinations in Angina
- Nitrates + beta blockers
- Nitrates + calcium channel blockers
- Dihydropyridine calcium channel blockers + beta blockers
- Nitrates + calcium channel blockers + beta blockers

MISCELLANEOUS DRUGS
They are:
- Ranolazine
- Ivabradine
- Trimetazidine

Antianginal Drugs

Ranolazine

Actions
- It is indicated in both monotherapy and combination therapy of angina.
- It inhibits sodium channels of myocardium.
- Thereby, it reduces the calcium overload of myocardial cells.
- It is also a pFox inhibitor and suppresses the fatty acid oxidative pathway in myocardium.
- Therefore, the myocardial energy is obtained from glucose oxidation instead of fatty acid oxidation.
- It is a cardioprotective drug.
- It does not affect heart rate or blood pressure and prolongs exercise duration.
- It is safe in asthmatic patients with coexisting angina.

Adverse Effects
- Dizziness, postural hypotension, headache
- QT prolongation

Contraindication
- Acute angina
- Drugs causing QT prolongation or *torsades de pointes*
- Liver and kidney disease.

Uses
- Stable angina
- Chronic angina
- Myocardial infarction
- Arrhythmia

Potassium Channel Openers in Angina
- They cause dilatation of both vascular and visceral smooth muscles.
- Nicorandil is a potassium channel blocker.

Nicorandil
- It dilates both arterioles and venules.
- It increases coronary blood flow.
- It is costly, but tried in angina due to its cardioprotective action.
- It does not result in tolerance.

Adverse Effects
- Headache
- Dizziness
- Flushing, palpitation
- Aphthous ulcers

Contraindication
- Co-administration with sildenafil
- Co-administration with sulfonylureas

Uses
- Resistant angina
- Hypertension

Trimetazidine
- It reduces fatty acid mediated metabolism of myocardial cells and converts it to glucose pathway.
- It increases the exercise capacity of heart.
- It causes dizziness and fatigue.

Ivabradine
- It decreases heart rate and myocardial oxygen utilization.
- It improves exercise tolerance in stable angina.

PHARMACOTHERAPY OF ANGINA

Stable or Exertional Angina
- Sublingual nitroglycerin 0.3 to 0.6 mg should be taken 5 minutes before exertion.
- In case of acute attack it relieves pain within 3 minutes.
- Absence of pain relief after 3 tablets in 15 minutes indicates myocardial infarction.

Prophylaxis
- 500 mg ranolazine twice daily(or)
- Cardioselective beta blockers (preferred in post MI) (or)
- 10 to 40 mg oral isosorbide dinitrate every 4 hours (or)
- Sustained release preparation of nitroglycerine (or)
- 20 mg oral isosorbide mononitrate once or twice (with 7 hours gap) daily.

Nocturnal Angina
Nitroglycerine ointment or transdermal nitroglycerine patch.

Variant Angina
- Nitrates
- Calcium channel blockers

Unstable Angina
- Beta blockers
- Nitrates

Therapy of Myocardial Infarction
Myocardial infarction (MI) is classified as MI without Non-ST segment elevation (NSTEMI) and MI with ST segment elevation (STEMI). Fibrinolytic agent is essential and life saving in STEMI and harmful in NSTEMI. Antiplatelet drugs and anticoagulants are the main line of treatment in NSTEMI.

The drugs used are:
- Sublingual nitroglycerin to relieve pain.
- Analgesics: Morphine 10 mg or pethidine 50 mg.
- Fibrinolytic: Life saving in STEMI if given within first 3 hours. Risk reduction is 10% if given within 12 hours. Single bolus dose of 0.5 mg/kg of tenecteplase is ideal. Streptokinase is an alternative drug. Fibrinolytic should be avoided in NSTEMI.
- Metoprolol 25 to 50 mg within first 24 hours.
- Antiplatelet: 300 mg of aspirin to be chewed initially. It is continued at lower dose of 75 to 150 mg after the acute phase. They should be continued on long term basis to prevent future attacks.
- Anticoagulants: 1 mg/kg subcutaneous enoxaparin every 12 hours is preferred. Heparin is an alternative drug.

Nursing Responsibilities in MI
- Maintenance of oxygen supply and assisted ventilation.
- Infusion of adequate fluids for the maintenance of blood volume.
- Pain not subsiding after three sublingual doses of nitroglycerine indicates the need for opioid analgesics morphine or pethidine.
- Patient should be told to chew the prescribed dose of aspirin as soon as MI is suspected.
- Biochemical estimation (arterial blood gas analysis) to rule out acidosis should be done.
- International normalized ratio (INR) value, the indicator of prothrombin time, should be monitored weekly and maintained between 2 to 3, in patients receiving anticoagulants.

CHAPTER 29

Diuretics

Diuretics reduce edema by promoting excretion of sodium and water.
The drugs are:
- Carbonic anhydrase inhibitors
- Osmotic diuretics
- Loop diuretics
- Thiazide diuretics
- Potassium sparing diuretics
- Inhibitors of nonspecific cation channel.

USES

Edematous States
- Cardiac failure
- Chronic renal failure
- Nephrotic syndrome
- Ascites
- Cerebral edema

Non-edematous States
- Hypertension
- Hypercalcemia
- Nephrolithiasis (renal stones)
- Diabetes insipidus

CARBONIC ANHYDRASE (CA) INHIBITORS
The drugs are:
- Acetazolamide
- Methazolamide

Actions
- They are sulfonamide derivatives.
- They are weak diuretics.
- They inhibit the carbonic anhydrase (CA) enzyme.

- They act in proximal and collecting tubule of kidney.
- They inhibit the reabsorption of sodium bicarbonate.
- They reduce the secretion of ammonium ions.
- This increases the urinary pH.
- It causes metabolic acidosis.
- They also inhibit the CA enzyme in eye, CNS, pancreas and gastric mucosa.

Adverse Effects
- Allergic reaction
- Hepatic encephalopathy
- Renal calculi
- Respiratory or metabolic acidosis.

Uses
- Edema
- Open angle glaucoma (dorzolamide, brinzolamide)
- Prophylaxis of mountain sickness
- Prophylaxis of familial periodic paralysis

OSMOTIC DIURETICS
The drugs are:
- Mannitol
- Glycerin
- Isosorbide
- Urea

Actions
- They are inert and are freely filtered by glomerulus.
- They act on loop of Henle and in proximal tubule.
- They expand extracellular fluid volume (ECF) through osmosis.
- This action reduces viscosity of blood and inhibits renin secretion.
- Therefore, they increase renal blood flow and GFR.
- This promotes the excretion of water and electrolytes along with it.

Adverse Effects
- Pulmonary edema
- Hyponatremia
- Headache, nausea, vomiting

Contraindications
- Anuria
- Pulmonary edema
- Active cranial bleeding
- Urea is contraindicated in liver disease.

Uses
- Cerebral edema
- Acute attack of glaucoma
- Pre and postoperative reduction of intraocular pressure in ocular surgery
- Dialysis disequilibrium syndrome.

LOOP DIURETICS
The drugs are:
- Furosemide
- Torsemide
- Axosemide
- Bumetanide
- Piretanide
- Tripamide
- Ethacrynic acid

Actions
- These drugs are 'high ceiling diuretics'.
- They act on the thick ascending loop of Henle.
- They inhibit $Na^+K^+2Cl^-$ symporter.
- So, they inhibit reabsorption of sodium, potassium and chloride.
- They also inhibit reabsorption of calcium and magnesium.
- Long-term therapy reduces uric acid excretion.
- They increase renal blood flow.
- They are direct vasodilators.
- They reduce preload and left ventricular filling pressure.

Adverse Effects
- Hypotension, circulatory collapse
- Hyponatremia, hypokalemia, hypomagnesemia, hypocalcemia
- Hyperglycemia, hyperlipidemia, hyperuricemia
- Tinnitus, deafness, vertigo
- Rash, photosensitivity

Contraindications
- Severe volume depletion
- Sulfonamide allergy
- Anuria

Uses
- Acute pulmonary edema
- Congestive heart failure
- Nephrotic syndrome
- Ascites of liver cirrhosis
- Forced diuresis in drug overdose
- Edema in chronic renal disease
- Hypercalcemia
- In life-threatening hyponatremia with hypertonic saline.

Furosemide
- It has short half-life and variable absorption.
- Hence, repeated doses are required.
- Its excretion is prolonged in renal disease.

Torsemide
- It can be administered once daily.
- It has long half-life and good oral absorption.
- It has higher therapeutic efficacy than furosemide.
- It is metabolized mainly by liver.
- Its excretion is prolonged in liver but not in kidney disease.

THIAZIDE DIURETICS
The drugs are:
- Hydrochlorothiazide
- Bendroflumethiazide
- Indapamide
- Metolazone
- Quinethazone
- Polythiazide

Actions
- They are moderately potent diuretics.
- They inhibit the Na^+Cl^- symporter.
- Some are also weak inhibitors of carbonic anhydrase enzyme.

- Their site of action is the early distal collecting tubule.
- They increase the excretion of sodium and chloride ions.
- The thiazides inhibiting carbonic anhydrase enzyme, increase the excretion of bicarbonate and phosphate ions.
- Serum uric acid level decreases on short-term administration and increases on long-term administration.
- Chronic administration decreases the calcium excretion.

Adverse Effects
- Hypotension
- Hyponatremia, hypokalemia, hypochloremia, hypomagnesemia
- Hypercalcemia, hyperuricemia, hyperglycemia
- Headache, vertigo, skin rash, photosensitivity, blood dyscrasias
- Erectile dysfunction

Uses
- Congestive heart failure
- Ascites of liver cirrhosis
- Nephrotic syndrome
- Chronic renal failure
- Hypertension
- Nephrogenic diabetic insipidus
- Calcium nephrolithiasis

Contraindication
Sulfonamide allergy

POTASSIUM SPARING DIURETICS
The drugs are:
- Spironolactone
- Canrenone
- Eplerenone
- Triamterene
- Amiloride

Actions
- They are low efficacy diuretics.
- They are not effective as monotherapy.
- They are combined with other diuretics.
- The site of action is late distal tubule.
- They increase the excretion of sodium and chloride.

- They decrease the excretion of potassium, calcium and magnesium.
- Spironolactone and eplerenone are aldosterone antagonists.
- Triamterene and amiloride block the epithelial sodium channels.
- They increase the serum uric acid level.

Adverse Effects
- Life-threatening hyperkalemia
- Nausea, vomiting.

Contraindication
Hyperkalemia

Uses
- Hypertension
- Edema

Triamterene
- Triamterene and its metabolite are active.
- In addition to its action on late distal tubule, it also acts on collecting duct.
- It should not be given in liver and kidney disease.
- It also causes dizziness, leg cramps, photosensitivity reactions, folic acid deficiency and megaloblastic anemia.

Amiloride
- In addition to its action on late distal tubule, it also acts on collecting duct.
- The aerosolized form is useful in cystic fibrosis.
- It is also used in lithium induced diabetes insipidus.
- It also causes headache and diarrhea.

Spironolactone
- It interacts with androgen and progesterone receptors.
- Hence, spironolactone causes gynecomastia, menstrual irregularities, hirsutism and impotence.
- It also causes gastric bleeding, diarrhea, headache and drowsiness.
- It can cause breast cancer and skin rash.

Contraindication
Peptic ulcer

Uses
- Hypertension
- Ascites of hepatic cirrhosis.
- Primary hyperaldosteronism induced resistant hypertension.
- Secondary aldosteronism induced refractory edema.
- Congestive heart failure (CHF).

Eplerenone
- It is a safe and more specific aldosterone antagonist.
- It does not interact with androgen or progesterone receptors.
- Hence, it does not cause gynecomastia, hirsutism and menstrual disturbances.
- It is indicated in myocardial infarction and CHF with LV dysfunction.

INHIBITORS OF NONSPECIFIC CATION CHANNEL
The drugs are:
- Carperitide
- Nesiritide

Actions
- Carperitide is an atrial natriuretic peptide and nesiritide is a brain natriuretic peptide.
- They prevent sodium reabsorption.
- They act at inner medullary collecting duct.
- They are given intravenously and have short half-life.
- They are indicated only in acutely decompensated CHF.
- They increase creatinine level secondary to depletion of extracellular fluid volume.

Nursing Responsibilities
- Regular estimation of serum electrolytes is required and alterations in electrolytes level should be reported to the physician immediately.
- Weight of the patient should be recorded periodically to check change in fluid volume.

Antidiuretics
Vasopressin Analogs
The drugs are:
- Desmopressin

- Terlipressin
- Lypressin

Actions
- They act through vasopressin receptors.
- Their site of action is the collecting duct.
- They increase the water permeability and promote water conservation.
- They also cause vasoconstriction.

Adverse Effects
- Nausea, belching
- Urge to defecate
- Water intoxication
- Gangrene.

Uses
- Central diabetes insipidus.
- Desmopressin is used in nocturnal enuresis.
- Terlipressin is used in esophageal varices.
- Desmopressin is used in type I von Willebrand's disease.

Vasopressin Antagonists
They are:
- Conivaptan
- Tolvaptan.

Uses
- Syndrome of inappropriate ADH secretion (SIADH).
- Congestive heart failure

Treatment of Diabetes Insipidus (DI)

Types: Central DI and nephrogenic DI.
Differential test: Desmopressin test increases urine osmolality in central DI but has little or no effect in nephrogenic DI.

Treatment of Central DI
- Desmopressin—intranasal or oral route
- Thiazide diuretic chlorpropamide.

Treatment of Nephrogenic DI
- Thiazide diuretics
- Indomethacin
- Amiloride in lithium induced DI.

CHAPTER 30

Drugs in Heart Failure

Congestive heart failure (CHF) results in volume overload. Left heart failure presents as dyspnea, low cardiac output and high pulmonary venous pressure. Edema is the predominant feature of right heart failure. Systolic heart failure is commonly due to myocardial dysfunction. Reduction of the pumping capacity of the left ventricles decreases cardiac output. Diastolic heart failure results from excess preload due to renal failure, hypertension and cardiomyopathy. Treatment is aimed on improving the cardiac output and reducing the volume overload.

Drugs used are:
- Diuretics
- Aldosterone antagonists
- Vasodilators
- Cardiac glycosides
- Dopaminergic agonists
- Phosphodiesterase inhibitors.

DIURETICS IN CHF

The drugs are:
- Furosemide
- Torsemide
- Bumetanide

Actions

- They reduce extracellular fluid volume and ventricular filling pressure.
- They reduce the preload but do not reduce cardiac output.
- Loop diuretics are one of the first line drugs in the management of CHF with LV dysfunction.
- They should not be given in asymptomatic LV dysfunction.
- Furosemide, torsemide and bumetanide are the preferred loop diuretics.

Drugs in Heart Failure 189

- They reduce pulmonary venous congestion and peripheral edema.
- Thiazide diuretics, if given alone are ineffective.
- They are effective in refractory CHF only when combined with loop diuretics.

ALDOSTERONE ANTAGONISTS
They are:
- Spironolactone
- Eplerenone

Actions
- They reduce the circulating plasma aldosterone level.
- They are effective in CHF with LV dysfunction.
- Spironolactone and eplerenone are used.
- They cause significant reduction in sudden cardiac death.
- They cause life-threatening hyperkalemia.

VASODILATORS IN CHF
They are:
- Angiotensin converting enzyme (ACE) inhibitors
- Angiotensin receptor blockers (ARBs)
- Direct renin inhibitors
- Vasopressin antagonists
- Beta blockers
- Phentolamine
- Hydralazine
- Sodium nitroprusside
- Organic nitrates

Actions
- Arteriolar dilator hydralazine reduces the afterload.
- Venodilator organic nitrates reduce the preload.
- ACE inhibitors, ARBs, sodium nitroprusside, beta blockers reduce both pre and afterload.

ACE Inhibitors in CHF
- First line drugs in CHF as they reduce mortality.
- They are preferred in CHF patients with systolic dysfunction.

- They cause arterial vasodilatation and reduce the blood pressure.
- They reduce the afterload.
- They increase the cardiac output.
- They reduce mortality in asymptomatic LV dysfunction following MI.
- They improve the survival rate of CHF patients.
- Hyperkalemia should be watched for, when they are combined with aldosterone antagonists.
- They should be started at low dose to prevent iatrogenic hypotension.

ARBs in CHF

- They block AT_1 receptors which mediate the harmful effects of angiotensin in CHF.
- So, they are very effective in CHF due to systolic dysfunction.
- They are preferred in patients who do not tolerate ACE inhibitors.
- Hyperkalemia should be watched for, when they are combined with aldosterone antagonists.
- They are used in acute or chronic CHF with systolic dysfunction.
- They can cause angioedema.

Direct Renin Inhibitors in CHF

- Aliskiren reduces left ventricular remodeling in CHF.
- The duration of action is long.
- It is a competitive inhibitor of renin, blocking the conversion of angiotensin I to angiotensin II.
- It also reduces the plasma level of pro brain natriuretic peptide (BNP), a marker for active CHF.
- It can be safely combined with beta blocker/ACE inhibitor/ angiotensin receptor blocker.

Vasopressin Antagonists in CHF

- They inhibit the hyperresponsiveness to vasopressin commonly seen in CHF.
- Tolvaptan if combined with standard therapy improves the symptoms.
- It reduces right atrial pressure and pulmonary artery systolic blood pressure.
- The therapy should be given only in hospital setting as it requires monitoring of serum sodium level.

Nitrates in CHF
- They reduce the preload and left ventricular filling pressure.
- They reduce systemic and pulmonary vascular resistance.
- They increase coronary blood flow.
- They improve cardiac function.
- Intravenous nitroglycerine is effective in LV dysfunction following acute MI.
- Topical, sublingual, short-acting and long-acting oral preparation of organic nitrates can be used.

Hydralazine in CHF
- It reduces the systemic and pulmonary vascular resistance.
- It reduces the afterload.
- It causes moderate cardiac contraction.
- It increases the renal blood flow.
- So, it is used in CHF patients with renal impairment.
- It can cause hypotension, tachycardia and lupus like symptoms.

Sodium Nitroprusside in CHF
- It is given intravenously in CHF with systolic dysfunction.
- It reduces the afterload.
- It increases cardiac output and renal blood flow.
- It can cause hypotension and tachycardia.

Beta Blockers in CHF
- Beta blockers can be given only in stable heart failure.
- They improve left ventricular function and exercise tolerance.
- They reduce left ventricular hypertrophy.
- They decrease the incidence of tachyarrhythmia in CHF.
- Carvedilol and metoprolol are preferred.

CARDIAC GLYCOSIDES
They are called 'cardiac tonics' as they improve cardiac function without increasing oxygen requirement. The only cardiac glycoside used therapeutically is digoxin.

Digoxin
Actions
- It inhibits $Na^+K^+ATPase$ enzyme.
- It increases intracellular calcium in myocardial cells.

- It increases the force of contraction and cardiac output.
- It is a drug with low margin of safety.
- It reduces heart rate.
- It has diuretic effect.
- It reduces the edema associated with CHF.
- It is preferred in CHF due to left ventricular systolic dysfunction.
- It is a second line drug in patients who do not tolerate ACE inhibitors.

Adverse Effects
- Diarrhea, nausea, vomiting.
- Hypokalemia in chronic therapy
- Hyperkalemia in acute intoxication.
- Blurred vision
- Ectopic beats, AV block
- Ventricular arrhythmia

Digitalization
It is a cumulative drug. So, a loading dose is followed by maintenance doses. Response to therapy is usually seen around 7 days.

Treatment of Digitalis Overdose
- Stop the drug.
- IV lidocaine or phenytoin for digoxin induced ventricular arrhythmias.
- Oral or parenteral potassium supplementation. Intravenous potassium chloride 20 mmol/hour, prevents digoxin induced automaticity.
- Digoxin immune Fab that binds to digoxin in severe toxicity.

Contraindications
- Hypokalemia
- Acid-base imbalance
- Heart block

Drug Interactions
- The antiarrhythmic agent quinidine decreases digoxin clearance and increases its plasma level.
- Diuretics aggravate hypokalemia induced by digoxin.

Uses
- Congestive heart failure
- Paroxysmal supraventricular tachycardia (PSVT)

- Atrial fibrillation
- Atrial flutter

Nursing Responsibilities
- Pulse rate and ECG to be monitored regularly to avoid occurrence of arrhythmias.
- Initial signs of overdose of digitalis such as diarrhea should be watched for carefully and should be reported immediately.
- Patient should be instructed to take the medication regularly, at the same time daily.

DOPAMINERGIC DRUGS IN CHF
They are:
- Dopamine
- Dobutamine

Dopamine and dobutamine are positive inotropic agents and increase the force of contraction of heart.

Dopamine
- At low doses (≤ 2 µg/kg/min) it increases renal blood flow.
- At intermediate dose (2-5 µg/kg/min) it increases cardiac contraction.
- At higher doses (5-15 µg/kg/min) it increases blood pressure.
- Hence low dose dopamine is helpful to maintain renal blood flow in CHF patients.
- It has diuretic action and reduces edema associated with CHF.
- High dose causes tachycardia.

Dobutamine
- It increases the force of contraction of heart.
- It also causes peripheral vasodilatation.
- It is used in CHF patients with systolic dysfunction.
- Tolerance develops on prolonged administration.
- Side effects are tachycardia and arrhythmia.

PHOSPHODIESTERASE INHIBITORS
They are:
- Inamrinone
- Milrinone

Actions

- They inhibit degradation of cyclic AMP in cardiac and smooth muscles.
- They increase the force of cardiac contraction.
- They cause peripheral vasodilatation.
- They decrease the pre and afterload.
- They are known as 'inodilator' as they increase cardiac output.
- They are used in CHF due to systolic dysfunction.

Inamrinone and Milrinone

- They are selective phosphodiesterase 3 (PDE3) inhibitors.
- They promote cardiac contraction as well as relaxation.
- They cause dilatation of both arteries and veins.
- They decrease preload and afterload.
- Both drugs are given through intravenous route.
- They are started as loading dose and followed by continuous infusion.
- Inamrinone causes thrombocytopenia.
- Milrinone is more selective and short acting drug.
- Besides, milrinone does not cause thrombocytopenia.
- Hence, it is preferred for short-term use.

CHAPTER 31

Antihypertensive Drugs

Antihypertensive drugs reduce the risk of stroke. General measures such as reduction of body weight, increase in physical activity, restriction of salt intake and alcohol consumption can control the blood pressure.

The drugs are:
- Diuretics
- Angiotensin converting enzyme (ACE) inhibitors
- Angiotensin II receptor blockers (ARBs)
- Calcium channel blockers
- Sympatholytic drugs
- Centrally acting adrenergic agonists
- Direct renin inhibitors
- Vasodilators.

DIURETICS IN HYPERTENSION
- **Thiazide diuretics:** Hydrochlorothiazide, metolazone, indapamide, chlorthalidone
- **Loop diuretics:** Furosemide, bumetanide, torsemide, ethacrynic acid
- **Potassium sparing diuretics:** Triamterene, amiloride, spironolactone, eplerenone

Thiazide Diuretics
- Thiazide diuretics are preferred in hypertension.
- Chlorthalidone and indapamide are used.
- They are moderately effective.
- They cause moderate electrolyte depletion on long-term therapy.
- They are either used alone or in combination with other antihypertensive drugs.
- Initially, they reduce cardiac output.
- Long-term therapy reduces the blood pressure and normalizes cardiac output.

- They cause peripheral vasodilatation.
- Thiazides are not effective in patients with renal insufficiency.
- 4 to 6 weeks is necessary for full therapeutic benefit.

Chlorthalidone
- It has long half-life.
- Hence, once daily dose controls blood pressure even during night.

Hydrochlorothiazide
- It has similar efficacy to chlorthalidone.
- It is more suitable for combination therapy.
- It can cause severe hyponatremia.

Metolazone
The only thiazide diuretic effective in patients with renal insufficiency when glomerular filtration rate (GFR) falls below 30 mL/minute is metolazone.

Adverse Effects of Thiazides
- Hypokalemia, erectile dysfunction, gout.
- Hydrochlorothiazide can cause severe hyponatremia.

Loop Diuretics
- Furosemide and bumetanide are short acting drugs.
- Hence, multiple doses are necessary to control 24 hour blood pressure.
- Loop diuretics cause severe electrolyte imbalance.
- So, they are not preferred.
- They are useful in patients with azotemia.

Potassium Sparing Diuretics
- They are never given as monotherapy.
- They require frequent monitoring of potassium.
- Spironolactone and eplerenone reduce blood pressure (BP).
- They are preferred in hypertension associated with hyperaldosteronism.
- Triamterene does not reduce BP.
- Triamterene reduces thiazide induced hypokalemia.

Contraindication
- Renal insufficiency
- Hyperkalemia

ANGIOTENSIN CONVERTING ENZYME INHIBITORS (ACE INHIBITORS)

All drugs in this group have similar actions and therapeutic uses. They prevent the conversion of angiotensin I to angiotensin II by inhibiting angiotensin converting enzyme.

Angiotensin I
↓ Angiotensin converting enzyme
↓ (ACE) ← (↓ by ACE inhibitors)
Angiotensin II

The drugs are:
- Captopril
- Enalapril
- Ramipril
- Lisinopril
- Fosinopril
- Quinapril
- Moexipril
- Perindopril
- Benazepril
- Trandolapril

Actions
- They decrease the level of angiotensin II.
- They increase the level of bradykinin.
- They cause peripheral vasodilatation.
- They reduce blood pressure.
- They improve renal blood flow.
- They do not increase GFR.
- They maintain coronary and cerebral blood flow.
- They should be started as a low dose and increased gradually.
- Otherwise, they can result in hypotension.
- They exert renoprotective action.
- Oral bioavailability of captopril and moexipril is low in the presence of food.

Adverse Effects
- Cough
- Hypotension
- Hyperkalemia
- Alteration of taste sensation or 'dysgeusia'
- Teratogenicity. They belong to category 'C'

- Angioedema
- Skin rash

Uses
- **Hypertension:** One of the first line drugs.
- **Congestive heart failure (CHF):** First line drug for grade I to grade IV.
- **Myocardial infarction (MI):** Useful both in recurrent as well as evolving MI.
- Diabetic nephropathy
- Scleroderma crisis

Contraindications
- Coadministration of potassium sparing diuretics.
- Coadministration of digoxin.
- Bilateral renal artery stenosis.

Nursing Responsibilities
- Potassium supplements or food rich in potassium should be avoided in patients on ACE inhibitors.
- BP to be monitored after the first dose to prevent first dose induced hypotension.

Captopril: It contains sulfydryl moiety. It causes skin rash frequently.
Enalapril: It is a prodrug. It is converted to enalaprilat. It is also available as enalaprilat intravenous preparation.
Lisinopril: It is not a prodrug. It is more potent than enalapril.
Benazepril: It is also a prodrug. It is more potent than lisinopril.
Fosinopril: It is a prodrug. Its excretion is not altered in renal impairment.
Trandolapril: It is a prodrug. Its elimination is reduced in liver and kidney disease.
Ramipril: It is a prodrug. It is mainly excreted through kidney. Ramipril is preferred in those with high-risk for cardiovascular complications.
Perindopril: It is a prodrug. It is excreted mainly through kidney.
Quinapril: It is a prodrug. It is highly bound to tissues.
Moexipril: It is a prodrug. Dose should be reduced by 50% in renal impairment.

ANGIOTENSIN II RECEPTOR BLOCKERS (ARBS)
They are losartan, candesartan, irbesartan, telmisartan, valsartan, olmesartan, eprosartan.

Actions
- They selectively bind to AT_1 receptors.
- They inhibit angiotensin II mediated action.
- Their efficacy is comparable to ACE inhibitors.
- They have better safety profile.
- The incidence of cough and angioedema is minimal.
- They prevent diabetic nephropathy.
- They are given orally.
- Telmisartan and valsartan are eliminated only by liver.
- All other drugs are eliminated by both liver and kidney.
- Losartan and irbesartan are used in diabetic nephropathy.
- Losartan is also used for prophylaxis of stroke.
- Valsartan is used in CHF.

Adverse Effects
- Hyperkalemia
- Hypotension
- Teratogenicity
- Anaphylaxis, agranulocytosis, alopecia

Uses
- Hypertension
- Congestive heart failure
- Diabetic nephropathy
- Prophylaxis of stroke
- Left ventricular failure (LVF) following myocardial infarction.

Nursing Responsibilities
Hyperkalemia, hyponatremia should be watched for during therapy.

CALCIUM CHANNEL BLOCKERS IN HYPERTENSION
They are verapamil, amlodipine, nicardipine, nifedipine, nisoldipine, felodipine, clevidipine, diltiazem.

Actions

- Calcium channel blockers are one of the main line drugs.
- They inhibit the calcium channels of vascular smooth muscles.
- They cause peripheral vasodilatation.
- They reduce blood pressure.
- Dihydropyridines are potent vasodilators but can cause reflex tachycardia.
- Verapamil and diltiazem result in minimal reflex tachycardia.
- They are less effective in hypertension.
- Amlodipine is preferred.
- It has long-duration of action and can be given once daily.
- Amlodipine causes minimal reflex tachycardia.
- Sublingual preparation of nifedipine does not result in higher plasma concentration than oral formulation.
- Immediate release preparation of nifedipine causes reflex tachycardia.
- Hence, it should be avoided in therapy of hypertension.
- Intravenous preparation of clevidipine is used in perioperative hypertension.

Use

Systolic hypertension.

SYMPATHOLYTIC DRUGS

- **Beta receptor blockers:** Atenolol, metoprolol, propranolol
- **Alpha receptor blockers:** Prazosin, terazosin
- **Mixed α β receptor blockers:** Labetalol, carvedilol
- **Adrenergic neuron blockers:** Reserpine, guanadrel

Beta Receptor Blockers in Hypertension

- They are effective in hypertension.
- They cause peripheral vasodilatation and reduce blood pressure.
- They reduce heart rate and cardiac output.
- They also reduce the level of renin and angiotensin II.
- Cardioselective beta blockers are preferred in hypertension coexisting with bronchial asthma.
- Propranolol and atenolol increase total triglycerides and decrease high-density lipoproteins (HDL) cholesterol.
- They are given either once or twice daily.
- Sudden discontinuation aggravates the condition.

Antihypertensive Drugs

Drug Interactions
- Nonsteroidal anti-inflammatory drugs (NSAIDs) reduce the antihypertensive effect of beta blockers.
- Non selective beta blockers increase the risk of hypoglycemia in diabetes patients on insulin therapy.

Adverse Effects
- Fatigue
- Alteration of serum lipid level.
- Bradycardia

Precautions
- Bronchial asthma
- Diabetes mellitus
- Congestive heart failure

Alpha Receptor Blockers in Hypertension
- The selective α_1 blockers are preferred.
- They are combined with other antihypertensive agents.
- Initially, they cause reflex tachycardia.
- However, heart rate returns back to normal on long-term therapy.
- They do not alter the renal blood flow.
- They reduce low density lipoprotein (LDL) cholesterol and triglycerides.
- They increase HDL cholesterol.
- They cause postural hypotension after the first dose called 'first dose effect'.
- Patients develop tolerance to first dose effect on subsequent administration.

Adverse Effects
- Orthostatic hypotension
- Nasal stuffiness
- Erectile dysfunction

Contraindication
Congestive heart failure

Mixed α β Blockers in Hypertension
- Labetalol and carvedilol block β and α_1 receptors.
- Labetalol is given intravenously in hypertensive emergency.

- It reduces blood pressure quickly.
- Carvedilol is used in congestive heart failure with systolic dysfunction and in hypertension.

Adverse Effects
- Fatigue
- Bradycardia
- Hypotension.

Contraindication
Decompensated congestive heart failure.

Precautions
- Diabetes mellitus.
- Bronchial asthma.

Adrenergic Neuron Blockers in Hypertension

Guanadrel
- It acts as a 'false neurotransmitter'.
- It accumulates into the adrenergic storage vesicles and released instead of norepinephrine.
- This causes peripheral vasodilatation and reduces blood pressure.

Adverse Effects
- Severe postural hypotension
- Retrograde ejaculation

Drug Interactions
The effect of guanadrel is inhibited by:
- Tricyclic antidepressants
- Cocaine
- Ephedrine
- Amphetamine
- Chlorpromazine

Use
No longer preferred and very rarely used in hypertension.

Reserpine

Actions
- It is less expensive.
- It depletes catecholamines from the storage vesicles.
- Long-term therapy reduces blood pressure and cardiac output.

Adverse Effects
- Depression
- Suicidal tendencies

Use
Rarely used in hypertension.

CENTRALLY ACTING ADRENERGIC DRUGS IN HYPERTENSION
They are clonidine, methyldopa.

Methyldopa
Actions
- It is a prodrug.
- It is converted to α-methylnorepinephrine, a pseudotransmitter which is released instead of norepinephrine on neuronal stimulation.
- The oral absorption of methyldopa is rapid.
- Although it has short half-life, its duration of action extends upto 24 hours.
- It is not teratogenic.
- So, preferred in hypertension during pregnancy.

Adverse Effects
- Sedation
- Depression
- Dryness of mouth
- Hyperprolactinemia
- Galactorrhea
- Gynecomastia
- Hepatotoxicity
- Hemolytic anemia

Uses
- Mild to moderate hypertension.
- Hypertension associated with pregnancy.

Nursing Responsibilities
- BP to be monitored to rule out hypotension.
- Dose should not be missed and nursing personnel should ensure that the patient takes drug regularly.

Clonidine

Actions
- Clonidine stimulates α_2 receptors.
- It inhibits the release of noradrenaline.
- It causes peripheral vasodilatation.
- It reduces cardiac output and blood pressure.
- It is completely absorbed with 100% oral bioavailability.
- It is also available as transdermal formulation that delivers the drug for about a week.
- If stopped abruptly, it results in rebound hypertension.
- Abrupt discontinuation of transdermal application can also lead to rebound hypertension and withdrawal syndrome.

Adverse Effects
- Rebound hypertension
- Postural hypotension
- Sedation
- Dry mouth, dry eyes and dry nasal mucosa
- Erectile dysfunction
- Nightmares
- Depression
- Restlessness

Contraindication
Coadministration with tricyclic antidepressants.

Uses
- Hypertension.
- Diagnosis of pheochromocytoma.

Off Label Uses
- Withdrawal syndrome due to alcohol, opioid and tobacco discontinuation.
- Diarrhea in diabetics with autonomic neuropathy
- Menopausal hot flushes
- Restless leg syndrome
- Postherpetic neuralgia
- Mania, psychosis

Nursing Responsibilities
- Patient should be advised not to forget even one dose of clonidine.
- BP should be monitored periodically.

DIRECT RENIN INHIBITOR IN HYPERTENSION
Aliskiren
- It is a competitive inhibitor of renin.
- It inhibits the synthesis of angiotensin II.
- It can be given either as monotherapy or as a combination with other antihypertensives.
- It can cause diarrhea, cough, angioedema, headache and dizziness.

VASODILATORS IN HYPERTENSION
- **Arteriolar dilator:** Hydralazine, minoxidil, diazoxide, fenoldopam.
- **Arteriolar venular dilator:** Sodium nitroprusside.
- They dilate either arterioles or both arterioles and venules.
- They cause rapid fall of blood pressure as they act directly on blood vessels.

Hydralazine
Actions
- It dilates arterioles but not the venules.
- It reduces systolic blood pressure.
- This results in reflex tachycardia.
- It increases myocardial contraction.
- It increases plasma renin activity and causes fluid retention.
- It does not result in postural hypotension.
- It reduces BP equally in both standing and supine positions.

Adverse Effects
- Hypotension
- Tachycardia
- Palpitation
- Angina
- Dizziness
- Headache
- Drug induced lupus syndrome
- Serum sickness
- Polyneuropathy

Precautions
- Coronary artery disease (CAD).
- Patients with myocardial ischemia.
- Elderly individuals.

Uses
- With beta blockers or diuretics as second line drug in hypertension.
- Second line drug in pregnancy induced hypertensive emergency.
- Congestive heart failure with nitrates.

Nursing Responsibilities
- In patients with hydralazine induced polyneuropathy, pyridoxine should be given as it reverses this condition.
- Periodic monitoring of blood pressure is essential to prevent hypotension.
- Onset of side effects should be reported to the attending physician.

Minoxidil

Actions
- Its metabolite dilates the arterioles.
- It is also a potassium channel opener.
- It does not relax venules.
- It increases the blood flow to heart, gastrointestinal tract (GIT) and skeletal muscles.
- It increases cardiac output by 3 to 4 times.
- It also results in reflex tachycardia.
- It increases renal blood flow.
- It increases renin secretion.

Adverse Effects
- Edema
- Tachycardia
- Cardiac failure
- Pericardial effusion
- Hypertrichosis or increased hair growth
- Glucose intolerance
- Steven-Johnson syndrome
- Electrocardiogram (ECG) changes

Contraindications
- Coronary artery disease
- Myocardial infarction
- Renal failure
- Cardiac failure
- Diabetic patients on sulfonylureas

Uses
- Refractory and severe hypertension.
- Topical application for male pattern baldness.

Nursing Responsibilities
- Periodic chest X-ray is necessary to rule out pericardial effusion.
- Periodic monitoring of body weight is necessary to rule out edema.

Sodium Nitroprusside

Actions
- It acts by releasing nitrous oxide.
- It has quick onset but short-duration of action.
- It dilates both arterioles and venules.
- Therefore, it reduces both preload and afterload.

Adverse Effects
- Hypotension
- Lactic acidosis
- Hypothyroidism

Contraindication
Chronic obstructive pulmonary disease.

Uses
- Hypertensive emergencies
- Acute aortic dissection
- Refractory congestive heart failure with pulmonary edema
- To reduce cardiac workload after myocardial infarction
- To induce controlled hypotension during anesthesia

Nursing Responsibilities
- Nitroprusside bottle should not be exposed to light and should be covered in opaque wrapping as it decomposes in light.
- It should be freshly prepared every time before infusion.
- Blood pressure should be closely monitored during infusion to prevent hypotension.

Diazoxide
- It causes marked reduction in blood pressure.
- It causes reflex tachycardia.

Uses
- Hypertensive emergency (rarely used now)
- Hypoglycemia
  Fenoldopam: See Section II, Chapter 10

HYPERTENSIVE EMERGENCY
- Blood pressure above 200/120 mm Hg is a hypertensive emergency.
- BP should be lowered by 30% in the first few hours.
- Then it should be reduced gradually.
- Drugs should be administered intravenously.
- Drugs used are labetalol, nicardipine, esmolol, fenoldopam, sodium nitroprusside, hydralazine and phentolamine.

HYPERTENSIVE URGENCY
- In hypertensive urgency, diastolic blood pressure is elevated above 120 mm Hg.
- Oral clonidine is the most effective drug.

PERIOPERATIVE HYPERTENSION
Drugs used are esmolol or clevidipine.

ORTHOSTATIC HYPOTENSION
Midodrine or phenylephrine is used.

CHAPTER 32

Antiarrhythmic Agents

Disturbance in cardiac impulse generation or its propagation can cause arrhythmia. Disturbance in impulse generation results in bradyarrhythmia while improper propagation results in heart block. Tachyarrhythmias occur due to triggered automaticity of heart or due to reentry phenomenon. Antiarrhythmic drugs act either to prevent or to treat the condition.

Drugs used in the treatment of arrhythmia are broadly classified into:

Class I – Sodium channel blockers: Class I agents are again subclassified into class IA, IB and IC.

    Class IA – Rate of recovery of sodium channels is moderate; from 1 to 10 seconds: Quinidine, procainamide, disopyramide

    Class IB – Rate of recovery of sodium channels is short; less than 1 second: Lidocaine, mexiletine

    Class IC – Rate of recovery of sodium channels is high; more than 10 seconds: Propafenone, flecainide

Class II – Beta blockers: Propranolol, sotalol, esmolol

Class III – Potassium channel blockers: Amiodarone, dronedarone, dofetilide, ibutilide

Class IV – Calcium channel blockers: Verapamil, diltiazem

Others – Adenosine, atropine, digoxin, magnesium, vernakalant.

ADENOSINE

Actions

- It binds to adenosine receptors.
- It inhibits automaticity and conduction velocity.
- It prolongs the refractory period of atrioventricular (AV) node.
- It has a very short half-life.
- The action terminates within seconds.
- Hence, it requires a rapid bolus dose.
- It is a safe drug as its side effects are short lived.

Adverse Effects
- Dyspnea
- Bronchoconstriction
- Atrial fibrillation

Drug Interactions
- Dipyridamole potentiates the action of adenosine.
- Theophylline and caffeine increase the dose requirement of adenosine.

Uses
- Re-entrant supraventricular arrhythmias.
- Controlled hypotension during surgical procedures.
- Diagnosis of coronary artery disease.

Nursing Responsibilities
- The administration of intravenous bolus dose of adenosine should be rapid.
- Patients should be prevented from taking beverages before the administration of adenosine.

QUINIDINE

Actions
- It blocks the cardiac sodium and potassium currents.
- The rate of recovery of sodium channels is moderate.
- It decreases the excitability of cardiac cells.
- It decreases the automaticity.
- It prolongs action potential duration and refractory period.
- It has vagolytic action.
- It is an enzyme inhibitor and decreases the metabolism of coadministered drugs.
- Enzyme inducers such as phenobarbitone and phenytoin reduce the plasma level of quinidine.

Adverse Effects
- Diarrhea
- *Torsades de pointes* or prolonged QT syndrome
- Cinchonism
- Thrombocytopenia
- Ventricular tachycardia

Drug Interactions
- It increases the plasma level of propafenone.
- It increases the concentration of digoxin by reducing its clearance.
- It decreases the conversion of codeine to morphine.

Uses
- To maintain sinus rhythm in atrial flutter and atrial fibrillation.
- To prevent recurrence of ventricular fibrillation and ventricular tachycardia.

Nursing Responsibilities
- Since diarrhea causes hypokalemia which can result in *torsades de pointes*, it should be reported immediately to the attending physician.
- Electrolyte level should be monitored in patients with diarrhea to rule out hypokalemia.
- Platelet count should be monitored.
- To avoid the risk of hypotension, blood pressure should be monitored during intravenous administration of quinidine.

PROCAINAMIDE

Actions
- It does not have vagolytic and α adrenergic blocking property.
- It blocks both sodium and potassium currents in heart.
- It prolongs the action potential, refractory period and conduction velocity.
- It reduces the automaticity of heart.
- Intravenous administration of procainamide is better tolerated than quinidine.
- Patients tolerate short-term intravenous administration than long-term oral therapy.
- Procainamide has a short duration of action as it is eliminated quickly.
- Lupus syndrome occurs early, in patients with slow acetylation status.

Adverse Effects
- Hypotension
- Nausea
- Aplastic anemia

- Lupus syndrome
- *Torsades de pointes*

Use
Supraventricular and ventricular arrhythmias.

Nursing Responsibilities
- Sustained release oral preparation is preferred as it prolongs the therapeutic benefit.
- Monitoring of blood pressure (BP) during intravenous administration is essential as it can cause hypotension.
- Monitoring of blood count and antinuclear antibody is essential.

DISOPYRAMIDE
Actions
- It blocks the cardiac sodium channels.
- It does not prolong the action potential duration.
- It does not block α receptors.
- It has marked anticholinergic action.
- It is well absorbed orally.

Adverse Effects
- Anticholinergic side effects such as glaucoma, urinary retention, constipation and dry mouth.
- Heart failure
- *Torsades de pointes*

Uses
- To maintain sinus rhythm in atrial flutter and atrial fibrillation.
- To prevent recurrent ventricular fibrillation and ventricular tachycardia.

LIDOCAINE AS ANTIARRHYTHMIC AGENT
Actions
- It blocks the cardiac sodium channels.
- It is not useful in the treatment of atrial arrhythmia.
- Lidocaine decreases the automaticity of cardiac cells.
- It is not effective orally as it undergoes high first pass metabolism.

- Intravenous route of administration is preferred.
- Plasma concentration falls rapidly after single intravenous loading dose.
- Hence, a loading regimen is required till a steady state concentration is reached.
- This is followed by infusion of maintenance dose.

Adverse Effects
- Seizure
- Nystagmus
- Tremor
- Dysarthria

Use
Ventricular arrhythmia.

Nursing Responsibilities
- Patient should be monitored for seizures during rapid intravenous administration of large doses.
- The speed of maintenance dose infusion should be optimal and should not be either too slow or too fast.

MEXILETINE
- It is an analog of lignocaine.
- It is useful for chronic therapy.
- It blocks cardiac sodium currents.
- Unlike lidocaine, it does not undergo high first pass metabolism.
- So, it can be given orally.

Adverse Effects
- Tremor
- Nausea

Use
Ventricular arrhythmias

Nursing Responsibilities
Patients should be advised to take mexiletine with food.

FLECAINIDE

Actions
- It blocks the cardiac sodium channels.
- The rate of recovery of sodium channels is delayed.
- It also blocks potassium and calcium currents in heart.
- It prolongs the action potential duration in atrium.
- It maintains sinus rate in patients with supraventricular arrhythmias.
- It is well absorbed orally.

Adverse Effects
- Blurring of vision
- Arrhythmia
- Congestive heart failure in patients with left ventricular failure (LVF)
- Heart block

Contraindications
- Myocardial infarction.
- Patients with conduction abnormalities.

Uses
- To maintain sinus rhythm in supraventricular arrhythmia.
- Sustained ventricular tachycardia.

Nursing Responsibilities
- Heart rate to be monitored as flecainide can cause lethal arrhythmias.
- Blurring of vision to be reported to the attending physician as it indicates high dose.

PROPAFENONE

Actions
- It blocks cardiac sodium and potassium channels.
- It also blocks beta receptors in some patients.
- It undergoes variable first pass metabolism.
- It is given orally two times a day.
- It is available as sustained release formulation.

Adverse Effects
- Re-entrant ventricular tachycardia
- Bradycardia
- Bronchospasm

Use
Supraventricular tachycardia.

Nursing Responsibilities
Liver and kidney function test should be done.

PROPRANOLOL
See Section II, Chapter 12

SOTALOL
Actions
- It is a nonselective beta blocker.
- It is under orphan drug status.
- It prolongs conduction velocity and refractory period.
- It decreases automaticity.

Adverse Effects
- *Torsades de pointes.*
- Early after depolarization.
- Other adverse effects: See Section II, Chapter 12

Uses
- Atrial flutter
- Atrial fibrillation
- Ventricular tachyarrhythmias

Nursing Responsibilities
It is necessary to monitor serum potassium level.

ESMOLOL
- It is a selective β_1 blocker.
- It has a very short duration of action.
- Hence, adverse effects disappear very quickly.
- It is given intravenously for the control of rapidly conducted atrial fibrillation.

AMIODARONE

Actions
- It is structurally similar to thyroid hormone.
- It also inhibits the cardiac calcium and potassium currents.
- It also blocks the sodium channels.
- In addition, it blocks the adrenergic receptors.
- It decreases conduction velocity.
- It prolongs the action potential.
- It suppresses automaticity.
- It is highly lipophilic and accumulates in many tissues.
- Besides, it has prolonged duration of action.
- So its adverse effects also disappear slowly.
- Since it is insoluble in water, the solvent dimethyl sulfoxide is added in intravenous preparation.
- This solvent is responsible for the adverse effects of intravenous preparation.
- Hypotension occurs following intravenous administration due to the solvent.
- Fall in BP can also be due to vasodilatation and improper cardiac function.
- Generally, oral loading dose does not result in adverse effects.
- Rarely, oral loading dose can cause nausea which disappears on dose reduction.
- Long-term treatment causes severe side effects due to its tissue accumulation.

Adverse Effects
- Hypotension on intravenous administration.
- Nausea during oral loading dose.
- Pulmonary fibrosis.
- Corneal microdeposits.
- Peripheral neuropathy.
- Hepatotoxicity.
- Hypothyroidism.
- Hyperthyroidism.
- Photosensitivity.
- It prolongs QT but rarely causes *torsades de pointes*.

Uses
- To maintain sinus rhythm in patients with atrial fibrillation.
- Immediate arrest of ventricular tachycardia or fibrillation.

Nursing Responsibilities
- BP should be checked during intravenous administration.
- If nausea occurs following oral loading dose, it should be reported to the attending physician.
- Periodic chest X-ray and pulmonary function test is necessary and any abnormality should be reported to the physician immediately.
- It is vital to do thyroid function test to rule out any abnormality in thyroid status.
- Liver function test should be done to rule out drug induced hepatic dysfunction.
- If patient misses to take one or two doses during chronic therapy he/she should be given reassurance to continue the drug.

DRONEDARONE
Actions
- It is a derivative of amiodarone.
- When compared to amiodarone, it has lower efficacy but better safety.
- It blocks potassium, calcium and sodium currents.
- It also blocks the adrenergic receptors.

Adverse Effects
- Nausea, vomiting, diarrhea
- Asthenia
- Abdominal pain

Drug Interaction
- Enzyme inhibitors such as ketoconazole inhibit its metabolism increasing its plasma level.
- Digoxin and metoprolol increase its concentration.

Contraindication
Heart failure

Uses
- Atrial flutter
- Atrial fibrillation

IBUTILIDE
Actions
- It blocks the cardiac potassium current.
- It prolongs the action potential.
- It is not effective orally.
- It is administered as rapid infusion.

Adverse Effect
Torsades de pointes.

Use
Conversion of atrial flutter or fibrillation to normal sinus rhythm.

DOFETILIDE
Actions
- It blocks cardiac potassium current.
- It should not be used in patients with renal failure.

Adverse Effect
Torsades de pointes

Use
To maintain sinus rhythm in atrial fibrillation.

DIGOXIN AS ANTIARRHYTHMIC AGENT
Actions
- Digoxin is a drug with low therapeutic index.
- As antiarrhythmic agent, it inhibits calcium current in AV node and potassium current in atrium.
- It causes hyperpolarization and increases the refractory period of AV node.
- Since its rate of distribution is slow, even after intravenous administration, the onset of its antiarrhythmic action is delayed.

Adverse Effects
- Atrial tachycardia
- Ventricular bigeminy
- Nausea, blurred vision, cognitive impairment
- Hypokalemia, hypomagnesemia, hypercalcemia
- ST segment depression, PR prolongation

Treatment of Digoxin Induced Alterations in Cardiac Rhythm
- Magnesium for tachycardia and AV block.
- Atropine for bradycardia.
- In digitalis induced arrhythmia, anti-digoxin Fab to bind with digoxin to promote its excretion.

Uses
- Re-entrant arrhythmias involving AV node.
- Atrial fibrillation to control ventricular response.

Nursing Responsibilities
See Section VI, Chapter 30

MAGNESIUM
It is given through intravenous route.

Uses
- Recurrent episodes of *torsades de pointes*.
- Digitalis induced arrhythmias.

VERNAKALANT
- It inhibits potassium, sodium and L-type calcium current of atrium.
- It prolongs the refractory period of atrium.
- It is given through intravenous route.
- It is used to convert atrial fibrillation to sinus rhythm.

SECTION VII

Blood

- Coagulants
- Anticoagulants
- Fibrinolytic Drugs
- Antiplatelet Agents
- Hypolipidemic Drugs
- Treatment of Shock
- Iron Deficiency Anemia
- Megaloblastic Anemia and Hematopoietic Growth Factors

CHAPTER 33

Coagulants

Substances that control hemorrhagic state and promote clotting of blood are called coagulants. They are:
- Vitamin K
- Fibrinogen
- Antihemophilic factor
- Adrenochrome monosemicarbazone
- Desmopressin
- Rutin
- Ethamsylate

VITAMIN K

Actions
- It is a fat soluble vitamin necessary for the synthesis of clotting factors.
- Vitamin K_1 or phytonadione is the only natural vitamin from plant source used in therapy.
- K_2 or menadione is a synthetic preparation.
- Phytonadione is safer than menadione.
- Vitamin K is involved in the synthesis of factors II (prothrombin), VII, IX and X.
- Since it is a fat soluble vitamin, bile salts promote its intestinal absorption.
- Malabsorption, obstructive jaundice, liver disease and chronic therapy of broad spectrum antibiotics cause vitamin K deficiency.

Adverse Effect
Menadione causes kernicterus and hemolysis in newborn.

Uses
- Vitamin K deficiency.
- In premature infant to increase the levels of prothrombin and other clotting factors.
- Overdose of oral anticoagulants.

- American pit viper bite
- Hepatocellular disease
- Malabsorption

FIBRINOGEN AND ANTIHEMOPHILIC FACTOR
They are given in the treatment of hemophilia.

ADRENOCHROME
- It reduces microcapillary bleeding.
- It is used in epistaxis, hematuria and bleeding.

RUTIN
- It is a plant product.
- It reduces capillary bleeding.
- It has uncertain efficacy.

ETHAMSYLATE
- It exerts antihyaluronidase activity.
- It is used to control bleeding after abortion, melena, menorrhagia, postpartum hemorrhage, epistaxis and hematuria.
- It can cause rash and headache.

VASOPRESSIN AGONISTS
The drugs are:
- Desmopressin
- Terlipressin
- Vasopressin
- Lypressin

Actions
- They act on vasopressin receptors and cause vasoconstriction.
- In addition, desmopressin increases factor VIII and von Willebrand factor.

Adverse Effects of Desmopressin
- Tachyphylaxis
- Water intoxication

Uses of Desmopressin
- Type I von Willebrand's disease.
- Moderate and not severe hemophilia A.
- Central diabetes insipidus.
- Nocturnal enuresis.
- Cirrhosis or drug induced bleeding disorders.

Adverse Effects of Vasopressin and Terlipressin
- Headache, nausea, belching.
- Urge to defecate.
- Facial flushing, urticaria.
- Gangrene.
- Rhinorrhea, pruritus and irritation after intranasal administration.

Uses of Terlipressin
- Bleeding esophageal varices.
- Acute hemorrhagic gastritis.
- Cyclophosphamide induced hemorrhagic cystitis.
- Bleeding during surgical procedures.

Contraindication
Psychogenic polydipsia as it can cause hyponatremia.

Drug Interactions
- Lithium, ethanol and demeclocycline reduce the diuretic effect of desmopressin.
- Tricyclic antidepressant (TCA), morphine, non-steroidel anti-inflammatory drugs (NSAIDs) and chlorpropamide can potentiate the diuretic effect of desmopressin.

Nursing Responsibilities
Bleeding and clotting time should be monitored for patients on coagulants to prevent overdose.

STYPTICS
Actions
- These compounds are applied locally to arrest bleeding.
- They control mild oozing from capillaries.

- Thrombin available as dry powder can be applied on the bleeding surface.
- Gelatin foam, fibrin, oxidized cellulose are absorbable styptics.
- 0.1% adrenaline is also used as local hemostatic agent.
- Occasionally, the astringent tannic acid is used to arrest bleeding.

Uses
- Epistaxis
- Bleeding gum

Nursing Responsibilities
- Manual pressure can arrest local bleeding and should be tried.
- Absorbable styptics need not be removed as they are absorbed within 4 weeks.
- Adrenaline should be cautiously used as styptic in hypertensives and elders.

SCLEROSING AGENTS
- These irritants promote fibrosis and arrest bleeding.
- Sodium tetradecyl sulfate and polidocanol are sclerosing agents.
- They are injected into varicose veins or hemorrhoids.

CHAPTER 34

Anticoagulants

Drugs that prolong bleeding time by inhibiting coagulation are known as anticoagulants. They are classified as oral and parenteral agents. Some are effective both *in vivo* and *in vitro*, while others are effective only *in vivo*.

Anticoagulants effective *in vivo*
- **Parenteral agents:** Heparin, low molecular weight heparinoids (LMWH), fondaparinux, desirudin, lepirudin, bivalirudin, argatroban, drotrecogin α.
- **Oral agents:** Dicumarol, warfarin, acenocoumarol, phenindione, dabigatran etexilate, rivaroxaban

Anticoagulants effective *in vitro*
- Heparin, sodium citrate, sodium edate, sodium oxalate

HEPARIN

Actions
- It is a parenteral anticoagulant.
- It can be administered either intravenously or subcutaneously.
- It can be used both *in vivo* and *in vitro*.
- It is obtained from porcine intestinal mast cells.
- It does not have intrinsic anticoagulant action.
- It binds to antithrombin and inhibits factors IIa, IXa, Xa, XIa, XIIa and XIIIa.
- It inhibits platelet aggregation at higher doses and prolongs bleeding time.
- By increasing plasma lipoprotein lipase, it clears lipemic plasma.
- Rebound hyperlipidemia occurs on cessation of therapy.
- Since it does not cross placenta, it is the preferred anticoagulant during pregnancy.
- Overdose of heparin is treated by protamine sulfate.

Adverse Effects
- Bleeding
- Thrombocytopenia

- Osteoporosis
- Hepatic dysfunction
- Hyperkalemia
- Venous thromboembolism

Contraindications
- Bleeding disorders
- Coadministration of antiplatelet drugs.
- Hepatic dysfunction

Uses
- Prophylaxis of postoperative deep vein thrombosis.
- Prophylaxis of postoperative pulmonary embolism.
- Venous thrombosis.
- Initial management in acute myocardial infarction or unstable angina.
- During coronary balloon angioplasty.
- Disseminated intravascular coagulation (DIC).
- Cardiopulmonary bypass surgery.

Nursing Responsibilities
- Bleeding and clotting time should be monitored.
- If hematuria occurs, it should be reported to the attending physician.
- Do not mix heparin with other drugs in the same syringe or in the same infusion.
- During subcutaneous (SC) administration of heparin, it should be injected without rubbing.
- Heparinized blood sample should never be sent for estimation of blood count, fragility test or compliment fixation test.
- The rate of infusion of heparin should be assessed by activated thromboplastin time (aPTT) or whole blood clotting time.
- Do not give heparin through intramuscular route.

LOW MOLECULAR WEIGHT HEPARIN (LMWH)
They inhibit factor Xa and has minimal inhibitory effect on factor IIa. They do not inhibit platelet aggregation and rarely cause thrombocytopenia.

The drugs are:
- Enoxaparin
- Reviparin
- Dalteparin
- Nadroparin
- Ardeparin
- Tinzaparin

Advantages
- They have better subcutaneous bioavailability.
- They have longer duration of action.
- They are administered once daily through subcutaneous route.
- They do not require monitoring of aPTT or clotting time.
- They have a minimal risk for osteoporosis or thrombocytopenia even after prolonged therapy.
- They do not cross placenta.

Disadvantages
- In case of overdose, their action cannot be fully reversed by protamine.
- They should not be administered in patients with heparin induced thrombocytopenia.
- They accumulate in patients with renal impairment causing bleeding.

Uses
- Prophylaxis of postoperative deep vein thrombosis.
- Prophylaxis of postoperative pulmonary embolism.
- Venous thrombosis.
- Preferred to heparin in myocardial infarction (MI) or unstable angina.
- In patient's undergoing dialysis.
- Coronary balloon angioplasty.

Contraindication
Renal dysfunction

Nursing Responsibilities
Compulsory monitoring of aPTT is not required for patient's receiving LMWHs.

FONDAPARINUX

Actions
It inhibits factor Xa and does not inhibit factor IIa.

Advantages
- It has 100% bioavailability through subcutaneous administration.
- Since it has long-duration of action, it can be given once daily.
- It has very minimal risk of thrombocytopenia.
- The risk of osteoporosis is minimal even on long-term treatment.
- It does not require laboratory monitoring of aPTT.
- It does not cross placenta.

Disadvantage
- It is not a suitable anticoagulant during coronary balloon angioplasty as it can cause catheter thrombosis.
- Its actions cannot be reversed by protamine.

Contraindication
Renal dysfunction

Uses
- Venous thrombosis, pulmonary embolism.
- Prophylaxis in patient undergoing knee or hip surgery.
- Initial management of MI.

Nursing Responsibilities
Frequent monitoring of platelet count is not necessary.

Idraparinux
- It is a derivative of fondaparinux.
- It has longer duration of action than fondaparinux.
- So it can be administered subcutaneously once in a week.

OTHER PARENTERAL ANTICOAGULANTS

Direct Thrombin Inhibitors
The drugs are lepirudin, desirudin, bivalirudin, argatroban and drotrecogin α.

Anticoagulants

Lepirudin
- It is present in salivary glands of leech.
- It is administered through intravenous route.
- It is indicated as an alternate anticoagulant in patient's with heparin induced thrombocytopenia.
- It has a risk of prolonged anticoagulant effect.
- No antidote available for reversing its action in drug overdose.

Nursing Responsibilities
It requires daily monitoring of aPTT.

Desirudin
- It can be administered subcutaneously.
- It is used for the prophylaxis of deep vein thrombosis in patient undergoing elective hip replacement surgery.
- It should be used cautiously in renal dysfunction.

Bivalirudin
- It is an alternative to heparin in coronary angioplasty or cardiopulmonary bypass surgery.
- It is given through intravenous route.
- It should be used with caution in renal dysfunction.

Argatroban
Actions
- It is a reversible thrombin inhibitor.
- It is administered through intravenous route.
- It has immediate onset of action.
- It prolongs aPTT and prothrombin time.
- Hence aPTT should be monitored.
- It is an alternate anticoagulant in patients with heparin induced thrombocytopenia.

Drotrecogin a
- It inactivates factors Va and VIIIa.
- It also has anti-inflammatory property.
- It is indicated in patients at high-risk for sepsis following shock and oliguria.
- It should be given within 48 hours of onset of organ dysfunction.

TREATMENT OF HEPARIN OVERDOSE
Protamine Sulfate
Actions
- It is a heparin antagonist obtained from sperm of salmon fish.
- It is effective in the management of heparin overdose.
- It does not reverse the effect of fondaparinux.
- It reverses the effect of LMWHs partially.
- It is used to rapidly terminate the action of heparin after cardiac or vascular surgery.
- It binds tightly to heparin, neutralizing its anticoagulant effect.
- It causes anaphylaxis in diabetics on insulin containing protamine.
- On its own, it can act as a weak anticoagulant in the absence of heparin.

ORAL ANTICOAGULANTS
Warfarin
Actions
- It antagonizes the action of vitamin K.
- Thereby it prevents the synthesis of the coagulation factors II, VII, IX and X.
- It inhibits vitamin K epoxide reductase that converts vitamin K epoxide to reduced vitamin K.
- The time required to suppress each coagulation factor is not the same.
- Hence the onset of therapeutic action of warfarin is delayed by several days.
- Its dose should be fixed according to international normalized ratio (INR) and international sensitivity index (ISI) derived as per prothrombin time.
- The normal range of INR is 2 to 3.
- Since it is highly protein bound, it is prone for various interactions with other highly protein bound drugs.
- It crosses placenta and attains almost equal concentration in foetus.
- Hence it is not preferred for pregnancy associated conditions.
- It is not secreted through milk and can be safely administered in lactating women.

Drug Interactions
- Cholestyramine reduces its intestinal absorption.
- Enzyme inducers such as barbiturates, rifampin and carbamazepine stimulate its metabolism.
- Amiodarone, azole antifungals, metronidazole, cimetidine, disulfiram, clopidogrel, co-trimoxazole, zafirlukast and isonicotinic acid hydrazide (INH) inhibit its metabolism.
- Loop diuretics and sodium valproate increase its plasma level.

Contraindications
- Pregnancy
- Renal and hepatic dysfunction.
- Heparin induced thrombocytopenia as it increases the risk of gangrene.

Adverse Effects
- Bleeding
- Warfarin syndrome – birth defects in newborn.
- Necrosis of skin.
- Bluish discoloration of plantar aspect of toes (purple toe syndrome).
- Alopecia, dermatitis and urticaria.
- Gangrene in patient's with heparin induced thrombocytopenia.

Uses
- Following administration of heparin, to prevent deep vein thrombosis or pulmonary embolism.
- Prevention of venous thromboembolism.
- Prevention of coronary ischemia in patients with acute MI.
- In patients with prosthetic heart valves.
- Chronic atrial fibrillation.

Nursing Responsibilities
- INR and ISI values should be monitored daily till the dose is stabilized.
- ISI value is variable and mentioned in each kit.
- Interaction between warfarin and coadministered drugs should be monitored.
- Skin lesions on extremities, penis and breast should be closely monitored.

- Hematuria, melena and excess menstrual bleeding indicate overdose of anticoagulants and should be immediately reported to the attending physician.

Dabigatran Etexilate
Actions
- It is a prodrug.
- It is converted to dabigatran.
- It reversibly blocks the active site of thrombin.
- It does not require routine monitoring of coagulation factors.
- It is superior to warfarin in efficacy for prevention of stroke in patient with atrial fibrillation.
- It is also effective in venous thromboembolism.

Rivaroxaban
- It inhibits factor Xa.
- It has good oral bioavailability.
- It is used for prevention of thrombosis in patient undergoing elective surgery of lower limb.

Nursing Responsibilities
It does not require monitoring of prothrombin time.

CHAPTER 35

Fibrinolytic Drugs

The drugs are:
- Plasminogen
- α_2-antiplasmin
- Streptokinase
- Tissue plasminogen activator (tPA)
- Alteplase
- Reteplase
- Tenecteplase

ACTION OF FIBRINOLYTIC DRUGS
- Tissue plasminogen activator (tPA) is secreted by endothelial cells during injury and bind to fibrin, activating plasminogen to plasmin which lysis fibrin.
- The plasminogen inactivators 1 and 2 (PAI-1 and PAI-2), inactivate tPA.

Adverse Effects
Bleeding is the major toxicity.

Contraindications
- Prior intracranial hemorrhage
- Ischemic stroke
- Active bleeding
- Coagulation disorders
- Uncontrolled hypertension
- Pregnancy
- Active peptic ulcer

Uses
To lyse thrombi in acute myocardial infarction and in coronary thrombosis.

PLASMINOGEN
It enhances fibrinolysis by binding with fibrin.

α_2-ANTIPLASMIN
- It inactivates plasmin.
- It produces a systemic lytic state.
- It impairs fibrin polymerization and promotes bleeding.

STREPTOKINASE
- It is obtained from β- hemolytic streptococci.
- It causes allergy and anaphylaxis.
- So it is rarely used now.
- It is inactive as such and gets activated by forming a complex with plasminogen.

TISSUE PLASMINOGEN ACTIVATOR
- It is effective only in the presence of fibrin.
- It has 100 times rapid action on plasminogen bound to fibrin.

ALTEPLASE
- It is obtained through doxyribonucleic acid (DNA) recombinant technology.
- It is used to lyse coronary thrombi.
- It is given as bolus intravenous (IV) followed by two maintenance doses.

RETEPLASE
- It is obtained through DNA recombinant technology.
- It has long-duration of action due to long half-life.
- It should be given as two bolus doses at 30 minutes interval.

TENECTEPLASE
- It can be given as a single bolus dose.
- Unlike alteplase and reteplase, it is resistant to PAI-1 and PAI-2.

Nursing Responsibilities
Hypersensitivity reactions should be watched for during the administration of streptokinase.

INHIBITORS OF FIBRINOLYSIS

The drugs are:
- Aminocaproic acid
- Tranexamic acid

Aminocaproic Acid

Actions
- It inhibits fibrinolysis.
- It prevents the interaction between fibrin and plasmin.
- It can be administered both orally as well as intravenously.

Adverse Effects
- Myopathy
- Muscle necrosis

Uses
To reduce bleeding after tooth extraction or prostatic surgery in hemophilic patients.

Disadvantage
It confers limited benefit as it can induce thrombosis.

Tranexamic Acid

Actions
- It can be administered orally and intravenously.
- It prevents the interaction between fibrin and plasmin.
- It is used to prevent excessive menstrual bleeding.

Uses
- Heavy menstrual bleeding.
- Bleeding after tooth extraction or other procedures in hemophilic patients.

Nursing Responsibilities
Renal function should be monitored for patients receiving aminocaproic acid or tranexamic acid.

CHAPTER 36

Antiplatelet Agents

The drugs are:
- Aspirin
- Dipyridamole
- Clopidogrel
- Ticlopidine
- Prasugrel
- Cangrelor
- Ticagrelor
- Abciximab
- Eptifibatide
- Tirofiban

ASPIRIN

Actions

- At low dose, aspirin inhibits the enzyme thromboxane A_2.
- This inhibits platelet aggregation.
- Its action at low dose in platelets is permanent as it inhibits thromboxane A_2 for 7 to 10 days, the life span of platelets.
- At high doses, it is ineffective as it inhibits prostacyclin.

DIPYRIDAMOLE

Actions

- It is also a vasodilator.
- It inhibits phosphodiesterase enzyme.
- It increases cyclic adenosine monophosphate (AMP) level.
- It is given with warfarin to prevent embolism of prosthetic heart valves.

TICLOPIDINE

Actions

- It inhibits $P2Y_{12}$ purinergic receptor irreversibly in platelets.
- It thereby inhibits platelet aggregation.

- It has short half-life but it has long-duration of action.
- Therefore it acts as a 'hit and run' drug.
- The maximum therapeutic benefit occurs only after 8 to 11 days of therapy.
- A loading dose promotes faster onset of action.
- Its therapeutic effect persists for few more days after its discontinuation.

Adverse Effects
- Nausea, vomiting and diarrhea
- Severe neutropenia
- Agranulocytosis
- Rarely, thrombotic thrombocytopenic purpura

Use
Secondary prevention of stroke.

Nursing Responsibilities
Complete blood count should be monitored in patient on ticlopidine.

CLOPIDOGREL
Actions
- It is a prodrug.
- It is an irreversible inhibitor of $P2Y_{12}$ purinergic receptor in platelets.
- Although slow acting, it is more potent and less toxic than ticlopidine.
- It acts synergistically with aspirin.

Uses
- Unstable angina.
- After angioplasty and coronary stent implantation.
- Prevention of recurrent myocardial infarction (MI) and stroke.

PRASUGREL
Actions
- It is a prodrug.
- It has quick onset of action.
- It inhibits platelet aggregation.

- It is an irreversible inhibitor of $P2Y_{12}$ purinergic receptor in platelets.
- It has superior antiplatelet action than clopidogrel.
- Its effect persists even after its discontinuation.

Adverse Effect

Life-threatening bleeding episodes.

Contraindications

Previous history of cerebrovascular disease.

Nursing Responsibilities

Patients should be advised to stop taking antiplatelet agent atleast 1 week prior to any elective surgery.

GLYCOPROTEIN IIb/IIIa INHIBITORS

Glycoprotein IIb/IIIa serves as a receptor for von Willebrand factor and fibrinogen. Abciximab, eptifibatide and tirofiban act as antiplatelet agents by inhibiting the binding of fibrinogen and von Willebrand factor to glycoprotein IIb/IIIa.

Abciximab

Actions
- It prevents restenosis and recurrent MI.
- It has long-duration of action.
- It is administered intravenously.
- Its effect persists for 24 hours after discontinuation of the drug.

Adverse Effects
- Bleeding
- Thrombocytopenia

Nursing Responsibilities

Platelet count should be monitored frequently to rule out thrombocytopenia.

Eptifibatide

Actions
- It should be administered intravenously.
- It is less effective than abciximab.
- It has short-duration of action.

- So it is given with heparin and aspirin.
- It is used in acute coronary syndrome and after angioplasty.

Adverse Effect
Bleeding

Nursing Responsibilities
Platelet count to be monitored to rule out thrombocytopenia.

Tirofiban

Actions
- It is given intravenously with heparin.
- It has short-duration of action.
- It is useful in unstable angina and MI.
- Bleeding is the main adverse effect.

Nursing Responsibilities
Tirofiban and eptifibatide should be prepared for infusion as per the manufacturer's instruction.

Newer Drugs

Cangrelor and ticagrelor are newer antiplatelet agents with reversible $P2Y_{12}$ purinergic receptor antagonism.

Cangrelor

- It is short-acting drug and administered intravenously.
- Its activity subsides within 1 hour of stopping the infusion.

Ticagrelor

- It is orally acting drug.
- It has short-duration of action.
- It has rapid onset of action but greater efficacy.
- It causes predictable platelet inhibition than clopidogrel.

CHAPTER 37

Hypolipidemic Drugs

The drugs are:
- Statins
- Bile acid sequestrants
- Niacin
- Peroxisome proliferator activated receptor alpha (PPARα) agonists
- Ezetimibe

STATINS
They are:
- Mevastatin
- Lovastatin
- Simvastatin
- Pravastatin
- Fluvastatin
- Atorvastatin
- Rosuvastatin
- Pitavastatin

Actions
- They are very effective in the treatment of hyperlipidemia.
- They reduce cholesterol biosynthesis by inhibiting 3-hydroxy-3 methyl-glutaryl-coenzyme A (HMG-CoA) reductase enzyme.
- They reduce total cholesterol and low density lipoprotein cholesterol (LDL-C) levels.
- Higher doses of potent statins reduce triglyceride levels.
- Few statins increase the high-density lipoprotein cholesterol (HDL-C) levels.
- They increase endothelium mediated nitric oxide synthase.
- They reduce platelet aggregation.
- They also exert anti-inflammatory action.
- They have antioxidant property.
- They undergo high first pass metabolism.

Adverse Effects
- Hepatotoxicity
- Myopathy

Contraindication
Pregnancy

Uses
Hypercholesterolemia

Nursing Responsibilities
- Aspartate aminotransferase (AST) and alanine aminotransferase (ALT) should be monitored to rule out hepatotoxicity.
- Myalgia should be immediately reported to the attending physician.

Lovastatin
- It is more effective if taken with evening meal.
- The starting dose is 20 mg and dose is increased every 3 to 6 weeks.
- The maximum permitted dose is 80 mg/day.

Simvastatin
- A daily dose of 20 mg is effective.
- It should be taken only at bed time.
- Daily dose can be increased to 40 mg as prophylaxis in high-risk patients.
- In patients receiving cyclosporine, niacin or fibrates, the daily dose should not exceed 20 mg.

Pravastatin
- It is started as 20 mg/day and increased to 80 mg/day.
- It should be taken only at bed time.
- It should never be coadministered with bile acid sequestrants.

Fluvastatin
- It should be administered only at bed time.
- The starting dose is 20 to 40 mg/day.
- Bile acid sequestrants should not be coadministered with it.

Atorvastatin
- It has a long half-life.
- It can be administered at any time of the day.
- A daily dose of 10 mg/day is effective.
- It can be increased upto 80 mg/day.

Rosuvastatin
- It has long half-life.
- It can be administered at any time of the day.
- The preferred oral dose is 5 to 10 mg/day.

BILE ACID SEQUESTRANTS
They are:
- Cholestyramine
- Colestipol
- Colesevalam

Actions
- They bind to bile acids preventing their absorption and promoting their excretion.
- They decrease hepatic cholesterol level.
- They increase hepatic bile acid synthesis.
- They cause hypertriglyceridemia.
- They cause dose dependent reduction in LDL-C level.
- These drugs are very safe as they are not absorbed.
- They are not effective as monotherapy.
- Large doses of cholestyramine and colestipol are required for therapeutic benefit.
- The dose of cholestyramine is 8 to 12 g and colestipol is 10 to 15 g.
- The maximum daily dose of colesevalam is 4.375 g.

Adverse Effects
- Dyspepsia, bloating
- Hyperchloremic acidosis

Drug Interaction
- Cholestyramine and colestipol reduce the absorption of digoxin, warfarin, furosemide, thiazides, propranolol, thyroxine and statins.

- Colesevalam does not interfere with absorption of fat soluble vitamins and many drugs such as digoxin, lovastatin, metoprolol, warfarin, etc.

Nursing Responsibilities
- Cholestyramine and colestipol powder should be mixed with water before oral administration.
- Since the mixture is gritty its taste is usually unpleasant.

NIACIN
Actions
- It is water soluble B complex vitamin.
- It inhibits lipoprotein lipase.
- It decreases the synthesis of triglycerides.
- It also reduces the synthesis of very low density lipoprotein cholestro (VLDL-C).
- It increases HDL-C level.

Adverse Effects
- Flushing
- Dyspepsia
- Pruritus
- Rashes
- Acanthosis nigricans
- Dry skin
- Hepatotoxicity
- Hyperglycemia
- Toxic ambylopia and toxic maculopathy

Use
Hypertriglyceridemia

Contraindications
- Pregnancy
- Peptic ulcer
- Gout

Nursing Responsibilities
- Patient should be advised to avoid hot beverages such as coffee or tea.

- Patient on niacin should be encouraged to take aspirin regularly.
- Skin moisturizers and lotions containing salicylic acid help to prevent niacin induced dry skin and black spots respectively.
- Liver function and blood sugar should be monitored.

PEROXISOME PROLIFERATOR ACTIVATED RECEPTOR (PPAR) AGONISTS

They are:
- Clofibrate
- Ciprofibrate
- Bezafibrate
- Fenofibrate
- Gemfibrozil

Actions
- They stimulate PPARα mediated fatty acid oxidation.
- They also stimulate clearance of triglycerides.
- They reduce VLDL-C.
- They increase the plasma HDL-C level.

Adverse Effects
- Rash, urticaria
- Hair loss, myalgia
- Fatigue, headache
- Impotence, anemia
- Myopathy
- Gallstones with clofibrate.

Contraindications
- Pregnancy
- Children

Drug Interactions
Clofibrate, fenofibrate and bezafibrate compete with oral anticoagulants for binding sites with albumin and displace it causing bleeding.

Uses
- Hypertriglyceridemia
- Chylomicronemia syndrome.

Nursing Responsibilities

It is necessary to monitor serum creatinine kinase once in 3 months in patients taking both statins and fibrates.

EZETIMIBE

Actions

- It reduces intestinal cholesterol absorption.
- It does not interfere with intestinal triglyceride absorption.
- It is more effective in reducing plasma LDL-C levels if combined with statins.
- Food does not interfere with its absorption.
- Rarely it causes allergy.
- It can be taken at any time of the day.

CHAPTER 38

Treatment of Shock

Shock is characterized by low blood pressure and circulatory failure resulting in impaired tissue perfusion.

TYPES
- Hypovolemic shock
- Cardiogenic shock
- Anaphylactic shock
- Septic shock
- Neurogenic shock

Management: Ventilator assistance, intravenous (IV) fluids and volume expanders without inducing volume overload are common measures. Selective measures are:

Hypovolemic Shock
Vasopressor such as noradrenaline or dopamine.

Septic Shock
- Antibiotics
- Sodium bicarbonate to correct acidosis
- Anti-endotoxin
- Drotrecogin α.

Anaphylactic Shock
- Adrenaline – life saving drug
- Corticosteroids
- Antihistamines.

Neurogenic Shock
- Vasopressor such as noradrenaline
- Volume expanders
- IV fluids
- Ephedrine.

Cardiogenic Shock
- Dopamine or dobutamine.
- Noradrenaline when BP is low.
- Nitroglycerine if BP is stable.

Nursing Responsibilities
- Administration of IV fluids and maintenance of ventilation is essential.
- Do not infuse IV fluids rapidly, otherwise volume overload can occur.
- Other vital functions such as blood pressure and urine output should be monitored.

VOLUME EXPANDERS
   I. Whole blood or plasma
  II. Colloidal plasma expanders
 III. Crystalloid plasma expanders

Whole Blood
- It is indicated in hemorrhage, anemia and agranulocytosis as well as in erythroblastosis foetalis.
- It should be stored between 2 and 6°C.
- Anticoagulants used for preservation are citrate phosphate dextrose (CPD) or citrate phosphate dextrose adenine (CPDA).
- Autologous transfusion is safe and more compatible as it is devoid of immunological reactions.
- Blood transfusion can promote renal insufficiency due to clogging of renal tubules by hemolysed RBCs and can cause unnecessary exposure to anticoagulants.
- Rigor, fever, allergy, circulatory overload, air embolism, transmission of infection such as HIV, syphilis, hepatitis B or C and malaria are the potential risks.
- Hemolysis, hypocalcemia, acute respiratory distress syndrome (ARDS), iron and citrate overload are other complications.
- Failure to rewarm the blood to room temperature before transfusion can result in hyperkalemia.

Nursing Responsibilities
- Blood grouping, Rh compatibility and cross matching should be done before each transfusion.
- Blood should be stored at temperature below 6°C.

- It should not be stored below 2°C.
- Discard the blood exposed to room temperature beyond 30 minutes.
- Blood in CPD preservative can be used within 21 days and that in CPDA preservative can be used before 35 days.
- Rigor, oliguria, hemoglobinuria and pain in loins during transfusion should be immediately reported to the attending physician.
- Monitoring of serum iron level during repeated blood transfusion is necessary.

Packed Red Cells
- It is administered when the oxygen carrying capacity of blood has to be increased without altering the blood volume.
- It is indicated in patients with aplastic or refractory anemia.
- It is also given in blood dyscrasia such as thalassemia and hemolytic anemia.
- One unit of packed cell increases the hemoglobin concentration by 1%.
- It is relatively safe with fewer incidences of allergy or anaphylaxis.

Nursing Responsibilities
- Discard the unused packed cells 12 hours after its preparation.
- Packed cells of O negative persons is suitable to persons with other blood groups.
- Maximum volume should not exceed 500 mL.
- In anemic patients, do not give more than 10 to 15 drops per minute.

Plasma
- Fresh plasma should be administered immediately while frozen plasma can be used later.
- They both contain albumin, globulin and coagulation factors.
- It is used in patients with coagulation factor deficiency.
- It can be prepared even from expired blood.
- It is either prepared from a single donor or from multiple donors.
- Plasma prepared from multiple donors can be frozen and stored upto 5 years.

Nursing Responsibilities
- Frozen plasma should be stored at -30°C.
- Use the frozen plasma immediately after thawing.

- It can be stored between 1 and 6°C after thawing but should be administered within 24 hours.
- Plasma obtained from blood group AB is **neutral** and **universal** for all other blood groups.

Human Serum Albumin
- It is non toxic.
- It does not interfere with coagulation.
- It is used for hypoproteinemia.
- It is also used as a vehicle for packed cells transfusion.

Nursing Responsibilities
It should be administered slowly at the rate of 1 mL/min.

Plasma Expanders
An ideal plasma expander should:
- Be stable for long periods.
- Have oncotic pressure similar to plasma.
- Remain for long period in circulation.
- Be excreted eventually.
- Should not be antigenic.
- Not alter the intrinsic physiologic functions of the body.
- Not interfere with blood grouping or cross matching.
- Be readily available.

Colloidal Plasma Expanders
- They are dextran, hydroxyethyl starches, polyvinyl pyrolidine and gelatin polymers.
- They are compounds with high molecular weight.
- They remain in circulation for a long time.
- They increase the oncotic pressure.
- Thereby they increase the blood volume.

Dextran
- It is obtained from beetroot.
- Dextran 40 is 10% solution with molecular weight of 40,000.
- It is excreted within 1 week after administration.
- Dextran 70 is 6% solution with a molecular weight of 70,000.
- It is stored for a long period in reticuloendothelial cells.
- After autoclaving, they can be stored upto 10 years.
- Their oncotic pressure is similar to plasma.
- They inhibit the rouleaux formation of RBCs and improve the microcirculation.

- They do not interfere with blood grouping, cross matching and in determining Rh compatibility.
- They interfere with platelet function and can cause hemorrhage.
- Fifty percent of dextran 40 is excreted through kidney.
- It can cause oliguric renal failure by blocking renal tubules.

Contraindications
- Dextran allergy
- Heart failure
- Renal failure
- Thrombocytopenia
- Low fibrinogen level.

Nursing Responsibilities
- They should always be administered through intravenous route and never through subcutaneous route.
- Urine output should be monitored in the first 3 to 6 days of initiation of therapy.

Hydroxy Ethyl Starches
- They are resistant to hydrolysis by amylase.
- They are not antigenic.
- They have long-duration of action.
- They do not result in clotting abnormality.
- They do not cause renal failure.

Polyvinyl Pyrolidine (PVP)
- It is used less frequently.
- Its molecular weight is 35,000 to 40,000.
- It is administered intravenously as 40% solution with normal saline.
- 75% of PVP is excreted rapidly through kidney and 10% is excreted through bile.
- Rest is stored in reticuloendothelial cells, skin and skeletal muscle.

Nursing Responsibilities
- It interferes with blood grouping.
- It should not be administered with penicillin.

Gelatin Polymers (Haemacel)
- It is a polypeptide.
- It has a half-life of 4 to 5 hours.
- It is stable at room temperature at potential hydrogen (pH) 7.2 for a period of 3 years.

Treatment of Shock

Nursing Responsibilities
- It does not interfere with blood grouping and cross matching.
- During infusion, it may cause rigor, flushing or urticaria.
- BP should be monitored during infusion.

Crystalloid Plasma Expanders
- They are not restricted within blood vessels.
- Normal saline and 5% dextrose are crystalloid plasma expanders.

Normal Saline
- 0.9% normal saline is isotonic with plasma.
- One litre of normal saline increases 300 mL of blood volume.
- It is given in hypovolemic shock, hemorrhage, vomiting or diarrhea.
- It is useful as a vehicle for administration of drugs through intravenous route.

Nursing Responsibilities
- It should be administered slowly.
- Fever and rigor can occur during infusion.
- Noradrenaline should never be administered with normal saline infusion.

5% Dextrose
- One litre of 5% dextrose increases blood volume by 100 mL.
- It is used in renal impairment.

Nursing Responsibilities
Noradrenaline can be administered with dextrose infusion.

Iron Deficiency Anemia

- Iron deficiency is the most common cause of anemia.
- Blood loss, malabsorption, inadequate iron intake, hookworm infestation and pregnancy are some of the causes of iron deficiency.
- Deficiency of iron results in hypochromic microcytic anemia.
- Iron is an essential component of heme enzymes, hemoglobin and myoglobin.
- Hence, iron deficiency affects oxygen delivery as well as muscle metabolism.
- Iron present in dietary source is in the form of ferric ion.
- It is converted to ferrous ion in the duodenum.
- Divalent metal transporter I transports ferrous ion into intestinal mucosal cells.
- There it is oxidized to ferric state.
- The ferric ion complexes with apoferritin to form ferritin for temporary storage.
- Mucosal ferric ion released into circulation is reduced to ferrous state.
- It is again reoxidised to ferric state by ceruloplasmin.
- In blood, the ferric ion is transported by transferrin.
- The storage form of iron is ferritin.
- Ferritin is stored in intestinal mucosal cells, liver, spleen and bone marrow.
- Meat is a rich source of iron.

ORAL IRON THERAPY

- Only ferrous salts should be used.
- Ferrous sulfate, ferrous gluconate and ferrous fumarate are inexpensive and very effective orally.
- The required dose is 200 to 400 mg of elemental iron daily.
- Treatment should be continued upto 6 months.
- Nausea, abdominal cramp, constipation and diarrhea are the adverse effects of oral iron preparation.

- They can be minimized either by lowering the dose or by administering them immediately after food.

PARENTERAL IRON THERAPY
- It is reserved for patients who are unable to tolerate or absorb oral iron.
- Small bowel resection, inflammatory bowel disease and malabsorption syndrome are some indications for parenteral iron therapy.
- Iron dextran, iron sucrose, ferumoxytol and sodium ferric gluconate complex are parenteral iron preparations.
- Iron dextran can be given as deep intramuscular injection or as intravenous infusion.
- Iron sucrose and ferric gluconate are preferred mainly in anemia due to chronic renal disease.
- Headache, lightheadedness, nausea, vomiting, fever, arthralgia, urticaria, bronchospasm and anaphylaxis can occur.
- Iron sucrose complex and sodium ferric gluconate complex have minimal potential to cause hypersensitivity reaction.
- Sodium ferric gluconate is given IV in hemodialysis patients.
- This preparation is preferred for parenteral iron therapy.

ACUTE IRON TOXICITY
- Activated charcoal is not effective as it does not bind to iron.
- Whole bowel irrigation with polyethylene glycol (PEG) to promote excretion of drug through feces.
- Deferoxamine should be administered parenterally. Other details: See Section XII, Chapter 80.

CHRONIC IRON TOXICITY
- Chronic iron overload is called hemochromatosis.
- In this condition, the excess iron is deposited in heart, liver, pancreas and other organs.
- This can result in death due to organ failure.
- Parenteral iron chelator deferoxamine is less effective.
- Oral iron chelator, deferasirox is more preferred.

Nursing Responsibilities
- Anemia should be corrected immediately in children as it causes learning and behavioral problems in them.

- Iron deficiency anemia is a common occurrence in pregnant women and in infants deprived of breastfeeding.
- Ascorbic acid or vitamin C increases the oral absorption of iron.
- A test dose of 0.5 mL should be injected intramuscularly before administering intramuscular (IM) iron dextran.
- A test dose of 0.5 mL of iron dextran diluted in saline should be given intraveneous (IV) before infusion of iron dextran.
- Parenteral iron should not exceed the required iron dose to prevent iron overload.
- Advice the patients to continue the oral iron therapy for 3 to 6 months even after correction of blood picture to replenish the iron storage.
- As a precautionary measure, stool examination for melena should be done in patients passing black stools to rule out gastrointestinal tract (GIT) bleeding.
- Always give iron as 'z track' by deep intramuscular injection to minimize pain.
- Always give a test dose of iron dextran before giving IM or IV iron.
- Never use the universal antidote, activated charcoal in acute iron poisoning as it does not bind to iron
- Iron overload is common in patients with thalassemia major due to repeated blood transfusion.
- Parenteral iron chelator deferoxamine is less effective and oral iron chelator, deferasirox should be administrated in chronic iron toxicity.

Megaloblastic Anemia and Hematopoietic Growth Factors

Deficiency of vitamin B_{12} and folic acid cause megaloblastic anemia.

VITAMIN B_{12}

- The source of vitamin B_{12} is liver, egg and dairy products.
- Deoxyadenosylcobalamin and methylcobalamin are the active forms of vitamin B_{12}.
- Vitamin B_{12} is called as extrinsic factor.
- The intrinsic factor secreted from stomach helps for its absorption.
- It complexes with intrinsic factor and is absorbed in distal ileum.
- It is transported by transcobalamin to liver, its storage site.
- It is necessary for the conversion of homocysteine to methionine and for the conversion of methyltetrahydrofolate to tetrahydrofolate.
- Deficiency of vitamin B_{12} occurs due to ileal resection, chronic pancreatitis and bacterial overgrowth of small intestine.
- Macrocytic, megaloblastic anemia, neurological symptoms such as paresthesia and weakness are classic symptoms of vitamin B_{12} deficiency.
- Schilling test that shows the absorption of radioactively labeled vitamin B_{12} helps to diagnose diminished intestinal absorption of the vitamin.
- Parenteral therapy is required if oral absorption is impaired.
- Hydroxocobalamin is preferred to cyanocobalamin for parenteral therapy.

FOLIC ACID

- Folic acid or pteroylglutamic acid is necessary for the synthesis of amino acids, purines and deoxyribonucleic acid (DNA).
- Folic acid and its cofactors are necessary for 'one carbon transfer reactions' of DNA synthesis.
- Yeast, liver, kidney and green leafy vegetables are the important sources of folic acid.

- It is absorbed in proximal jejunum.
- It is stored in liver.
- Inadequate intake, pregnancy, alcoholism, liver disease and drugs such as methotrexate cause folic acid deficiency.
- Oral folic acid 1 mg daily is required to correct the deficiency.

HEMATOPOIETIC GROWTH FACTORS

- They help in the proliferation of hemetopoietic progenitor cells in bone marrow.
- They are erythropoietin, granulocyte-colony stimulating factor (G-CSF), granulocyte macrophage colony-stimulating factor (GM-CSF), romiplostim and interleukin-11.

Erythropoietin

- It stimulates erythroid proliferation and differentiation.
- It causes release of reticulocytes from bone marrow.
- Patients with renal disease respond well to erythropoietin.
- Patients with bone marrow disorders do not respond well to erythropoietin.
- It can cause hypertension and thrombosis.
- It is administered thrice weekly intravenously.
- Darbepoetin-α can be administered once in 2 weeks or once in a month either subcutaneously or intravenously.

Myeloid Growth Factors

- Granulocyte-colony stimulating factor and granulocyte-macrophage colony-stimulating factor are available for clinical use.
- G-CSF is filgrastim and GM-CSF is sargramostim.
- They stimulate proliferation and differentiation of myeloid progenitor cells.
- G-CSF stimulates and proliferate neutrophil progenitor cells.
- GM-CSF stimulates proliferation and differentiation of granulocytic erythroid and megakaryocyte progenitor cells.
- They are effective in cancer chemotherapy induced neutropenia, congenital neutropenia, cyclic neutropenia and aplastic anemia.
- Pegfilgrastim is a polyethylene product of filgrastim with long half-life and can be administrated once after each cycle of cancer chemotherapy.

- G-CSF and pegfilgrastim cause bone pain.
- GM-CSF causes arthralgia, myalgia, fever and edema.
- It can also cause pleural and pericardial effusion.

Megakaryocyte Growth Factors
- Interleukin-11, its recombinant form oprelvekin and romiplostim are used.
- They stimulate the growth of megakaryocytic progenitor cells.
- They are used in secondary prevention of thrombocytopenia in patients receiving cancer chemotherapy.
- Romiplostim is also effective in chronic idiopathic thrombocytopenia.
- Romiplostim causes headache.
- Interleukin-11 causes fatigue, headache and dizziness.

Nursing Responsibilities
- Patients with neurological symptoms should be advised to stick on to regular vitamin B_{12} therapy otherwise the neurological symptoms can progress to ataxia.
- Neurological symptoms of megaloblastic anemia cannot be corrected by folic acid alone but require the administration of vitamin B_{12}.

SECTION VIII

Hormones and Hormone Antagonists

- Growth Hormone, Prolactin, Gonadotropins and GnRH Agonists
- Thyroid Hormone and Antithyroid Drugs
- Corticosteroids
- Insulin and Oral Hypoglycemic Drugs
- Estrogens and Progestins
- Androgens
- Agents Involved in Bone Turnover
- Uterine Stimulants and Relaxants

CHAPTER 41

Growth Hormone, Prolactin, Gonadotropins and GnRH Agonists

RECOMBINANT HUMAN GROWTH HORMONE (SOMATROPIN)

Actions
- Somatropin is growth hormone preparation through recombinant (DNA) technology.
- It promotes growth of bones and organs.
- It increases bone mineral density and promotes fusion of epiphysis.
- It inhibits glucose utilization.
- It stimulates lipolysis and gluconeogenesis.
- It increases muscle mass.
- Growth hormone releasing hormone (GHRH) regulates the release of growth hormone from hypothalamus.
- Dopamine, α_2 adrenergic agonists, serotonin, hunger or hypoglycemia, exertion, stress and protein rich meals stimulate growth hormone release.
- Similarly free fatty acids and β adrenergic agonists inhibit its release.
- It is administered subcutaneously once daily.
- It has 70% bioavailability.
- Excessive secretion of growth hormone causes gigantism in children and acromegaly in adults.
- Inadequate secretion of growth hormone causes dwarfism.

Adverse Effects
- Myalgia, headache, lethargy
- Hyperglycemia

Contraindication
Retinopathy

Uses
- Pituitary dwarfism
- Muscle wasting in acquired immunodeficiency syndrome (AIDS)
- Turner's syndrome

Nursing Responsibilities
Frequently change the site of subcutaneous injection to prevent lipodystrophy.

SOMATOSTATIN
Actions
- It inhibits the secretion of growth hormone, insulin, glucagon, prolactin, thyroid stimulating hormone (TSH) and gastric acid.
- It reduces hepatic, renal and splanchnic blood flow.
- It reduces gastrointestinal secretion.
- Its duration of action is very short and lasts only for few minutes.
- Hence its analogs lanreotide or octreotide are used clinically.

OCTREOTIDE AND LANREOTIDE
Actions
- Octreotide is a somatostatin analog.
- It has 100% bioavailability on subcutaneous administration.
- It is given three times daily.
- It inhibits the secretion of growth hormone.
- It also reduces the secretion of serotonin and incretins.
- Octreotide is used in secretory diarrhea associated with metastatic carcinoid tumor, adenoma, cancer chemotherapy, human immunodeficiency virus (HIV) infection and diabetes mellitus.
- It is also used in dumping syndrome and acute variceal bleeding.
- Long-acting slow release formulation can be administered intramuscularly once a month.
- Lanreotide is administered through intramuscular route.
- Long-acting slow release lanreotide preparation can be administered intramuscularly once in 14 days.
- Lanreotide autogel formulation is also available.

Adverse Effects
- Nausea, abdominal pain, diarrhea, bloating
- Hypothyroidism
- Hypo or hyperglycemia
- Gallstones.

Growth Hormone, Prolactin, Gonadotropins and GnRH Agonists

Uses
- Acromegaly
- Secretory diarrhea in carcinoid tumor, adenoma, cancer chemotherapy, HIV infection and diabetes mellitus
- Acute variceal bleeding
- Diagnostic imaging of pituitary adenoma
- Prophylaxis and treatment of acute pancreatitis.

Nursing Responsibilities
Complaints of severe back pain should be reported to the attending physician as it can indicate the presence gallstones.

Pegvisomant
- It is a growth hormone antagonist.
- It is administered subcutaneously for therapy of acromegaly.

Nursing Responsibilities
Pegvisomant should not be used in patients with hepatic dysfunction.

PROLACTIN
Actions
- Suckling reflex induces prolactin secretion.
- Its role is only physiological and it is not used therapeutically.
- It induces growth and development of breast during pregnancy.
- Dopamine and its agonist bromocriptine inhibit its release.
- Antagonists of dopamine such as metoclopramide and chlorpromazine increase its release.
- Increased secretion causes galactorrhea and amenorrhea in women.
- In men, hyperprolactinemia causes erectile dysfunction and loss of libido.

BROMOCRIPTINE
Actions
- It is a dopamine receptor agonist.
- It is a semisynthetic ergot alkaloid.
- Being a dopamine agonist, it decreases the release of prolactin.
- Nausea, vomiting and decreased gastrointestinal tract (GIT) motility occur as a result of increased dopamine level.

- It has poor oral bioavailability due to high first pass metabolism.
- A slow release oral formulation is available.
- It can also be administered intravaginally.

Adverse Effects
Nausea, vomiting, postural hypotension, hallucination, headache.

Uses
- Prolactinoma
- Acromegaly
- Parkinsonism.

Nursing Responsibilities
Patient should be advised to be careful while standing for longtime as it can cause postural hypotension.

CABERGOLINE
Actions
- It is an ergot alkaloid.
- It is a selective and potent dopamine agonist.
- Long-acting and administered twice weekly.
- The incidence of nausea and vomiting is low.
- So it is preferred to bromocriptine.

Adverse Effects
- Dizziness
- Hypotension
- Valvular heart disease.

Uses
- Hyperprolactinemia
- Acromegaly
- Prolactinoma.

QUINAGOLIDE
- It is a non-ergot dopamine agonist.
- Its efficacy is moderate and is between bromocriptine and cabergoline.
- It is administered once daily.

PERGOLIDE
- It is an ergot derivative and dopamine agonist.
- It is used in Parkinsonism.
- It is used off-label in the treatment of hyperprolactinemia.
- It can cause valvular heart disease.

GONADOTROPINS
Actions
- Gonadotropins act on gonads.
- Gonadotropin releasing hormone (GnRH) regulates gonadotropin release.
- It is secreted in a pulsatile manner.
- GnRH pulse generator is active during late foetal life and during puberty.
- Follicle stimulating hormone (FSH), luteinizing hormone (LH) and human chorionic gonadotropin (hCG) are gonadotropins.
- While pulsatile release of GnRH promotes action of LH and FSH, continuous release reduces their action.
- In men, LH stimulates synthesis of testosterone and FSH promotes sperm maturation.
- In women, FSH stimulates growth of ovarian follicle and LH stimulates ovulation.
- Defective secretion causes hypogonadism and infertility.
- Gonadorelin is a synthetic GnRH and can be administered subcutaneous (SC) or intravenous (IV).
- It can be used for both diagnostic as well as therapeutic purposes.

Uses
Diagnostic
- Gonadorelin is used to differentiate the hypothalamic and pituitary defects of hypogonadotropic hypogonadism.
- To determine if the precocious puberty in children is due to central or peripheral etiology.

Therapeutic
- Female infertility as pulsatile therapy to mimic physiological cycle.
- **Main advantage:** Lower risk of multiple fetus and minimal need to monitor follicle size and plasma estradiol levels.

Follicle Stimulating Hormone (FSH)
- It stimulates growth of ovarian follicle in women.
- In men, it promotes maturation of sperms.
- Urofollitropin is a combination of FSH and monoclonal antibodies.
- Recombinant FSH (rFSH) preparations are follitropin α and follitropin β.
- They are pure, safe and more effective.
- They are administered subcutaneously.

Luteinizing Hormone (LH)
- It promotes maturation and rupture of ovarian follicles.
- It does not cause ovarian hyperstimulation.

Menotropin
- It is obtained from urine of postmenopausal women.
- It has LH activity and promotes follicular maturation.
- Recombinant human LH is called as lutropin-α.
- It is used in *in vitro* fertilization (IVF) protocol.

Adverse Effects
- Ovarian hyperstimulation
- Pleural effusion
- Ascites
- Multiple birth.

Uses
- Assisted fertilization alongwith hCG.
- Induce ovulation in women with polycystic ovarian disease (PCOD).

Human Chorionic Gonadotropin (hCG)
- It is obtained from urine of pregnant women.
- It induces ovulation.
- It is administered through intramuscular route.

Diagnostic Uses of Gonadotropins
- Pregnancy test.
- To detect ectopic pregnancy, choriocarcinoma, hydatidiform mole.
- To calculate ovulation time.
- To differentiate central and peripheral causes of hypogonadotropic hypogonadism.

Therapeutic Uses of Gonadotropins
- Assisted reproduction. FSH should be administered prior to hCG
- Male infertility
- Cryptorchidism.

Nursing Responsibilities
- Pregnancy can be detected within few days of missed menstrual period by evaluating hCG level.
- To find out if ovulation has occurred, LH level of urine should be measured everyday.

GnRH AGONISTS
They are:
- Leuprolide
- Goserelin
- Histrelin
- Nafarelin
- Triptorelin

Actions
- They have prolonged duration of action.
- Depot preparations release the drug continuously and reduce gonadotropins secretion.
- Intermittent pulse therapy stimulates gonadotropin secretion.
- Leuprolide is available as depot preparation that can be administered SC or intramuscular (IM).
- It can also be administered as subcutaneous injection.
- Depot preparation is effective in uterine fibroid, endometriosis, precocious puberty and prostate cancer.
- Goserelin is available for subcutaneous implantation.
- It is effective in advanced prostate cancer, breast cancer and endometriosis.
- Histrelin is also available as subcutaneous implant.
- It is used in prostate cancer and precocious puberty.
- Nafarelin is available as nasal spray and effective in precocious puberty as well as endometriosis.
- Triptorelin is available as depot preparation.
- This depot preparation is administered as IM injection.
- Triptorelin is used in advanced prostate cancer.

Adverse Effects
- Hot flashes
- Osteoporosis
- Vaginal dryness
- Erectile dysfunction.

GnRH ANTAGONISTS
The drugs are ganirelix and cetrorelix.

Actions
- They suppress LH surge.
- They prevent premature ovulation.
- They have 90% bioavailability on subcutaneous administration.

Adverse Effects
- Hypersensitivity reactions
- Anaphylaxis

Use
Assisted reproduction

CHAPTER 42

Thyroid Hormone and Antithyroid Drugs

SYNTHESIS AND ACTIONS OF THYROID HORMONE
- Iodine from diet is transported to thyroid gland as iodide ion.
- Iodide is oxidized and combines with tyrosyl residues to form mono and diiodotyrosyl residues.
- Two diiodotyrosyl residues combine to form thyroxine (T_4).
- One diiodotyrosyl residue combines with one monoiodotyrosyl residue to form triiodothyronine (T_3).
- These reactions are catalyzed by thyroid peroxidase.
- Both T_3 and T_4 are stored within thyroglobulin and secreted into circulation through proteolysis.
- T_3 is the biologically active form and secreted as such from thyroid gland.
- Deiodination of T_4 and T_3 occurs in peripheral tissues.
- T_4 is also converted to inactive T_3 or 'reverse T_3' (rT_3).
- Thyroxine binding globulin binds mainly to T_4 and sparsely with T_3.
- While bound hormone is clinically inactive and not available for metabolism or excretion, free hormone is clinically active.
- Half-life of thyroxine is 6 to 8 days.
- Half-life is short in hyperthyroidism and increased in hypothyroidism.
- Thyroid stimulating hormone (TSH) regulates the function of thyroid gland and thyrotropin releasing hormone (TRH) controls release of TSH.
- The level of circulating TSH is high during sleep.
- Thyroid hormone is necessary for brain development.
- Deficiency of thyroid hormone during the first 6 months after birth results in cretinism.
- Cretinism can be either sporadic or endemic.
- Sporadic cretinism is due to defect in synthesis of thyroid hormone.
- Endemic cretinism is due to iodine deficiency.

- Thyroid hormone causes skeletal muscle contraction and produces heat.
- Tachycardia reduced peripheral resistance, cardiac hypertrophy, insulin resistance and impaired glucose tolerance occur in hyperthyroidism.
- Bradycardia increased peripheral resistance, pericardial effusion, decreased glucose absorption, reduced peripheral glucose utilization, decreased insulin secretion and hypercholestrolemia occur in hypothyroidism.

Levothyroxine T_4

- It is a synthetic preparation of thyroxine and preferred in replacement therapy.
- It is highly protein bound and so has prolonged half-life of 7 days.
- It can be administered orally once daily and is converted in the body to T_3.
- High oral absorption if given in empty stomach.
- Replacement therapy should be continued lifelong.

Uses
- Adult hypothyroidism (myxoedema)
- Myxoedema coma
- Nontoxic goiter
- Hypothyroidism of pregnancy
- Congenital hypothyroidism.

Adverse Effects
Overdose can result in thyrotoxicosis causing tremor, tachycardia, restlessness, insomnia, intolerance to heat and sweating.

Nursing Responsibilities
- Patients should be instructed to take levothyroxine on empty stomach at same time daily in the morning.
- The patient should be advised to use the same brand of thyroxine.

Liothyronine
- It is a synthetic preparation of T_3 with 100% oral bioavailability.
- The onset of action is rapid but the duration of action is short.
- It requires to be administered frequently.
- It is expensive.
- So, it is not suitable for long-term therapy.
- Since its onset of action is quick it is effective in myxoedema coma.

HYPOTHYROIDISM
- Common cause is autoimmune or Hashimoto's thyroiditis.
- Clinical features are goiter, intolerance to cold, lethargy, fatigue, paucity of mental functions, dry skin, weight gain, infertility, delayed reflexes, non-pitting edema, constipation, depression.

Hypothyroidism of Pregnancy
- The dose of levothyroxine in hypothyroid women should be increased during pregnancy.
- Hypothyroidism during pregnancy causes foetal distress and impaired neural development.
- The incidence of miscarriage is also high.
- The requirement of levothyroxine increases from 5th week of gestation.
- The dose should be increased upto 16 or 20th week.
- Dose should be reduced after delivery.

Myxoedema Coma
- It is a medical emergency requiring immediate therapy.
- Clinical features are hypothermia, respiratory depression, impaired consciousness, bradycardia and delayed reflexes.
- It also causes dilutional hyponatremia, acidosis, increased creatinine kinase and lactate dehydrogenase.
- Evaluation of TSH and serum free thyroxine is necessary.

Treatment
- Covering patients with blankets to maintain body warmth.
- Respiratory support.
- Correction of hyponatremia and acidosis.
- Intravenous T_4 (levothyroxine) or T_3 (liothyronine) or T_4 and T_3.
- Corticosteroids.

HYPERTHYROIDISM
- It can occur due to Graves' disease or toxic nodular goiter.
- Graves' disease is an autoimmune disorder.
- It occurs mostly in women than in men.
- Clinical features are increased appetite, excessive production of heat, tachycardia, loss of weight, warm and moist skin.

Antithyroid Drugs

- **Inhibit hormone synthesis:** Propylthiouracil, methimazole, carbimazole
- **Ionic inhibitors:** Thiocyanate, perchlorate, nitrates
- **Inhibit hormone release:** Iodide, iodine, lithium
- **Destruction of thyroid tissue:** Radioactive iodine I_{131}, I_{125}, I_{123}
- **Inhibit peripheral conversion of T_4 to T_3:** Amiodarone.

THIOUREYLENE DERIVATIVES

The drugs are:
- Propylthiouracil
- Carbimazole
- Methimazole

Propylthiouracil

Actions

- It inhibits peroxidase enzyme and prevents iodination of tyrosine residues and coupling of MIT and DIT.
- It also inhibits the peripheral conversion of T_4 to T_3.
- Due to these multiple mechanisms, propylthiouracil is preferred in thyroid storm.
- It is rapidly absorbed with quick onset of action.
- Its duration is short and needs to be administered at least 3 times daily.
- The metabolism is not altered in hepatic and renal disease.
- It crosses placenta and is secreted in milk.
- It should not be used for children.

Adverse Effects

- Agranulocytosis
- Urticaria
- Nausea, arthralgia, paresthesia, headache, loss of hair
- Skin pigmentation, drug fever
- Hypothyroidism
- Hepatitis.

Uses

- Graves' disease
- Subtotal thyroidectomy—preoperative preparation of thyroid gland
- Thyroid storm

Carbimazole, Methimazole

Actions
- Carbimazole is converted to methimazole after absorption.
- It inhibits peroxidase enzyme and prevents the synthesis of thyroid hormones.
- It does not block the peripheral conversion of T_4 to T_3.
- Therefore, it is not preferred in thyroid storm where a quick blockade of thyroxine action is required.
- It is long-acting and can be administered once daily.
- It crosses placenta and is secreted in milk.
- The metabolism of methimazole is altered in hepatic dysfunction but not in renal dysfunction.

Adverse Effects
- Agranulocytosis
- Skin pigmentation, joint stiffness, drug fever

Use
Graves' disease

IONIC INHIBITORS
The drugs are:
- Thiocyanate
- Perchlorate
- Fluoroborate

Actions
- Thiocyanate inhibits organification of iodine.
- Perchlorate is more effective in inhibiting iodine uptake by thyroid gland but can cause aplastic anemia.
- Perchlorate is used in the diagnosis of iodide organification.

IODIDE

Actions
- It inhibits synthesis of iodotyrosines and iodothyronines.
- It decreases release of thyroid hormone from the gland.
- It reduces the vascularity of the gland making it firm.
- It increases the colloid content of follicles.
- It increases the amount of bound iodine.
- The maximum therapeutic benefit occurs within 15 days.

- This benefit is transient and symptoms reappear with continuous therapy.

Adverse Effects
- Hypersensitivity, fever, arthralgia
- Angioedema on IV administration of sodium iodine
- Anorexia, bloody diarrhea
- Headache, pulmonary edema, enlargement of salivary glands
- Depression
- Brassy taste, sore throat, gum and teeth soreness, hypersalivation, sneezing and coryza indicate 'iodism' in patients on chronic therapy.

Uses
- Preoperative preparation of hyperthyroid patients.
- Potassium iodide is given in radiation emergency.
- With propranolol in thyrotoxic crisis.

Lugol's Solution
- It contains 5% iodine and 10% potassium iodide.
- It is given as 2 to 6 drops daily in radiation emergency.

Lithium
It reduces secretion of T_4 and T_3 from thyroid gland.

Radioactive Iodine

Actions
- The radioisotopes of iodine used are I^{123} and I^{131}.
- I^{123} has short half-life and emits γ rays.
- It is used for diagnostic thyroid imaging and 24 hours iodine uptake by thyroid gland.
- I^{131} has a half-life of 8 days.
- I^{131} emits both γ rays and β particles.
- γ rays passes through tissues and help in diagnosis.
- β particles destroy the parenchyma cells and are useful in therapy.
- Both I^{123} and I^{131} are given orally and are absorbed rapidly.
- They accumulate into colloid and are released slowly.
- I^{131} is used for Graves' disease that recurs after subtotal thyroidectomy.
- I^{131} is used in toxic nodular goiter.

- It is also used for diagnosis of hyperthyroidism.
- It is contraindicated in pregnancy.
- It is administered orally as sodium iodide solution or capsule.
- It is cheap and selective only to thyroid gland but not to other tissues.
- It may take 2 to 3 months for the maximal therapeutic benefit.

HYPERTHYROIDISM IN PREGNANCY
- Both propylthiouracil and methimazole can be used in first trimester.
- Methimazole is preferred during 2nd and 3rd trimester.

Nursing Responsibilities
- Estimation of serum TSH, free T_3 and T_4 level once in every 2 to 4 months is necessary.
- Patient on antithyroid drugs should be advised to report immediately if they develop fever or sore throat and evaluated for blood dyscrasia as it may indicate agranulocytosis.
- Liver function should be monitored during propylthiouracil therapy.
- Hypothyroid patient should be advised to stop smoking.
- Patients with hypothyroidism should be advised to avoid cabbage in their diet.

CHAPTER 43

Corticosteroids

The two steroidal hormones produced in adrenal cortex are corticosteroids and androgens. Glucocorticoids and mineralocorticoids are the two types of corticosteroids. Glucocorticoids alter carbohydrate metabolism and mineralocorticoids modulate salt and water balance while androgens contribute to male sexual characters.

GLUCOCORTICOIDS
They are:
- Hydrocortisone
- Prednisolone
- Methylprednisolone
- Triamcinolone
- Dexamethasone
- Betamethasone

Actions
- They promote gluconeogenesis and reduce the peripheral utilization of glucose.
- They inhibit glucose uptake in adipose tissue, skin and fibroblasts.
- They increase blood glucose levels.
- They decrease muscle mass and result in negative nitrogen balance.
- They also promote lipolysis and redistribution of fat.
- They reduce the number of circulating lymphocytes, monocytes, eosinophils and basophils.
- They suppress inflammation and have immunosuppressive property.
- Glucocorticoids are required for normal functioning of skeletal muscles.
- They increase blood pressure and elevate mood.
- Corticotropin releasing hormone (CRH) modulates the release of glucocorticoids.

Adverse Effects
- Sudden discontinuation causes flare-up of the underlying condition for which the steroids were prescribed.
- Acute adrenal insufficiency on abrupt cessation after prolonged therapy.
- Hypertension, hyperglycemia, osteoporosis, osteonecrosis.
- Posterior subcapsular cataract.
- Cushing's syndrome.
- Immunosuppression, stunted growth.
- Myopathy, insomnia, nervousness.

Use
Glucocorticoids are used in many conditions.

Replacement Therapy In
- Acute adrenal insufficiency.
- Chronic adrenal insufficiency.

Therapeutic In
- Rheumatoid arthritis
- Systemic lupus erythematosus
- Polyarteritis nodosa
- Wegener's granulomatosis
- Nephrotic syndrome
- Angioneurotic edema, hay fever, serum sickness
- Contact dermatitis, urticaria
- Bronchial asthma
- Chronic obstructive pulmonary disease (COPD)
- *Pneumocystis carinii* pneumonia in AIDS patients
- Ocular inflammation
- Eczema
- Chronic ulcerative colitis, Crohn's disease
- Autoimmune hepatitis
- Cerebral edema
- Lymphoma
- Acute lymphocytic leukemia
- Sarcoidosis
- Thrombocytopenia
- Hemolytic anemia
- Organ transplantation

Contraindications
- Peptic ulcer
- Congestive heart failure (CHF)
- Osteoporosis
- Tuberculosis
- Diabetes mellitus
- Hypertension
- Herpes simplex infection
- Epilepsy
- Psychosis

Hydrocortisone
- It has quick onset and short-duration of action.
- It has significant mineralocorticoid property.
- It is used for replacement therapy in adrenocortical insufficiency.
- It is also used in inflammatory conditions and allergy.

Prednisolone
- It has more glucocorticoid than mineralocorticoid activity.
- It has intermediate duration of action.
- It can be administered daily.
- It is used for replacement therapy as well as in allergy, autoimmune and inflammatory conditions.

Methylprednisolone
- It is more potent than prednisolone and has more glucocorticoid property.
- It has intermediate duration of action.
- It is given as pulse therapy to suppress immunological reaction in rheumatoid arthritis.

Triamcinolone
- It has more glucocorticoid than mineralocorticoid activity.
- It can be administered through intraarticular route.

Dexamethasone
- It has pronounced glucocorticoid activity and lacks minimal mineralocorticoid activity.
- Dexamethasone suppression helps in the diagnosis of Cushing's syndrome.

- It is long-acting with half-life of more than 35 hours.
- It is given in cerebral edema as it causes minimal fluid retention.

Betamethasone
- It is long-acting and lacks mineralocorticoid activity.
- It is used in cerebral edema.

DEFLAZACORT
- It has glucocorticoid but not mineralocorticoid activity.
- It is preferred in children.
- It is used in inflammatory and immunological conditions.
- It causes few side effects.

MINERALOCORTICOIDS
Actions
- They promote sodium and water retention and potassium excretion.
- They cause aldosterone mediated hypertension, cardiac fibrosis and cardiac failure.
- Hypokalemia induced by mineralocorticoids interfere with normal functioning of skeletal muscles.

The mineralocorticoids are:
- Aldosterone
- Desoxycorticosterone acetate (DOCA)

Fludrocortisone
- Fludrocortisone has glucocorticoid activity.
- It is used for replacement therapy in Addison's disease.
- It is also effective in congenital adrenal hypoplasia.
- Desoxycorticosterone acetate has pure mineralocorticoid activity and is used in Addison's disease.
- Aldosterone is seldom used due to its poor oral bioavailability.
- Mineralocorticoids cause volume expansion, edema, hypokalemia, hypertension, cardiac fibrosis and CHF.

Cushing's Syndrome
- Clinical features are obesity, hyperglycemia, edema, hypertension, osteoporosis, menstrual disturbances, hirsutism and myopathy.
- A characteristic buffalo hump or moon face occurs in Cushing's syndrome.

Treatment
Surgical resection in case of tumor of adrenal glands with replacement therapy.

Addison's Disease
- Clinical features are hypoglycemia, weakness, hyperpigmentation of skin and mucous membrane, hypotension, hyponatremia, hyperkalemia.
- Hydrocortisone is the main line of treatment.
- However, fludrocortisone can be added to therapy.

Acute Adrenal Insufficiency
- It is a life-threatening condition.
- Clinical features are hyponatremia, hypotension, hyperkalemia, nausea, vomiting and lethargy.
- Isotonic sodium chloride infusion with 5% glucose and hydrocortisone should be given.
- Hydrocortisone is adequate to correct both glucocorticoid and mineralocorticoid deficiency.
- In unconfirmed adrenal insufficiency, dexamethasone is preferred as it does not interfere with the diagnostic 'cosyntropin stimulation' test.

Nursing Responsibilities
- Patients should be informed that replacement therapy should continue lifelong.
- Patients should be told to take steroids either twice daily as two-third of dose in morning and one-third in evening or once daily at bedtime according to physician's advice.
- Patients on replacement therapy with steroids should be advised to report to their physicians if they suffer from fever or infection as they require dosage increments during these times.
- Bone X-ray is required in a patient on steroids to rule out osteoporosis.
- Supplemental doses are required at times of stress such as fever, infection, surgery or trauma.
- Patients on alternate day therapy of steroids should be told to take the medication before 9AM daily.
- Patients should be warned not to stop the medication abruptly as it may result in acute adrenal insufficiency.
- Patients should be advised to report blurring of vision or black stools as they indicate side effects of steroids.

Insulin and Oral Hypoglycemic Drugs

- The two principal forms of Diabetes mellitus are type I and type II.
- Type I Diabetes is due to autoimmune process and is of sudden onset.
- It is not hereditary and the primary defect is the development of antibodies to pancreatic islet cells.
- Insulin should be administered and oral hypoglycemic drugs are not effective.
- The onset of type II Diabetes is gradual.
- Family history is often present and it usually starts after 40 years.
- Either insulin resistance or insulin deficiency can be present.
- Oral hypoglycemic drugs are often effective but some may require insulin.

INSULIN

Actions

- It is secreted by the β cells or pancreatic islet cells.
- The gastrointestinal tract (GIT) hormones, pancreatic hormones and autonomic neurotransmitters regulate the secretion of insulin.
- Glucose, fatty acids and amino acids promote the release of insulin.
- The metabolic actions of insulin are primarily anabolic.
- It increases peripheral uptake of glucose.
- It promotes glycogen synthesis and protein synthesis.
- It also inhibits gluconeogenesis in liver, muscle and adipose tissue.
- It increases uptake of amino acids and synthesis of proteins in muscle.
- It inhibits release of free fatty acids and glycerol from adipose tissues.
- In the absence of insulin, glycogenolysis, gluconeogenesis and reduced peripheral utilization of glucose occurs leading to hyperglycemia.

Insulin Preparations

Short-Acting Insulin Analogs
- Insulin aspart
- Insulin lispro
- Insulin glulisine

Short-Acting Insulins
Regular insulin

Intermediate Acting Insulins
- Neutral protamine Hagedorn (NPH) insulin
- Insulin detemir

Long-Acting Insulins
- Insulin glargine
- Ultralente

Short-Acting Insulin Analogs
- They are adsministered subcutaneously 15 minutes before meals.
- The absorption is three times faster and the onset of action is rapid.
- The incidence of hypoglycemia is minimal.
- They result in better glycemic control than regular insulin.
- They reduce the incidence of nocturnal hypoglycemia.
- They can be administered after food in patients with gastroparesis.
- They can also be administered through continuous subcutaneous insulin infusion (CSII) pump.

Short-Acting Insulin
- Regular insulin should be administered subcutaneously 30 minutes before food.
- It is absorbed slowly from the site of administration and has delayed onset of action.
- It can also be administered intravenously in diabetic ketoacidosis.

Intermediate Acting Insulin
- Protamine in neutral protamine hagedorn (NPH) insulin retards absorption.
- So the onset is delayed and duration of action is upto 16 hours.
- It is administered twice daily before breakfast and before dinner.
- It can be mixed with short-acting insulin.
- It can cause allergic reactions.
- The onset of action of insulin detemir is slow and the duration of action is delayed compared to NPH.

Long-Acting Insulin
- Insulin glargine is a clear solution at acidic pH of 4.
- Due to its stability at this potential of hydrogen (pH), its absorption is predictable and prolonged.
- It cannot be mixed with short-acting insulins of neutral pH due to its acidic pH.
- It causes sustained peakless insulin level even after multiple administrations.
- Besides, absorption does not depend upon the site of injection.
- Hence, it results in minimal hypoglycemic episodes.
- It increases the risk of retinopathy.
- Ultralente has slow onset and prolonged peak with unpredictable action.
- Hence, ultralente is not preferred.

Insulin Formulations
Stable, mixed, combinations of protamine lispro/lispro, protamine aspart/aspart and NPH/regular are available.

Newer Insulin Delivery Devices
Insulin can be administered through
- Insulin syringes, pen devices
- Continuous insulin infusion pumps
- Propellant driven mechanical pumps
- Surgically implanted insulin pumps that deliver insulin intraperitoneally.

Adverse Effects
- Hypoglycemia
- Lipodystrophy
- Allergy, insulin resistance.

Uses
- Type I Diabetes mellitus
- Diabetic ketoacidosis
- Type II Diabetes mellitus.

ORAL HYPOGLYCEMIC DRUGS
They are given in type II Diabetes mellitus. They are classified as:
- Sulfonylureas
- Meglitinides
- Biguanides

- Thiazolidinediones
- Alpha-glucosidase inhibitor
- Dipeptidyl peptidase- 4 inhibitors

Sulfonylureas

First Generation
- Tolbutamide
- Tolazamide
- Chlorpropamide

Second Generation
- Glipizide
- Glyburide
- Gliclazide
- Glimepiride

Actions
- They stimulate insulin release from pancreatic beta cells.
- They block adenosine triphosphate (ATP) sensitive potassium channels to release insulin.
- They reduce hepatic metabolism of insulin.
- They promote tissue response to insulin.
- Second generation drugs are preferred to first generation drugs.
- The required dose of second generation drugs is low and their duration of action is long.
- They should be taken before food.
- Glyburide can reduce beta cell mass resulting in secondary failure.
- The incidence of hypoglycemia is high with glyburide.
- Glimepiride reduces the incidence of cardiotoxicity.
- The incidence of hypoglycemia is minimal with glimepiride.

Adverse Effects
- Hypoglycemia
- Nausea, vomiting, agranulocytosis, aplastic anemia
- Cholestatic jaundice

Meglitinides
- Repaglinide
- Nateglinide

Actions
- They are oral insulin secretogogues.
- They promote insulin release from pancreas.

- They release insulin by blocking adenosine triphosphate (ATP) mediated potassium channels.
- They should be taken before food.
- Repaglinide is absorbed quickly and undergoes rapid elimination.
- It can be either given alone or combined with other oral hypoglycemic agents.
- It should be used cautiously in patients with hepatic dysfunction.
- Given orally, nateglinide has faster onset.
- The incidence of hypoglycemia with nateglinide is minimal.
- It can result in secondary failure.

Adverse Effect
Hypoglycemia

Biguanides
Metformin

Actions
- Metformin increases insulin sensitivity and improves insulin action.
- It promotes peripheral utilization of glucose.
- It reduces hepatic glucose production.
- Further, it inhibits gluconeogenesis.
- It causes weight reduction.
- It induces ovulation in patients with polycystic ovarian syndrome (PCOD).
- It should be administered after food.

Adverse Effects
Anorexia, metallic taste, abdominal discomfort, vitamin B_{12} deficiency, lactic acidosis.

Uses
- Type II Diabetes mellitus
- Polycystic ovarian syndrome

Thiazolidinediones
Pioglitazone.

Actions
- Pioglitazone is an agonist of peroxisome proliferator activated receptor-γ (PPAR-γ).
- It increases insulin sensitivity in peripheral tissues.

- It reduces hepatic glucose production and increases hepatic glucose uptake.
- It increases glucose entry into skeletal muscles.
- It increases high density lipoprotein cholestrol (HDL-C) and lowers triglycerides.
- It should be taken after food.
- Maximum therapeutic benefit occurs over 1 to 3 months.

Adverse Effects
- Peripheral edema
- Macular edema, congestive heart failure (CHF)
- Weight gain
- Bone fracture.

Use
Type II Diabetes mellitus

α Glucosidase Inhibitors
- Acarbose
- Voglibose
- Miglitol

Actions
- Polysaccharide are converted to monosaccharide by alpha glucosidase enzyme.
- Alpha glucosidase inhibitor prevent such conversion in intestine.
- Thereby, they reduce the absorption of carbohydrates.
- They can be used alone or in combination with biguanides or thiazolidinediones.
- They should not be combined with insulin, sulfonylurea or with meglitinides.
- Such a combination can cause hypoglycemia.

Adverse Effect
Flatulence, abdominal cramps, diarrhea.

Use
Type II Diabetes mellitus

Dipeptidyl Peptidase-4 Inhibitor
- Gliptin
- Sitagliptin
- Vildagliptin

- Alogliptin
- Saxagliptin

Actions
- Glucose dependent insulinotropic polypeptide (GIP) and glucagon like peptide (GLP) are inactivated by dipeptidyl peptidase enzyme.
- Dipeptidyl peptidase-4 inhibitors increase the duration of action of GLP and GIP.
- These incretins increase the release of insulin.
- They also reduce glucagon level.
- Hence, they improve glycemic control.
- They are effective orally.

Adverse Effect
Rarely pancreatitis

Use
Type II Diabetes mellitus

HYPOGLYCEMIC AGENTS GIVEN THROUGH SUBCUTANEOUS ROUTE

They are classified as:
- Glucagon like peptide-1 analogs
- Amylin analogs

Glucagon like Peptide-1 (GLP-1) Analogs
- Taspoglutide
- Liraglutide
- Albiglutide

Actions
- GLP-1 the incretin released on ingestion of glucose stimulates insulin synthesis.
- They analogs have longer duration of action than native GLP-1.
- They are administered through subcutaneous route before food.

Adverse Effects
- Nausea and vomiting
- Rarely pancreatitis.

Amylin Analog
- Pramlintide is an amylin analog.

- It reduces glucagon release, delays gastric emptying and causes satiety.
- It is administered subcutaneously before food.
- It causes loss of weight.

Adverse effects
- Nausea
- Hypoglycemia.

Diabetic Ketoacidosis
- It is characterized by hyperglycemia, acidosis and ketonuria.
- Diuresis, dehydration, hypotension and shock can occur.
- Acidosis results in hyperventilation and dehydration.
- It is further complicated by vomiting and reduced glucose entry into brain causing unconsciousness.

Treatment
- Intravenous regular insulin – bolus dose of 0.1 unit/kg followed by 1 unit/kg/hour.
- Normal saline infusion till blood pressure is stabilized and then switched over to half normal saline.
- Five percent glucose with half normal saline once blood sugar level reaches 300 mg/dL.
- Potassium chloride 10 to 20 mEq/hour after 4 hours of insulin infusion to prevent hypokalemia.
- Sodium bicarbonate, if acidosis and ketonuria persist and if blood pH is below 7.1.
- Antibiotics and phosphates, if necessary.

Nursing Responsibilities
- Do not mix short-acting insulin preparation with glargine in the same syringe.
- Do not shake insulin suspension vigorously.
- Discard the insulin preparation if it turns cloudy.
- Inject insulin in thigh, arm or abdomen.
- Advice the patient to rotate the injection site every month.
- Instruct the patient to store insulin vials in refrigerator.
- Keep prefilled insulin syringe in the refrigerator with needle pointing upwards.
- Teach patients on insulin, meglitinides, sulfonylureas or GLP-1 analogs to recognize the symptoms of hypoglycemia such as tachycardia, palpitation, headache, sweating or dizziness.
- Advice the patients to take glucose, honey or orange juice immediately if they have symptoms of hypoglycemia.

CHAPTER 45

Estrogens and Progestins

MENSTRUAL CYCLE
- Follicular phase and luteal phase covers one menstrual cycle.
- Gonadotropin releasing hormone (GnRH) required for synthesis of follicle stimulating hormone (FSH) and luteinizing hormone (LH) is released from hypothalamus in a pulsatile manner.
- Follicle stimulating hormone (FSH) and LH stimulate ovary to produce estrogen and progesterone.
- The pulsatile release of FSH is needed for growth of ovarian follicle.
- Midcycle LH surge stimulates ovulation.
- Ovulation is the rupture of matured ovarian follicle which turns into corpus luteum.
- Follicle stimulating hormone is required for maturation of ovarian follicle and LH for maintenance of corpus luteum.
- Estrogens stimulate proliferation and differentiation of uterine endometrium.
- Secretory phase of uterus is mediated by progesterone.
- If pregnancy does not occur, the corpus luteum shrinks.

ESTROGENS
Actions
- Estrogens are derived from androstenedione or testosterone, through the action of aromatase enzyme.
- Estradiol, estrone and estriol are the three forms of estrogen.
- Estradiol is the main secretory form of estrogen from ovary of premenopausal women.
- They are necessary for the growth and development of female reproductive tract.
- They are also necessary for the development of female secondary sexual characters.
- They maintain the balance between bone formation and bone resorption.

- Growth of long bones and epiphyseal fusion are mediated by estrogen.
- They reduce total cholesterol as well as low-density lipoprotein cholesterol (LDL-C) and increase high-density lipoprotein cholesterol (HDL-C).
- They increase nitrous oxide level causing vasodilatation and inhibit atherogenesis.
- They reduce secretion of bile acid and form gallstones.
- They stimulate both fibrinolytic and coagulation pathways.
- They can be administered through oral, parenteral, topical and transdermal routes.
- They are lipophilic and well absorbed after oral administration.
- Oil based ester preparations available for intramuscular injection can be administered once weekly or once monthly.
- They are also available for vaginal administration.
- They are extensively bound to plasma proteins and undergo enterohepatic circulation.
- They are contraindicated during pregnancy.

The synthetic estrogen preparations are:
- Diethylstilbestrol
- Ethinylestradiol
- Estropipate
- Estradiol
- Estradiol cypionate
- Mestranol
- Estradiol valerate

Adverse Effects
- Endometrial cancer
- Breast cancer
- Gallstones
- Thromboembolism
- Dementia
- Migraine
- Nausea, vomiting, edema.

Uses
- Hormone replacement therapy
- Turner's syndrome
- Dysfunctional uterine bleeding

- Contraception
- Carcinoma prostate

SELECTIVE ESTROGEN RECEPTOR MODULATORS (SERM)

They are agonist-antagonists facilitating action of estrogen in some tissues and blocking their actions in others.
The drugs are:
- Clomiphene
- Tamoxifen
- Toremifene
- Raloxifene

Clomiphene

Actions
- It has slight estrogenic agonist activity.
- It has moderate estrogen antagonistic activity.
- It inhibits pituitary gonadotropins.
- It stimulates ovarian follicular maturation and rupture.
- Thereby, it causes ovulation.
- So, it is used as an ovulation inducing agent.
- It is well absorbed after oral administration.
- It is excreted primarily through feces.
- It has long half-life of 7 days due to its lipophilicity, high protein binding and enterohepatic circulation.

Adverse effects
- Polycystic ovary
- Multiple pregnancy
- Hot flashes, vertigo.

Uses
- Infertility
- Polycystic ovarian disease (PCOD)
- Oligozoospermia
- Assisted *in vitro* fertilization.

Tamoxifen

Actions
- It has estrogenic, anti-estrogenic and mixed actions.
- It facilitates estrogen action in bone and endometrium.

- It inhibits bone resorption and reduces the incidence of fractures.
- It inhibits estrogen induced proliferation in breast.
- It inhibits proliferation of breast cancer cells.
- It stimulates proliferation of endometrial cells.
- It reduces total cholesterol and LDL-C but does not alter HDL-C.
- It is well absorbed orally.
- It undergoes enterohepatic circulation.
- It is excreted through feces.

Adverse Effects
- Endometrial carcinoma
- Pulmonary embolism
- Primary hepatocellular carcinoma
- Deep vein thrombosis
- Hot flashes, nausea, cataracts.

Uses
- Carcinoma breast
- Infertility

Toremifene
- It has similar pharmacological actions as tamoxifen.
- It does not cause hepatocellular carcinoma.
- It is used in the treatment of estrogen receptor (ER)-positive breast cancer in postmenopausal women.

Raloxifene
Actions
- It acts as estrogen agonist in bone.
- It reduces bone resorption.
- The overall reduction in fracture incidence is 50%.
- It reduces proliferation of breast cancer cells.
- So, it is effective in ER-positive but not in ER-negative breast cancer.
- It reduces total cholesterol and LDL-C but does not alter HDL-C.
- It does not stimulate proliferation of endometrial cells.
- Hence, it does not result in endometrial carcinoma.
- It is absorbed quickly after oral administration.
- It is excreted mainly through feces.
- It does not reduce hot flashes in menopausal women.

Adverse Effects
- Deep vein thrombosis
- Pulmonary embolism
- Hot flashes, leg cramps

Use
Osteoporosis in postmenopausal women.

SELECTIVE ESTROGEN RECEPTOR DOWNREGULATORS (SERD)

Fulvestrant

Actions
- It is a complete antagonist of estrogen.
- It has high affinity to estrogen receptors.
- It inhibits proliferation of breast cells.
- Its onset of action is quick and its duration of action is long.
- It is given monthly as intramuscular depot injection.
- It reaches maximum plasma concentration after 7 days.

Adverse Effects
- Hot flashes, asthenia
- Headache, pharyngitis, nausea
- Back pain.

Use
Estrogen receptor (ER) or progesterone receptor (PR) positive metastatic breast cancer in postmenopausal women.

Tibolone
- It has estrogen, progesterone and weak androgen like action.
- It is used for 'hormone replacement therapy'.
- It does not cause endometrial proliferation.
- It causes weight gain, spotting and increased facial hair.

AROMATASE INHIBITORS

They inhibit the synthesis of estrogen and cause total estrogen deprivation in tissues.
They are:
- Anastrozole
- Letrozole
- Exemestane

Anastrozole

Actions
- It is a reversible type II aromatase inhibitor.
- It is rapidly absorbed after oral administration.
- Given once daily, it accumulates in the body.
- It reaches a steady state concentration in 7 days.
- It reduces bone mass due to estrogen deprivation in bones.
- The incidence of endometrial cancer and thromboembolic events are lower compared to tamoxifen.

Adverse Effects
- Fracture due to osteoporosis
- Musculoskeletal disorders.

Uses
- In ER/PR positive early stage breast cancer as adjuvant hormonal therapy in postmenopausal women.
- Advanced ER/PR positive breast cancer in postmenopausal women.

Letrozole

Actions
- It inhibits synthesis of estrogen by 99%.
- Its oral bioavailability is around 99.9%.
- It is more effective than tamoxifen in breast cancer.
- It increases bone resorption.

Adverse Effects
- Nausea, hot flashes
- Hair thinning
- Arthralgia, myalgia, arthritis
- Osteoporosis.

Use
Early stage as well as late stage breast cancer in postmenopausal women.

Exemestane

Actions
- It is a potent and irreversible inhibitor of aromatase enzyme.
- It is known as 'suicide substrate'.
- It inhibits of aromatase activity by 98%.

- It is rapidly absorbed orally.
- Its gastrointestinal tract (GIT) absorption is facilitated by fatty meal.

Adverse Effects
- Nausea, fatigue, hot flashes
- Peripheral edema
- Diarrhea, arthralgia.

Use
Early and late stage ER/PR positive breast cancer in postmenopausal women.

Progestins

Actions
- Progesterone inhibits endometrial proliferation.
- It promotes development of secretory endometrium.
- It stimulates thick secretion by endocervical glands.
- It facilitates maintenance of pregnancy.
- It promotes proliferation of acini of mammary gland.
- It increases basal body temperature during ovulation.
- It causes depression and it induces sleep.
- It increases LDL-C and reduces HDL-C.
- It undergoes rapid first pass metabolism.
- It can be administered orally as well as parenterally.
- It is available as oily solution for intramuscular injection.
- It is also available as vaginal gel, vaginal insert and slow release intrauterine progesterone device.

Adverse Effects
- Headache, mood swing, increased body temperature
- Engorgement of breast, nausea, vomiting
- Increased risk of breast cancer
- Irregular menstrual bleeding.

Uses
- Hormone replacement therapy
- Contraception
- Maintenance of pregnancy
- Endometriosis
- Endometrial carcinoma
- Dysfunctional uterine bleeding

SYNTHETIC PROGESTERONE DERIVATIVES

The drugs are:
- Progesterone derivatives with selective activity
  - Medroxyprogesterone acetate
  - Hydroxyprogesterone caproate
  - Megestrol acetate
- 19-nortestosterone derivatives with androgenic activity
  - Norethindrone
  - Levonorgestrel
  - Norethynodrel
  - Ethynodiol diacetate
  - Desogestrel
  - Norgestimate
  - Gestodene
- Spironolactone derivatives with antiandrogenic and antimineralocorticoid activity
  - Drospirenone.

ANTIPROGESTINS

They are:
- Mifepristone
- Onapristone
- Ulipristal

Mifepristone

Actions

- It is progesterone receptor modulator (PRM).
- It is a competitive antagonist of progesterone.
- It facilitates decidual breakdown during early pregnancy.
- It causes detachment of blastocyst.
- It induces cervical softening.
- It facilitates expulsion of detached blastocyst.
- It reduces progesterone secretion by corpus luteum.
- It promotes uterine contraction.
- It interferes with ovulation.
- It also blocks the actions of glucocorticoid and androgen.

Adverse Effect

Vaginal bleeding

Use
Medical abortion

Onapristone
- It is a pure progesterone antagonist.
- It has similar actions and uses of mifepristone.

Ulipristal
Actions
- It is a selective progesterone receptor modulator.
- It is also a weak glucocorticoid antagonist.
- It inhibits proliferation of uterine endometrium.
- It inhibits LH release and LH mediated ovulation.
- It can inhibit ovulation upto five days or 120 hours of intercourse.
- It also inhibits the implantation of fertilized ovum in uterine endometrium.

Adverse Effects
- Abdominal pain
- Headache

Use
Emergency contraceptive

Nursing Responsibilities
- Apply estradiol transdermal patch on clean dry area in abdomen or trunk.
- Change the transdermal estrogen patch once or twice weekly.
- Insert the estrogen intravaginal ring into upper one-third of vagina.
- Change the intravaginal ring after 3 months.
- Patient should be instructed to apply the estrogen intravaginal cream with the help of an applicator.
- Persistent or recurrent vaginal bleeding in women on estrogen therapy should be reported to the gynecologist immediately.
- Monitor the blood pressure, blood sugar and lipid profile in patients on estrogen therapy.

CHAPTER 46

Hormonal Contraceptives

They cause reversible inhibition of conception. Oral and parenteral preparations are available for female contraception.

The types of oral female contraceptive pills are:
- Combination oral contraceptive
- Post coital contraceptive
- Mini pills or progestin only contraceptive

COMBINATION ORAL CONTRACEPTIVE

- They are available as monophasic, biphasic and triphasic formulations.
- These pills contain both an estrogen and a progestin.
- Monophasic pills contain fixed quantity of estrogen and progestin in each pill.
- The pack contains 21 hormonal pills.
- During the 7 days pill free period withdrawal bleeding occurs.
- Biphasic and triphasic pill pack contains varying amounts of estrogen and progesterone in the 21 hormonal pills.
- Ethinyl estradiol is the estrogen preparation commonly used.
- Progestin can be levonorgestrel, norgestrel or norethindrone.

Mechanism of Action

- Suppression of follicle stimulating hormone (FSH) and luteinizing hormone (LH) release.
- Inhibition of LH surge and ovulation.
- Thick cervical secretion hostile for sperm penetration.
- Unfavorable endometrium unsuitable for implantation.
- Increased uterine and fallopian tube contraction.

Adverse Effects

- Headache, nausea, vomiting
- Breast engorgement
- Acne, edema, weight gain
- Mood swing, hyperpigmentation of cheek

- Hyperglycemia, hypertension
- Deep vein thrombosis, pulmonary embolism
- Carcinoma of breast, vagina and cervix
- Gallstones, hepatoma.

Contraindications
- Coronary artery disease (CAD)
- Cerebrovascular disease
- Hypertension, Diabetes mellitus
- Hyperlipidemia
- Previous history of thromboembolism
- Gallbladder disease
- Malignancy, psychosis, undiagnosed vaginal bleeding
- Migraine

'Progestin Only' Contraceptive
- It contains low dose of either norethindrone or norgestrel.
- The success rate is lower than combination contraceptive pills.
- It alters cervical secretion causing thick mucus secretion preventing sperm entry.
- It inhibits implantation by altering the status of endometrium.
- It increases uterine and fallopian tube contractions.
- 'Progestin only' contraceptive should be taken daily at same time.

Adverse Effects
- Irregular spotting
- Breakthrough bleeding
- Headache, mood swings
- Amenorrhea after discontinuation.

POSTCOITAL CONTRACEPTIVE
Commonly used preparations contain:
- Levonorgestrel and ethinylestradiol combination
- Levonorgestrel
- Ulipristal

Levonorgestrel and Ethinylestradiol Combination
- Levonorgestrel 0.5 mg and ethinylestradiol 0.1 mg is less effective than levonorgestrel.
- This combination should be administrated twice within 72 hours.

- The incidence of nausea and vomiting is higher with this combination postcoital contraceptive.

Levonorgestrel
- Levonorgestrel should be administered within 72 hours of intercourse.
- It is either given as two doses of 0.75 mg or a single dose of 1.5 mg.
- It causes minimal side effects.
- It can delay the onset of subsequent menstrual cycle.

Ulipristal
- Ulipristal is effective upto 120 hours after intercourse.
- It is well tolerated and more effective postcoital contraceptive preparation.

Injectable Contraceptives
- They are either progestin alone preparation or estrogen progestin combination.
- Progestin alone preparation contain either medroxyprogesterone acetate or norethindrone enanthate.
- Fixed dose estrogen and progestin preparation is not advisable.

Progestin Alone Preparation
- Medroxyprogesterone acetate can be administered through intramuscular route at 3 months interval.
- Norethindrone enanthate is administered once in 2 months.
- It takes atleast 12 months for onset of menstrual cycle after the progestin alone injections are discontinued.

Mechanism
- By suppressing the ovulation.
- By making endometrium unsuitable for implantation
- By forming thick cervical secretion.

Adverse Effects
- Disruption of menstrual cycle
- Amenorrhea
- Excessive bleeding, headache
- Depression, weight gain, abdominal bloating
- Hot flashes
- Osteoporosis

Subdermal Implants
- 3-ketodesogestrel subdermal implant is very effective.
- It acts for longtime.
- It is implanted into the inner aspect of upper arm under local anesthesia.
- The hormone is released slowly into circulation upto 3 years.
- Ovulation occurs within 6 weeks of surgical removal of the implant.
- Since it is a progestin, it alters the cervical mucus and makes it unsuitable for sperm entry.
- It converts the uterine endometrium unsuitable for nidation.

Adverse Effects
- Menstrual irregularities such as amenorrhea, spotting or irregular profuse bleeding.
- Local irritation, weight gain.

Ormeloxifene

Actions
- It is a nonsteroidal oral contraceptive.
- It has selective estrogen receptor modulator activity.
- It antagonizes estrogen action on uterus and breast.
- It inhibits endometrial proliferation.
- It is administered twice weekly for 12 weeks and thereafter it is given once in a week.
- It is long-acting and fertility returns within few months after the discontinuation.

Adverse Effects
Headache, nausea, edema, weight gain.

Uses
- Contraception
- Dysfunctional uterine bleeding

Male Contraception
Gonadotropin releasing hormone (GnRH) analogs, antiandrogens, estrogens and progestins have been tried.

Gossypol

Actions
- It is obtained from cotton seed.
- It is given orally.
- It inhibits spermatogenesis and motility of sperm.
- Fertility resumes after couple of months on stopping therapy.
- Since it is a nonsteroidal compound it does not affect libido.

Adverse Effects
- Hypokalemia and muscular weakness
- Edema, diarrhea.

Use
Male contraception.

Nursing Responsibilities
- Women willing to take oral contraceptive pills (OCPs) should start it on 6th day of menstrual cycle.
- They should be advised to take the pills at same time daily.
- If 1 dose is missed, 2 pills should be taken on next day but if 3 doses are missed then the pills should be discontinued.
- Pain in leg, shortness of breath, blurring of vision, profuse bleeding or headache in women on OCP should be immediately reported to the gynecologist.
- Blood glucose and blood pressure should be monitored periodically in women on OCP.
- Progestin alone pill should be started on day one of menstruation.

CHAPTER 47

Androgens

The preparations are:
- Testosterone
- Testosterone enanthate
- Testosterone cypionate
- Testosterone undecanoate

Actions
- Testosterone is secreted from Leydig cells of testes.
- Follicle stimulating hormone (FSH) and luteinizing hormone (LH) regulate its secretion.
- Luteinizing hormone (LH) is also known as interstitial cell-stimulating hormone.
- It is necessary for the growth and development of male primary and secondary sexual characters.
- It is an anabolic hormone and stimulates growth of bone and skeletal muscles.
- It also stimulates the production and maturation of sperm.
- It increases the synthesis of erythrocytes.
- It is ineffective orally as it undergoes very high first pass metabolism.
- It is available as transdermal patch, buccal tablet and gel.

Adverse Effects
- Erythrocytosis
- Peripheral edema
- Hepatocellular carcinoma and cholestatic hepatitis.

Uses
- Replacement therapy in male hypogonadism
- Male senescence
- Delayed puberty
- Carcinoma breast
- Catabolic muscle wasting states in acquired immunodeficiency syndrome (AIDS)

- Refractory anemia
- Hereditary angioneurotic edema

Contraindications
- Carcinoma prostate
- Pregnancy
- Breast cancer in male

ANABOLIC STEROIDS

These compounds have higher anabolic and lower androgenic activity.
The preparations are:
- Oxandrolone
- Stanozolol
- Danazol
- Tetrahydrogestrinone.

Adverse Effects
- Virilization
- Hepatotoxicity
- Alteration in lipid profile.

Uses
- Catabolic muscle wasting states such as AIDS
- To improve athletic performance
- Refractory anemia
- Osteoporosis.

Danazol

Actions
- It has anabolic, weak androgenic and progesterone activity.
- It inhibits gonadotropin release from pituitary.
- It inhibits both ovarian and testicular function.

Adverse Effects
- Amenorrhea
- Hirsutism
- Acne
- Weight gain, edema.

Uses
- Endometriosis
- Menorrhagia
- Refractory hemolytic anemia
- Refractory immune thrombocytopenic purpura
- Fibrocystic breast disease
- Angioedema.

ANTIANDROGENS
- Androgen receptor antagonists:
  - Flutamide
  - Nilutamide
  - Bicalutamide
- 5α-reductase inhibitors:
  - Finasteride
  - Dutasteride
- GnRH antagonist:
  - Abarelix

Androgen Receptor Antagonists
Flutamide
Actions
- It blocks peripheral action of androgen thereby stimulating LH release.
- It is used with GnRH agonist in the treatment of metastatic prostate cancer.
- Flutamide is administered thrice daily.

Adverse Effects
- Hepatotoxicity
- Nausea, vomiting
- Breast or nipple tenderness

Uses
- Metastatic prostate cancer
- Hirsutism

Bicalutamide
Actions
- Bicalutamide is long-acting and can be administered once daily.
- It is less hepatotoxic than flutamide.

Adverse Effects
- Hot flashes
- Edema

Use
Carcinoma prostate

5α- Reductase Inhibitors

Finasteride
Actions
- Finasteride inhibits 5α-reductase necessary for the conversion of testosterone to dihydrotestosterone.
- It inhibits the enzyme in many tissues including prostate.
- It reduces the prostatic volume and facilitates urinary outflow.
- Maximum benefit occurs only after 6 months.

Adverse Effects
- Reduced libido
- Impotence
- Gynecomastia.

Uses
- Benign prostatic hypertrophy (BPH)
- Male pattern baldness.

Dutasteride
Actions
- Dutasteride is more effective in reducing dihydrotestosterone level.
- It has an extremely long half-life of 5 weeks.
- Hence, it is present in plasma long after its discontinuation.

Adverse Effect
Reduced libido

Uses
Benign prostatic hypertrophy (BPH).

GnRH Antagonist

Abarelix
It is used in carcinoma prostate.

Nursing Responsibilities
Patients should be advised to wash hands before and after applying testosterone gel.

PHOSPHODIESTERASE-5 INHIBITORS

The drugs are:
- Sildenafil
- Tadalafil
- Vardenafil

Actions
- They increase cyclic guanosine monophosphate (GMP) level by inhibiting phosphodiesterase -5 enzyme.
- They cause relaxation of smooth muscles of corpus cavernosum and penile arteries.
- This results in erection.
- They are well absorbed orally but fatty meal reduces absorption.
- The excretion is delayed in old age due to hepatic and renal dysfunction.
- Tadalafil has delayed onset longer-duration of action.
- Vardenafil causes prolonged QT syndrome.

Adverse Effects
- Hypotension
- Headache, flushing, dizziness
- Rash, diarrhea, dyspepsia
- Visual disturbances.

Contraindications
They should not be coadministered with:
- Nitrates
- α blockers, β blockers

Uses
- Erectile dysfunction
- Pulmonary arterial hypertension.

THERAPY OF ERECTILE DYSFUNCTION

Erectile dysfunction is characterized by persistent difficulty in sustaining erection.
The drugs used are:
- Phosphodiesterase-5 inhibitors: sildenafil
- Prostaglandin E_1: Alprostadil
- Papaverine/phentolamine.

- Alprostadil, papaverine and phentolamine can be administered directly into corpus cavernosum

THERAPY OF BENIGN PROSTATIC HYPERTROPHY
- Benign prostatic hypertrophy is a nonmalignant prostatic hypertrophy causing obstruction to urinary outflow.
- The symptoms are urinary hesitancy, urinary urgency, dysuria and frequent urination.

The drugs used are:
- **5α-reductase inhibitors:** Finasteride, dutasteride
- **α_1 adrenergic receptor antagonists:** Terazosin, doxazosin, tamsulosin, alfuzosin.

CHAPTER 48

Agents Involved in Bone Turnover

CALCIUM, PARATHORMONE, VITAMIN D, CALCITONIN

Calcium

Actions

Calcium is required for:
- Contraction of muscles
- Exocytosis
- Blood coagulation
- Skeletal remodeling
- Conductance in ionic calcium channels
- Dietary source is milk and dairy products.
- Serum calcium level is influenced by bone formation and bone resorption.
- Cholecalciferol (vitamin-D_3) promotes intestinal absorption of calcium.
- Similarly, renal tubular reabsorption of calcium is regulated by parathormone.
- Ninety percent of calcium is stored in bone in the form of hydroxyapatite crystals.
- It is involved in bone remodeling.
- It is available as gluconate, lactate, citrate, hydroxyapatite and carbonate salts for oral administration.
- It is available as calcium gluceptate, calcium gluconate and calcium chloride for intravenous (IV) infusion.

Hypercalcemia
- It occurs in primary hyperparathyroidism, malignancy, milk-alkali syndrome and vitamin D excess.
- Fatigue, depression, nephrolithiasis, polyurea, nausea, vomiting, bone and joint pain are the common symptoms.

Treatment
- Intravenous saline.
- Furosemide to increase renal excretion of calcium after repletion of fluid volume.

- Subcutaneous (SC) calcitonin for rapid reduction of calcium level.
- IV bisphosphonate to reduce bone resorption.
- Cinacalcet is effective in hypercalcemia associated with hyperparathyroidism.
- High dose corticosteroid (prednisolone) in hypercalcemia due to sarcoidosis.
- Oral sodium phosphate—in patients with hyperparathyroidism.
- Plicamycin—inhibits bone resorption.

Hypocalcemia
- Frequent causes are hypoparathyroidism, malabsorption.
- Tetany, convulsions and laryngeal spasm are frequent symptoms.

Treatment
- IV calcium gluconate followed by oral calcium with vitamin D for hypocalcemic tetany.
- Oral calcium salts for mild hypocalcemia.

Phosphate
Actions
- It is present in plasma, extracellular fluid (ECF), intracellular fluid (ICF), cell membrane, bone and collagen.
- It occurs both in organic and inorganic forms.
- The phosphate present in ECF is inorganic while that is seen in phospholipids is organic.
- It is bound to calcium as hydroxyapatite crystals in bone.
- It is available in most foods and vitamin D promotes its absorption.
- Eighty percent phosphate is reabsorbed in proximal convoluted tubule.
- Parathormone increases its excretion by inhibiting its tubular reabsorption.

Use
Acidification of urine.

Parathormone
Actions
- It is a polypeptide hormone.
- It maintains serum calcium level by influencing bone resorption, bone formation, synthesis of calcitriol, renal calcium excretion and reabsorption.
- Its actions on bone are both anabolic and catabolic.

- Chronic exposure to parathormone enhances bone resorption.
- Intermittent increase helps in bone formation.
- Parathormone is necessary for the synthesis of calcitriol or vitamin D_3.
- It converts vitamin D to its active form D_3 (calcitriol) which facilitates intestinal absorption of calcium.
- It promotes renal tubular reabsorption of calcium.
- High serum level of calcium reduces, while low serum calcium stimulates the release of parathormone.
- It inhibits the renal tubular reabsorption of phosphate increasing its excretion.
- It reduces magnesium excretion.

Teriparatide
Actions
- It is a recombinant form of parathormone.
- It increases bone density in postmenopausal women.
- It promotes bone formation and bone mineral density.
- It can be administered through subcutaneous or intravenous route.
- It is expensive.

Adverse Effect
It has a 'black box' warning for osteosarcoma.

Uses
- Osteoporosis in women with previous history of fracture.
- Hypogonadal osteoporosis in men.

Vitamin D
Actions
- It is a fat soluble vitamin as well as a hormone.
- It is called a hormone as it is synthesized in skin on exposure to sunlight and exerts its regulatory function in other areas of body.
- Cholecalciferol (vitamin D_3) and ergocalciferol (vitamin D_2) are the two active forms of vitamin D.
- Both D_2 and D_3 are absorbed in small intestine and bile is necessary for their absorption.
- It is stored in fat depots.
- It is excreted through bile.
- Vitamin D is hydroxylated to 25-hydroxycholecalciferol in liver.

- It is further hydroxylated to 1, 25-dihydroxycholecalciferol or calcitriol in kidney.
- Calcitriol increases intestinal absorption of calcium and phosphate.
- It promotes their reabsorption in kidney.
- Thereby, it promotes bone mineralization.
- The major dietary source of vitamin D is milk.
- Daily requirement is 400 IU for infants and children.
- The daily requirement in adults is 200 IU.
- Deficiency results in rickets in children and osteomalacia in adults.
- Since it inhibits proliferation of cells it can prevent cancer.
- It is available as calcitriol, dihydrotachysterol, hydroxycholecalciferol, ergocalciferol, paricalcitol, calcipotriol, oxacalcitriol and doxercalciferol.

Uses
- Nutritional rickets
- Hypoparathyroidism
- Osteomalacia
- Renal osteodystrophy
- Psoriasis vulgaris

Hypervitaminosis D
The signs and symptoms of hypervitaminosis D are similar to hypercalcemia.

Treatment
- Discontinuation of vitamin D administration.
- Furosemide to promote its excretion.
- Glucocorticoids to reduce its absorption.

Calcitonin

Actions
- It is a hypocalcemic hormone.
- Its release is regulated by serum calcium level.
- It inhibits bone resorption.
- It decreases serum calcium and phosphate level.
- It reduces serum alkaline phosphatase activity in Paget's disease.

Salmon Calcitonin
- Salmon calcitonin is used therapeutically as it has longer half-life.
- It is given once daily for the treatment of postmenopausal osteoporosis.
- It is available as nasal spray.

Adverse Effects
- Nausea, urticaria.
- Intranasal spray of salmon calcitonin can cause nasal dryness and irritation.
- Parenteral administration can cause injection site reactions, nausea and flushing of face.

Uses
- Paget's disease
- Postmenopausal osteoporosis
- Diagnosis of medullary thyroid cancer
- Hypercalcemia secondary to cancer

BISPHOSPHONATES
The drugs are:
- Alendronate
- Risedronate
- Pamidronate
- Ibandronate
- Zoledronate
- Etidronate
- Tiludronate

Actions
- They inhibit bone resorption.
- They are internalized into osteoclasts and promote osteoclastic apoptosis.
- They have poor oral bioavailability in the presence of food.
- They are available for oral administration and given either once daily or once weekly.
- Ibandronate is unique and can be administered once monthly.
- Zoledronate and pamidronate are available as intravenous formulation for hypercalcemia of malignancy.

Adverse Effects
- Oesophagitis on oral administration.
- Infusion causes flushing, nausea, vomiting, muscle and joint pain.
- Osteonecrosis of jaw.
- Renal damage with zoledronate infusion.

Uses
- Paget's disease
- Postmenopausal osteoporosis
- Corticosteroids induced osteoporosis
- Osteoporosis in cancer patients
- Intravenous bisphosphonates in hypercalcemia of malignancy.

Cinacalcet
- It is a calcimimetic drug.
- It inhibits parathormone secretion.
- It enhances the sensitivity of calcium-sensing receptors.
- It is used in secondary hyperparathyroidism due to chronic renal disease.
- It is effective on oral administration.
- It can cause hypocalcemia.

Paget's Disease
- It occurs usually after 60 years of age.
- It is characterized by increased bone resorption and abnormal bone replacement.
- The common sites are skull, pelvis, femur, spine and tibia.
- The bone becomes large, spongy and fragile.
- Altered bone structure can result in spinal cord compression and deafness.
- Serum alkaline phosphatase and urine hydroxyproline levels are high.

Treatment
- Bisphosphonates
- Salmon calcitonin

Osteoporosis
- It is characterized by increased bone loss and reduced bone mass.
- Common sites are distal radius, proximal femur and vertebral bodies.

- Bone mineral density (BMD) is an indicator for osteoporosis.
- Sufficient intake of calcium with vitamin D can reduce osteoporosis.

Treatment
- Bisphosphonates such as alendronate
- Calcitonin salmon nasal spray
- Teriparatide
- Raloxifene
- Denosumab, the monoclonal antibody.

Nursing Responsibilities
- Patients with hypocalcemia should be advised to avoid spinach, rhubarb, beet, bran and whole cereals.
- Since calcium reduces the absorption of tetracycline, they should not be given together.
- Patients should be asked to take chewable formulation of calcium as they have better oral bioavailability.
- Patients on oral bisphosphonates should be asked to take the drug in erect position with adequate water.
- Blurring of vision or any other vision problem in patients on bisphosphonates should be reported immediately.

CHAPTER 49

Uterine Stimulants and Relaxants

Drugs that cause uterine contraction are called oxytocics and drugs that cause uterine relaxation are called tocolytics.

UTERINE RELAXANTS OR TOCOLYTICS
The tocolytics are:
- Magnesium sulfate
- Nifedipine
- β-adrenergic agonists

Magnesium Sulfate
Actions
- It causes uterine relaxation.
- It is cheap and an effective uterine relaxant.
- It crosses placenta and can cause fetal hypotonia and sleepiness.

Adverse Effects
- Hypotension, flushing, headache, dizziness
- Hypothermia, renal failure, hypocalcemia.

Uses
- Preterm labor
- Seizures associated with eclampsia

Nifedipine
Actions
- Nifedipine the calcium channel blocker causes relaxation of uterine smooth muscles.
- It can be administered through sublingual, oral or intravenous routes.
- It is less likely to cause maternal side effects.

Adverse Effects
- Flushing, tachycardia
- Headache, dizziness
- Hypotension

Uterine Stimulants and Relaxants

Uses
- Preterm labor
- Hypertensive emergency.

β-Adrenergic Agonists
They are only second line drugs.
The drugs are:
- Ritodrine
- Terbutaline
- They stimulate β_2 receptors of uterus.
- They cause relaxation of uterine smooth muscle.
- They reduce both the amplitude and frequency of uterine contractions.

Adverse Effects
- Hypotension
- Pulmonary edema
- Tachycardia

Use
Preterm labor

Atosiban
- It is an antagonist of oxytocin receptors.
- It reduces the frequency of uterine contractions.

UTERINE STIMULANTS OR OXYTOCICS
The drugs are:
- Oxytocin
- Ergot alkaloids
- Prostaglandins

Oxytocin

Actions
- It is a posterior pituitary hormone.
- It causes uterine contraction and milk ejection reflex.
- It increases force and frequency of uterine contraction.
- The sensitivity of uterus increases as pregnancy advances.
- This is because the number of oxytocin receptors increases over time during pregnancy.
- It also transfers milk from alveolar ducts into sinuses of breast.

- It causes contraction of myoepithelium around alveolar channels and results in 'milk let out'.
- It is administered as intravenous infusion in the induction of labor.
- It can cause mild retention of water.

Adverse Effects
- Uterine rupture
- Edema.

Contraindications
- Cephalopelvic disproportion
- Placental abnormalities
- Previous uterine surgery
- Fetal distress.

Uses
- Induction of labor
- Postpartum hemorrhage
- Augmentation of labor.

Ergot Alkaloids

The ergot alkaloids used in induction of labor are:
- Ergonovine (ergometrine)
- Methylergometrine

Actions
- They increase the force and frequency of contraction.
- They cause sustained uterine contraction with minimal relaxation.
- They are not preferred for the induction of labor.
- They have quick onset of action.
- The action persists for prolonged period.
- Ergot derivatives ergotamine and dihydroergotamine causes vasoconstriction of cerebral vessels.
- Hence, they are used in the treatment of migraine.

Adverse Effects
- Hypertension on IV administration
- Nausea, vomiting, headache
- Convulsion.

Contraindications
Hypertension.

Uses
- Postpartum hemorrhage
- Migraine (ergotamine, dihydroergotamine)

Prostaglandins
The prostaglandins causing uterine stimulation are:
- Dinoprostone
- Carboprost
- Misoprostol

Actions
- The rigid and constricted cervix of pregnancy undergoes cervical ripening during labor.
- During cervical ripening the cervix dilates and becomes soft.
- Prostaglandins cause cervical ripening thereby facilitating smooth labor.
- They also stimulate uterine contractions during labor.

Dinoprostone
- It is approved by Food and Drug Administration (FDA) and used widely for this purpose.
- It is a prostaglandin E_2 (PGE_2) analog.
- It is available as vaginal gel and vaginal inserts.

Adverse Effect
Uterine rupture

Contraindications
- Glaucoma
- Myocardial infarction
- Bronchial asthma

Uses
- Induction of labor
- Termination of pregnancy
- Cervical priming

Misoprostol
- It is a prostaglandin E_2 (PGE_2) analog.
- It is cheaper, convenient and more effective.
- It causes intense and frequent uterine contraction.
- It is less preferred as it causes hyperstimulation of uterus.

Adverse Effects
- Uterine rupture
- Fetal distress.

Carboprost
- It is a prostaglandin $F_{2\alpha}$ ($PGF_{2\alpha}$) analog.
- It causes intense uterine contractions.
- Hence, it is used to manage postpartum hemorrhage.
- It is contraindicated in pelvic inflammatory disease.
- It causes vomiting, diarrhea and fever.

Nursing Responsibilities
- Renal function should be monitored during IV magnesium sulfate administration.
- Terbutaline is effective only during the first 48 hours of its administration.
- BP, heart rate and uterine contraction should be monitored after ergot administration.

SECTION IX

Gastrointestinal System

- Drugs in Peptic Ulcer and GERD
- Antiemetic Drugs
- Drugs in Constipation, Diarrhea and Other GIT Conditions

CHAPTER 50

Drugs in Peptic Ulcer and GERD

ACID PEPTIC DISEASE
- Peptic ulcer occurs due to imbalance between defensive and offensive factors.
- The major defensive factors are mucus and bicarbonate.
- Gastric acid, pepsin and *H.pylori* are the offensive factors.

The drugs are classified as:
- Proton pump inhibitors
- H_2 blockers
- Antacids
- Ulcer protective
- Anticholinergics
- Prostaglandins
- Miscellaneous agents.

PROTON PUMP INHIBITORS
The drugs are:
- Omeprazole
- Esomeprazole
- Lansoprazole
- Dexlansoprazole
- Rabeprazole
- Pantoprazole.

Actions
- They inhibit the 'proton pump' or $H^+K^+ATPase$ enzyme which is involved in acid synthesis.
- They are prodrugs and converted to active drugs in acidic environment.
- They should be administered 30 minutes before food.
- They are absorbed from small intestine and diffuse into gastric parietal cells.
- In the acidic pH of parietal cells they become active and bind irreversibly to the proton pump.

- They block the acid secretion permanently.
- The acid secretion resumes only after the synthesis of new proton pump.
- They are available as enteric coated formulation.
- The maximum clinical effect is seen only after 2 to 5 days of therapy.
- Pantoprazole, lansoprazole and esomeprazole are available as intravenous formulations for immediate action.

Adverse Effects
- Nausea, diarrhea, flatulence, abdominal pain, constipation
- Rashes, headache, myopathy, arthralgia.

Uses
- Gastric and duodenal ulcers
- Gastroesophageal reflux disease (GERD)
- Zollinger-Ellison syndrome
- Nonsteroidal anti-inflammatory drugs (NSAIDs) induced gastritis.

H_2 BLOCKERS
The drugs are:
- Cimetidine
- Ranitidine
- Famotidine
- Nizatidine.

Actions
- H_2 receptors of parietal cells are involved in acid secretion.
- These drugs are competitive inhibitors of H_2 receptors.
- They reduce the basal acid secretion.
- Hence, they are effective in suppressing nocturnal acid secretion.
- They are available for oral, intramuscular and intravenous administration.
- Cimetidine inhibits binding of testosterone with androgen receptors.
- Hence, it causes gynecomastia and impotence in men.
- It should not be given in male patients.

Adverse Effects
- Constipation
- Headache, drowsiness, fatigue
- Delirium, confusion, slurred speech

Uses
- Gastric and duodenal ulcers
- Uncomplicated gastroesophageal reflux disease (GERD)
- Stress ulcer.

ANTACIDS
The systemic and non-systemic antacids are:
- **Systemic antacid:** Sodium bicarbonate
- **Non-systemic antacids:** Calcium carbonate, aluminum hydroxide, magnesium hydroxide, magaldrate.

Actions
- Potency of antacids is generally measured with respect to their acid neutralizing capacity (ANC).
- ANC is the number of milliequivalents of gastric acid brought to pH 3.5 by a unit dose of antacid in 15 minutes.
- They do not reduce acid secretion but increase the pH.
- They neutralize gastric acid which reduces pepsin secretion.
- Although they promote healing of ulcer, they can result in acid rebound.
- By altering gastric pH, antacids interfere with absorption of many drugs.
- Simethicone, a surfactant is added to many antacid preparations to reduce foaming and esophageal reflux.
- Systemic antacids can cause systemic alkalosis as they are absorbed.
- The absorbed sodium causes edema and can worsen cardiac and renal function in patients with congestive heart failure (CHF) or renal failure.

Magnesium Salts
- They increase gastric motility but cause minimal acid rebound.
- If absorbed, they can interfere with renal function.

Aluminum Hydroxide
- It is slow acting, delays gastric motility as aluminum relaxes smooth muscles.
- If absorbed, it can cause osteoporosis, myopathy and encephalopathy.

Magaldrate
- It is hydroxymagnesium aluminate complex.
- It is converted to magnesium and aluminum salts.
- Magnesium salts increase motility while aluminum salts reduce motility.
- Hence aluminum and magnesium neutralize each other's action on GIT motility.

Calcium Carbonate
- It acts fast, releasing carbon dioxide which may cause distention and discomfort.
- It causes rebound acid secretion necessitating more frequent administration.
- Calcium may get absorbed to cause 'milk alkali syndrome'.
- Hypercalcemia, alkalosis and renal dysfunction are common in milk alkali syndrome.

ULCER PROTECTIVE
They cover the ulcer crater preventing its interaction with gastric acid.
They are:
- Sucralfate
- Colloidal bismuth subsalicylate.

Sucralfate
Actions
- In gastric acidic medium, sucralfate undergoes polymerization.
- This viscous and sticky gel adheres to gastric mucosal epithelium.
- It inhibits activity of pepsin, increases synthesis of prostaglandins and epidermal growth factor.
- It also binds with bile salts.
- It should be administered on empty stomach.

Adverse Effects
- Constipation
- Bezoars
- Aluminum overload in patients with renal dysfunction.

Drug Interactions
- Antacids should be taken only after 2 hours after sucralfate administration.

- Sucralfate inhibits absorption of many drugs such as phenytoin, cimetidine, fluoroquinolones and ketoconazole.

Uses
- Peptic ulcer
- Stress ulcer
- Aphthous ulcer
- Oral mucositis
- Bile reflux gastropathy
- Solitary rectal ulcers
- Radiation proctitis.

Colloidal Bismuth Subsalicylate

Actions
- It contains bismuth, salicylate and aluminum magnesium silicate.
- It has antisecretory, anti-inflammatory and antimicrobial effects.
- Bismuth subsalicylate precipitates at gastric pH and coats the ulcer crater.
- It detaches the *H.pylori* organism from its binding site into lumen.
- It causes black tongue and black stools due to bismuth sulfide formed as a result of interaction between bismuth and bacterial sulfides.

Adverse Effects
- Headache, dizziness, diarrhea
- Black tongue, black stools
- Salicylate absorption can aggravate Reye's syndrome.

Uses
- *H.pylori* regimen in peptic ulcer
- Traveler's diarrhea.

PROSTAGLANDINS

Actions
- Prostaglandins E_2 and I_2 (PGE_2 and PGI_2) bind to prostaglandin receptors of parietal cells.
- They reduce secretion of gastric acid.
- PGE_2 increases the secretion of mucin and bicarbonate.
- It also increases the mucosal blood flow.
- Prostaglandin E_1 analog misoprostol inhibits both basal and food induced gastric secretion.
- It should be given four times daily.
- Its main disadvantage is its need for frequent administration.

Adverse Effects
- Diarrhea
- Abdominal cramps
- Exacerbations of inflammatory bowel disease.

Use
NSAIDs induced gastritis.

ANTICHOLINERGICS
- Pirenzepine and telenzepine, the muscarinic M_1 receptor antagonists reduce acid secretion.
- They reduce basal acid secretion by acting on intramural ganglia.
- They are less effective and rarely used now.
- Besides, pirenzepine can cause blood dyscrasias.

Rebamipide
- It exerts cytoprotective action by increasing prostaglandin secretion.
- It also acts as an antioxidant by scavenging reactive oxygen species.

Ecabet
It acts by increasing PGE_2 and PGI_2 secretion.

Anti Helicobacter pylori Drugs
- *Helicobacter pylori*, a gram-negative rod thrives in acidic medium of stomach.
- It is found to be responsible for gastric and duodenal ulcer as well as gastric adenocarcinoma.
- Combination of two antibiotics, a proton pump inhibitor (PPI)/H_2 blocker is given for 14 days in triple therapy.
- An additional compound colloidal bismuth subsalicylate is added in quadruple therapy.

Triple Therapy
Proton pump inhibitor (PPI) bid + Clarithromycin 500 mg bid + Amoxicillin 1G bid/metronidazole 500 mg bid.

Quadruple Therapy
PPI bid + Metronidazole 500 mg tid + Colloidal bismuth subsalicylate 525 mg qid + Tetracycline 500 mg qid.

Nursing Responsibilities
- Peptic ulcer patients should be advised to avoid spicy food, alcohol, NSAIDs and smoking.
- Black tarry stool in such patients indicates bleeding peptic ulcer and they should be advised to report immediately.
- Patients should avoid spicy food and should be advised not to lie down immediately after a heavy meal.
- Suspension formulation of antacids is more effective than powder or tablet formulation.

Management of Bleeding Peptic Ulcer
- This complication can occur in 10% of peptic ulcer patients.
- The characteristic symptoms are hematemesis or malena.
- 'Coffee ground vomiting' in a patient with peptic ulcer indicates 'bleeding peptic ulcer'.
- Hemodynamic state should be assessed immediately in such patients.
- Patients presenting with shock and hypovolemia should be given blood transfusion and IV fluids.
- Blood transfusion is absolutely necessary in patients with low hematocrit value.
- Acidosis if present should be corrected by administration of sodium bicarbonate.
- Intravenous infusion of proton pump inhibitor for three days is necessary.
- The PPI pantoprazole 80 mg bolus followed by 8 mg/hour for 3 days is given.
- Either endoscopic therapy with thermocoagulation or application of endoscopic clips will arrest the bleeding.
- Subcutaneous adrenaline injection combined with endoscopic thermocoagulation is effective in bleeding peptic ulcer.

Nursing Responsibilities
- Assess hematocrit value and blood urea nitrogen (BUN) level.
- Check BP and pulse immediately to assess their hemodynamic status.
- Patients in shock should be immediately started with blood transfusion and IV fluids.
- Blood transfusion should target Hb > 7 mg/dL.
- Oral feeding should not be given for 72 hours.

- As soon as oral feeding is started, anti *H.pylori* drugs should be commenced.
- IV H_2 blockers are not effective in bleeding peptic ulcer.
- Patients on NSAIDs and low dose aspirin (for antiplatelet action) should be told to stop these drugs immediately.
- Endoscopy should be done within 24 hours to assess the risk of rebleeding.

Zollinger-Ellison Syndrome
- It is associated with gastric or duodenal gastrinoma that secrete huge amount of acid.
- High, twice daily dose of proton pump inhibitor is the main line of treatment.

GASTROESOPHAGEAL REFLUX DISEASE (GERD)
- GERD is characterized by esophageal erosion, stricture and Barrett's hyperplasia.
- Barrett's hyperplasia is the replacement of squamous cells by columnar epithelium.
- It is a chronic disorder and necessitates prolonged therapy.
- The severity of GERD is classified into three stages.
- Heart burn is the main symptom in stage I with 2 to 3 episodes per week.
- Frequent heart burn occurs in stage II. Esophagitis may or may not be present and associated with more than 3 episodes per week.
- Chronic symptoms with complications such as strictures are seen in stage III.

Treatment
Stage I
- Lifestyle modification such as diet and weight loss
- Antacids
- H_2 blockers.

Stage II
Intermittent, on demand therapy with PPI.

Stage III
Regular administration of PPI once or twice daily.

Antiemetic Drugs

These drugs are given for the suppression of nausea and vomiting. They are broadly classified as:
- Serotonin antagonists
- Antihistamines
- Dopamine antagonists
- Anticholinergics
- Cannabinoid
- Substance P/neurokinin receptor antagonists
- Miscellaneous:
    - Corticosteroids
    - Benzodiazepines.

SEROTONIN ANTAGONISTS
The drugs are:
- Ondansetron
- Granisetron
- Palonosetron
- Dolasetron.

Actions
- They are very effective antiemetic drugs.
- They block $5HT_3$ receptors at central and peripheral sites.
- They suppress the $5HT_3$ receptors present in area postrema and chemoreceptor trigger zone (CTZ).
- They also inhibit the action of serotonin released from gastric enterochromaffin cells, in response to anticancer drugs.
- Their effect persists even after their disappearance from plasma.
- They can be administered once daily.
- Except palonosetron, all other serotonin antagonists are effective in acute onset emesis but not in delayed onset emesis.
- Palonosetron is long acting so, is effective for delayed onset vomiting following chemotherapy or after radiation.
- They are available as oral and parenteral formulations.

Adverse Effects
- Dizziness, headache
- Diarrhea, constipation.

Uses
- Cancer chemotherapy induced emesis
- Radiation induced emesis
- Hyperemesis during pregnancy
- Postoperative emesis.

DOPAMINE ANTAGONISTS
- Phenothiazines
- Butyrophenones
- Benzamides.

Phenothiazines
They are:
- Chlorpromazine
- Prochlorperazine
- Perphenazine
- Fluphenazine.

Actions
- They act as antiemetic by blocking D_2 receptors in CTZ.
- They have anticholinergic and antihistaminergic property.
- They cause extrapyramidal side effects, hypotension, sedation and anticholinergic side effects.
- They are effective in emesis due to motion sickness.

Butyrophenones
They are:
- Haloperidol
- Droperidol.

Actions
- They inhibit emesis by blocking dopaminergic D_2 receptors.
- They cause extrapyramidal side effects, sedation and hypotension.
- Droperidol causes prolonged QT syndrome.

Benzamides
They are:
- Domperidone

- Metoclopramide

Actions
- They reduce emesis due to anticancer drugs and other drugs such as opioids.
- They are also used to reduce nausea and vomiting associated with GIT motility disorders.

ANTIHISTAMINES
The drugs are:
- Diphenhydramine
- Hydroxyzine
- Cyclizine
- Promethazine

Actions
- They inhibit the H_1 receptors on vestibular afferents in brainstem.
- They are effective in postoperative emesis and in motion sickness.

ANTICHOLINERGICS
Scopolamine
- Scopolamine is used as antiemetic in motion sickness.
- It is a muscarinic antagonist and inhibits the vestibular center.
- It is available as oral, subcutaneous and transdermal formulation.
- It is not effective in chemotherapy induced vomiting.
- It causes dry mouth, drowsiness and blurred vision.
- These adverse effects are minimal with transdermal application.

Other details: See Section II, Chapter 9

Nursing Responsibilities
Patient should be told to wash hands after handling hyoscine transdermal patch.

SUBSTANCE P/NEUROKININ RECEPTOR ANTAGONISTS
The drugs are:
- Aprepitant
- Fosaprepitant.

Actions
- They act by blocking substance P/neurokinin receptors in brain.
- They are effective in acute and delayed phase of chemotherapy induced emesis.

- They are administered one hour before chemotherapy followed by once daily dose on days 2 and 3.
- Fosaprepitant is available as parenteral formulation.

Adverse Effects
- Dizziness, hiccup, diarrhea
- Fatigue, asthenia.

Uses
Cancer chemotherapy induced vomiting.

CANNABINOIDS
The drugs are:
- Dronabinol
- Nabilone.

Dronabinol

Actions
- It is a lipid soluble naturally occurring cannabinoid.
- It is administered orally.
- It undergoes high first pass metabolism.
- It can also stimulate appetite.

Adverse Effects
- Palpitation, hypotension, blood red eyes
- Euphoria, anxiety, nervousness
- Paranoid delusion
- Abstinence syndrome.

Uses
- Prophylaxis for emesis induced by cancer chemotherapy
- AIDS induced anorexia

Nabilone
- It is a synthetic cannabinoid with high lipid solubility.
- It has similar adverse effects of dronabinol.
- The CNS side effects limit its therapeutic efficacy.
- It is used as prophylaxis in cancer chemotherapy induced emesis.

CORTICOSTEROIDS
- Dexamethasone is effective in NSAIDs, radiation and cancer induced emesis.

Antiemetic Drugs

- The possible mechanism is suppression of peritumoral inflammation.
- Dexamethasone inhibits synthesis of prostaglandins.

BENZODIAZEPINES
- Alprazolam and lorazepam are effective by inhibiting anxiety.
- They are effective due to their sedative and amnesic effects.

Therapy of cancer chemotherapy induced emesis
 A. For severe emesis:
   Combination of dexamethasone and palonosetron
 B. For moderate emesis:
   Ondansetron/Dronabinol/Prochlorperazine/Dexamethasone.

Treatment of Motion Sickness

Motion sickness occurs during travel and prophylaxis is very effective.
The drugs are:
- **Anticholinergics:** Scopolamine
- **Antihistamines:** Diphenhydramine, meclizine, cyclizine.

Drugs in Constipation, Diarrhea and Other GIT Conditions

LAXATIVES

The different types of laxatives are:
  A. Bulk forming laxatives
  B. Surfactant laxatives
  C. Stimulant laxatives
  D. Osmotic laxatives

- Water constitutes around 85% of stool volume and contributes to its consistency.
- The net water content in stool is a balance between fluid intake, intestinal secretions and luminal absorption.
- Laxatives cause evacuation of formed fecal material.
- Cathartics result in evacuation of unformed, watery stools.
- Effect of laxative is mild and slow but, effect of cathartic is quick and intense.

Laxatives Act by
- Increasing intraluminal water content
- Reducing intestinal absorption of water
- Stimulating motility.

Bulk Forming Laxatives
They are:
- Methylcellulose
- Psyllium preparations
- Bran
- Calcium polycarbophil

Actions
- Some undergo fermentation and increase the bacterial mass.
- Hence large amounts of water should be taken along with bulk laxatives.
- The others are hydrophilic substances and act by absorbing water.
- They are indigestible and swell up causing mechanical distention of bowel.

- They are mild laxatives and require 1 to 3 days for complete action.
- They soften the stools and also act as lubricants.
- Bran contains more than 40% dietary fiber.
- It increases stool weight.
- Psyllium husk obtained from ispaghula is hydrophilic and increases fecal mass.
- Methylcellulose and polycarbophil ferment poorly but absorb water and increase the intestinal bulk.

Contraindications
Megacolon.

Adverse Effects
- Bloating
- Abdominal colic.

Uses
- Constipation dominant irritable bowel syndrome
- Hemorrhoids
- Ulcerative colitis.

Surfactant Laxatives

They are stool wetting agents and require 1 to 3 days for producing soft stools.
The surfactant laxatives are:
- Docusates
- Poloxamers.

Actions
- They reduce surface tension, promote emulsification and produce soft stools.
- They stimulate intestinal fluid and electrolyte secretion.
- They also inhibit the intestinal absorption of water.
- Docusate sodium and docusate calcium are the two types of docusates.
- They lower surface tension and promote mixture of fatty and aqueous substances.
- They have lower efficacy and are available as capsule, syrup, tablet and liquid formulations.

Adverse Effects
- Flatulence
- Abdominal distention.

Uses
Constipation.

Stimulant Laxatives
The action is nonspecific, affects fluid secretion and alters intestinal motility.
The drugs are:
- Bisacodyl
- Senna
- Cascara
- Castor oil.

Actions
- They induce mild, low grade inflammation in the intestine.
- They increase the intestinal secretion of water and ions.
- They also stimulate the intestinal motility.
- While bisacodyl and senna act on large intestine, castor oil acts on small intestine.

Bisacodyl
- It is available as oral formulation as well as rectal suppository.
- Oral bisacodyl is given at bed time as it requires more than 6 hours for its effect.
- The onset of action of rectal suppository is rapid and it induces evacuation within one hour.
- Rectal suppository can cause proctitis and oral formulation can cause intestinal mucosal irritation.
- It can also result in electrolyte imbalance if given in higher doses.

Anthraquinone Laxatives
- Cascara and senna are derivatives of plants.
- They are stimulant laxatives.
- They act in large intestine.
- So, the onset of action is delayed by 6 to 12 hours.
- They produce soft and semisolid stool.
- They increase the water content of stool.
- Chronic use results in melanosis coli or melanin pigmentation of colon.

Castor Oil
- It is obtained from castor bean called *Ricinus communis*.
- In intestine it breaks down to protein ricin and triglyceride ricinoleic acid.

- Ricinoleic acid stimulates small intestine and causes evacuation within 2 to 6 hours.
- It is an intense cathartic and causes severe water and electrolyte depletion.

Phenolphthalein
- Its actions are similar to bisacodyl.
- It acts locally only in colon.
- It may cause abdominal cramps.
- It is carcinogenic and seldom used now.

Osmotic Laxatives
They draw water into intestinal lumen through their osmotic action. They are:
- Magnesium sulfate
- Magnesium hydroxide
- Magnesium citrate
- Sodium phosphate
- Polyethylene glycol solution
- Lactulose.

Actions
- They are poorly absorbed and act through their osmotic property.
- By drawing water into intestinal lumen, they increase and soften the fecal mass.
- This causes mechanical stretching of the intestine and stimulates peristalsis.
- Absorption of magnesium or sodium ions can result in systemic toxicity.
- Long chain polyethylene glycol (PEG) is poorly absorbed, draws water into intestinal lumen.
- It induces catharsis and is widely used.
- PEG-electrolyte preparations contain isotonic mixture of PEG and sodium or potassium salts.
- This reduces the systemic absorption of electrolytes.
- Lactulose is a synthetic disaccharide that is not broken down by intestinal disaccharidase.

Adverse Effect
Electrolyte depletion

Uses

- Constipation induced by opioids, vincristine
- Idiopathic chronic constipation
- Occasional constipation
- Lactulose in hepatic encephalopathy
- PEG for preparation of bowel prior to surgical, radiological and endoscopic procedures.
- For expulsion of worms
- PEG is also used in poisoning to promote the fecal evacuation of poisons.

AGENTS USED IN CONSTIPATION

Prokinetic Agents in Constipation

They stimulate intestinal motility by interacting with specific receptors.
They are:
- **5HT$_4$ receptor agonist:** Prucalopride
- **Prostanoid EP$_4$ agonist:** Lubiprostone
- **Guanyl cyclase C agonist:** Linaclotide
- **Opioid antagonist:** Methylnaltrexone, alvimopan.

Prucalopride

- It stimulates the descending colon and promotes evacuation of bowel.
- It is used in the treatment of chronic constipation.

Lubiprostone

- It increases intestinal secretion by stimulating intestinal chloride channels.
- It is used in chronic constipation and in constipation dominant irritable bowel syndrome (IBS-C).

Linaclotide

- It stimulates guanyl cyclase activity and increases intestinal secretion as well as motility.
- It is effective in chronic constipation and constipation dominant irritable bowel syndrome (IBS-C).

Opioid Induced Constipation

The opioid antagonists used in the management of opioid induced constipation are:
- Methylnaltrexone
- Alvimopan.

Drugs in Constipation, Diarrhea and Other GIT Conditions

Actions
- Opioids cause constipation when given as analgesic in cancer pain.
- Laxatives act nonspecifically and are ineffective in opioid induced constipation.
- Peripherally acting opioid antagonists are effective.

Methylnaltrexone
- It is a μ receptor antagonist and effective in opioid induced constipation in cancer patients.
- It does not interfere with opioid induced analgesia.

Alvimopan
- Alvimopan is a peripherally acting μ receptor antagonist that does not compromise opioid induced analgesia.
- Off-label use of alvimopan is opioid induced constipation.

Opioid induced postoperative paralytic ileus
- It occurs during the postoperative period within 1 to 3 days after surgery.
- The inhibitory action of μ opioid receptors along with local inflammation is responsible for this condition.

The drugs used are:
- Alvimopan
- Methylnaltrexone
- Dexpanthenol.

Dexpanthenol
- It is a congener of pantothenic acid.
- Pantothenic acid is a precursor of coenzyme A, the cofactor in the synthesis of acetylcholine.
- Dexpanthenol increases the synthesis of acetylcholine.
- Thereby, it promotes intestinal motility.
- It is given in immediate postoperative period to reduce the occurrence of paralytic ileus.
- Adverse effects are local irritation and mild hypotension.

Enema
Enema causes distention of bowel and induces the evacuation reflex.

Glycerin
- It is a hygroscopic and lubricating agent.
- It causes water retention that stimulates peristalsis.
- As a rectal suppository, it can cause burning sensation and bleeding.

Nursing Responsibilities
- Patient should be informed to refrain from taking laxatives frequently.
- Instruct the patient to take bulk forming laxatives or surfactant laxatives with plenty of water.
- Patient should be asked to swallow bisacodyl tablets as such.
- Patient should be told not to take castor oil at bed time.

ANTIDIARRHEAL AGENTS
- Alteration of intestinal motility and increased secretions into intestinal lumen increase net stool volume and cause diarrhea.
- To prevent dehydration and electrolyte imbalance, oral rehydration fluids should be given.
- Nonspecific agents reduce motility of bowel.
- Therefore, they should be avoided in infective diarrhea as they reduce the clearance of infective organisms.
- Besides they can also result in toxic megacolon.

The drugs used in diarrhea are:
 I. Hygroscopic, bulk forming agents
 II. Bile acid sequestrants
 III. Colloidal bismuth subsalicylate
 IV. Probiotics
 V. Opioids
 VII. Enkephalin inhibitors
 VII. Octreotide and somatostatin
 VIII. Alpha adrenergic agonists.

Hygroscopic, Bulk Forming Agents
They are:
- Carboxymethylcellulose
- Calcium polycarbophil
- Pectin-Kaolin mixture
- Attapulgite

Actions
- These compounds absorb water, modify stool texture and viscosity.
- These agents can also bind to bacterial toxins, drugs, nutrients and bile salts.
- They are effective in mild chronic diarrhea and in diarrhea associated with IBS.

Drugs in Constipation, Diarrhea and Other GIT Conditions

- Calcium polycarbophil absorbs water 60 times its weight.
- Kaolin is hydrated aluminium silicate and pectin is a plant polysaccharide.
- Pectin is an extract of inner portion of citrus fruits.
- Mixture of pectin kaolin is an effective antidiarrheal agent.
- Attapulgite is magnesium aluminum disilicate.
- It absorbs water 8 times more than its weight.

Bile Acid Sequestrants

They are:
- Cholestyramine
- Colestipol
- Colesevalam

Actions

- These agents bind to bile salts and bacterial toxins.
- Ileal resection interferes with enterohepatic circulation of bile salts which accumulate in colon.
- The bile salts induce diarrhea by increasing water and electrolyte secretion.
- Cholestyramine is a frequently used bile acid sequestrant.
- It is effective in bile salt induced diarrhea in patients who have undergone distal ileal resection.
- In patients with extensive ileal resection, it aggravates diarrhea.
- It is effective in mild antibiotic induced diarrhea and diarrhea due to *Clostridium difficile*.
- Generally, it is not indicated in infective diarrhea.
- Cholestyramine is also effective in pruritus due to biliary obstruction.

Colloidal Bismuth Subsalicylate

Actions

- Bismuth has anti-inflammatory, antimicrobial and antisecretory property.
- It is also effective in reducing nausea and abdominal cramps.
- It combines with *Vibrio cholerae* and *E.coli* organisms.
- It is an astringent and absorbent.
- It is not absorbed and binds to coadministered antibiotics and other anti-infective agents.

Adverse Effects
- Black tarry stools
- Black tongue
- Aggravation of Reye's syndrome.

Uses:
- Traveler's diarrhea
- Acute gastroenteritis
- Anti *H.pylori* regimen in peptic ulcer

Other details: See Section IX, Chapter 50

Probiotics
- Antibiotics alter the microbial flora of gut resulting in antibiotic induced diarrhea.
- Probiotics are mixture of beneficial lyophilized bacteria.
- They are safe and are given orally.
- Probiotics are noninfective and reverse the altered balance.
- They are also effective in infective diarrhea.

Opioids
The opioids used as antidiarrheal agents are:
- Loperamide
- Diphenoxylate
- Difenoxin.

Loperamide
Actions
- It has antisecretory activity and increases the tone of anal sphincter.
- It is orally active, more potent antidiarrheal agent than morphine and it does not accumulate in CNS.
- Hence, it does not cause addiction and is also devoid of other CNS side effects of opioids.
- However drug overdose can increase absorption and subsequent CNS mediated side effects.

Adverse Effect
Toxic megacolon

Uses
- Traveler's diarrhea
- Chronic, nonspecific diarrhea

Drugs in Constipation, Diarrhea and Other GIT Conditions

Diphenoxylate and Difenoxin
Actions
- Diphenoxylate is converted to its active metabolite difenoxin.
- Both the drug and its metabolite are effective in diarrhea.
- Diphenoxylate and difenoxin are extensively absorbed.
- So, they cause euphoria and other CNS side effects.
- Prolonged use in children can cause drug dependence.

Adverse Effects
- Toxic megacolon
- Constipation
- Anticholinergic side effects such as dry mouth, blurred vision, etc.

Use
Traveler's diarrhea

Enkephalinase Inhibitor
- Enkephalin, the endogenous opioid inhibits intestinal secretion.
- Enkephalinase inhibitor, racecadotril, promotes the activity of enkephalins.
- So, it is used in diarrhea.
- It does not interfere with gastrointestinal motility.

Octreotide and Somatostatin
Actions
- Somatostatin and its analog octreotide are effective in secretory diarrhea.
- They inhibit the secretion of serotonin.
- They also inhibit secretion of incretins.
- Octreotide can be administered either SC or IV.
- A long acting IM preparation of octreotide can be administered once a month.

Adverse Effects
- Nausea, bloating
- Pain at site of injection
- Gallstones
- Hypo or hyperglycemia.

Uses
- Secretory diarrhea induced by carcinoid tumor and adenomas
- Secretory diarrhea associated with HIV infection, cancer chemotherapy and diabetes mellitus

- Patients with dumping syndrome after gastric surgery or pyloroplasty.

Other details: See Section VIII, Chapter 41

α_2 Adrenergic Agonist

Actions
- α_2 adrenergic agonist clonidine promotes absorption and reduces intestinal secretion of fluid and electrolytes.
- Clonidine can be administered orally.

Adverse Effects
- Hypotension, fatigue
- Sedation, depression.

Uses
- Chronic diarrhea in diabetics
- Diarrhea due to opiate withdrawal.

Rehydration
- Oral and intravenous routes of administration are employed for rehydration.
- Severe dehydration necessitates administration of intravenous fluid.
- Otherwise, it can cause hypotension and shock.
- Electrolyte solution containing sodium, potassium, chloride and bicarbonate ions with 5% dextrose is recommended.
- An alternate is the ringer-lactate solution.
- Oral rehydration is given if fluid loss is minimal.
- Composition of oral rehydration fluid (ORS) is:
    - **Sodium chloride:** 2.6g
    - **Potassium chloride:** 1.5g
    - **Trisodium citrate:** 2.9g
    - **Glucose:** 13.5g
    - **Water:** 1 liter
- Since absorption of sodium and chloride is linked to glucose uptake in enterocytes, ORS which is the mixture of these substances promote absorption of water.
- ORS and IV fluids restore hydration, electrolyte balance and maintain pH.

Treatment of Diarrhea

Bacterial Diarrhea
- *Shigella species*: Norfloxacin, ciprofloxacin, ampicillin
- *Salmonella species*: Fluoroquinolones, cotrimoxazole, ceftriaxone
- *E.coli*: Fluoroquinolones, cotrimoxazole
- *Vibrio cholerae*: Doxycycline, fluoroquinolones
- *Clostridium difficile*: Metronidazole
- *Campylobacter jejuni*: Azithromycin

Protozoal Diarrhea
- *E.histolytica*: Metronidazole
- *Cyclospora species*: Cotrimoxazole
- *Cryptosporidium species*: Azithromycin

Traveler's Diarrhea
Rifaximin, the non-absorbable derivative of rifampin.

Nursing responsibilities:
- Patients having diarrhea should be instructed to drink oral rehydration mixture frequently or after each bout of diarrhea for adequate rehydration.
- They should be advised to take rice gruel, plain toasted bread, ripe banana and cooked apple.
- Patients should be told to avoid milk and milk products.

IRRITABLE BOWEL SYNDROME
- It is characterized by altered bowel movement and severe abdominal pain.
- There is significant disturbance to both sensory and visceral motor function.
- It is also called as 'motility disorder' as it causes constipation or diarrhea or both.
- The intense abdominal pain is mainly due to visceral hyperresponsiveness and hypersensitivity.
- IBS can be either constipation dominant or diarrhea dominant type.
- Pain is associated with altered stool consistency and evacuation reduces bowel pain.
- Treatment of IBS is nonspecific and symptomatic.

Nonspecific Drugs
- Tricyclic antidepressant is effective in reducing the chronic 'functional' visceral pain.
- Selective serotonin reuptake inhibitor (SSRI) reduces the functional constipation.
- The antispasmodic effect of the anticholinergic drug dicyclomine reduces the pain and fecal urgency.
- Anticholinergic agents such as cimetropium, glycopyrrolate and methscopolamine are also effective.
- Since they do not cross blood-brain barrier (BBB), they do not cause sedation or drowsiness.
- α_2 agonist clonidine reduces pain due to intestinal distention.
- Serotonin agonists such as buspirone, sumatriptan and somatostatin analog octreotide also reduce pain due to intestinal distention.
- Fedotozine, a selective opioid antagonist is useful in IBS with functional dyspepsia.
- Otilonium bromide blocks neurokinin and cholinergic receptors as well as calcium channels.
- Mebeverine HCl blocks potassium, sodium and calcium channels.

Specific Drugs
They are:
- Alosetron
- Tegaserod

Alosetron
- It is a serotonin antagonist.
- It reduces colonic transit time and increases fluid and electrolyte absorption.
- It reduces the visceral pain.
- It reduces fecal urgency and frequency.
- It is indicated only in women with 'diarrhea dominant IBS'.
- It can cause life-threatening ischemic colitis.

Tegaserod
- It is effective in 'constipation dominant IBS' in women.
- It is a serotonin agonist.
- It increases the colonic transit time.
- It reduces visceral pain and increases intestinal secretions.
- It promotes evacuation of bowel.
- It causes diarrhea resulting in dehydration and hypotension.

DRUGS IN INFLAMMATORY BOWEL DISEASE
- The two forms of inflammatory bowel disease are ulcerative colitis and Crohn's disease.
- Abdominal cramps and diarrhea occur in these conditions.
- Crohn's disease is transmural inflammation of terminal ileum.
- Ulcerative colitis is inflammation of colon and rectum.

The drugs used are:
- 5-aminosalicylates
- Glucocorticoids
- Immunosuppressants
- Monoclonal antibodies.

5-aminosalicylates
The drugs under this group are:
- Sulfasalazine
- Mesalamine
- Olsalazine
- Balsalazide

Actions
- They inhibit the production of interleukin and tumor necrosis factor-α (TNF-α).
- They promote free radical scavenging.

Sulfasalazine
- It is broken down by intestinal bacteria into sulfapyridine and 5-aminosalicylic acid (5-ASA).
- 5-ASA suppresses the inflammation.
- It is effective in mild to moderate ulcerative colitis.
- The adverse effects of sulfasalazine are mainly due to the sulfapyridine component.
- It causes nausea, fever, rash, Stevens-Johnson syndrome and hemolytic anemia.

Mesalamine
- It is 5-ASA and used for mild to moderate inflammatory bowel disease.
- Delayed release formulation of mesalamine acts throughout the length of small intestine and colon.
- pH sensitive mesalamine acts mainly in ileum and colon.
- It can be administered as retention enema or rectal suppository for psoriasis.

- The most frequent side effects are headache, dyspepsia and skin rash.

Olsalazine
- It contains two molecules of ASA.
- It is used for maintenance therapy of ulcerative colitis.
- It causes watery diarrhea, abdominal pain, rash, and joint pain.

Balsalazide
- It is used for mild to moderate ulcerative colitis.
- Intestinal bacteria causes breakdown of balsalazide into 5-ASA.
- It causes headache, abdominal pain and diarrhea.

Glucocorticoids
- Glucocorticoids are effective due to their anti-inflammatory property.
- Oral prednisolone is preferred in moderate to severe condition.
- Methyl prednisolone and hydrocortisone are used for intravenous therapy.
- Hydrocortisone is also available as retention enema and as foam suspension for proctitis.
- Budesonide is available as enteric coated formulation.
- Topical enema and suppository budesonide are effective in colitis of left side colon.
- Prolonged use causes severe side effects such as sepsis, infection due to cytomegalovirus and *Clostridium difficile*.
- Steroids are used for short-term remission.

Immunosuppressants
- Azathioprine, 6-mercaptopurine, methotrexate, cyclosporine are the immunosuppressants used.
- They are reserve drugs and the maximum benefit is seen after few weeks.
- 6-mercaptopurine, methotrexate and azathioprine cause bone marrow depression and cholestatic hepatitis.
- Cyclosporine causes renal toxicity and neurotoxicity.

Monoclonal Antibodies
- Infliximab, adalimumab, certolizumab and etanercept are used.
- They bind with TNF-α and inactivate it.
- Infliximab is very effective in refractory ulcerative colitis and Crohn's disease.

- It causes frequent respiratory infection, tuberculosis and other granulomatous infection.
- Natalizumab inhibits extravasation of lymphocytes and should never be combined with other immunomodulators.
- It can cause progressive multifocal leukoencephalopathy.

PROKINETIC AGENTS

These drugs increase the gastrointestinal tone and motility. The drugs are classified as:
- Dopamine antagonists
- Serotonin agonists
- Motilides
- Miscellaneous agents.

Dopamine Antagonists

They are:
- Metoclopramide
- Domperidone.

Metoclopramide

Actions
- Metoclopramide blocks dopamine (D_2), serotonin ($5HT_3$) and muscarinic receptors.
- It is also a serotonin receptor ($5HT_4$) agonist.
- It acts on upper GIT mainly.
- It increases the tone of lower esophageal sphincter.
- It stimulates contraction of gastric antrum and small intestine.
- Hence, it is a prokinetic agent.
- It inhibits vomiting by blocking the dopamine receptors in chemoreceptor trigger zone (CTZ).
- Oral formulation should be administered on an empty stomach.
- It is also available as parenteral administration for IM and IV use.

Adverse Effects
- Extrapyramidal symptoms such as dystonia especially in children
- Galactorrhea.

Uses
- Gastroparesis
- Postoperative ileus
- Persistent hiccup
- Nausea and vomiting due to GIT motility disorders

- Emesis due to cancer chemotherapy
- Symptomatic therapy of GERD.

Domperidone
- Domperidone blocks only the dopamine receptors in CTZ.
- It has the modest prokinetic action.
- It increases the upper GIT contractions.
- It does not cross the BBB.
- It does not result in extrapyramidal side effects.

Serotonin Agonists
They are:
- Cisapride
- Mosapride
- Itopride
- Prucalopride.

Cisapride, Mosapride and Itopride
- They increase the gastrointestinal motility by stimulating serotonin ($5HT_4$) receptors.
- They are effective in GERD and gastroparesis.
- Cisapride can prolong QT interval and can cause cardiac arrhythmias.
- This risk is minimal with its analog mosapride and itopride.

Prucalopride
- It is also a serotonin ($5HT_4$) agonist.
- In addition, it promotes cholinergic activity.
- It increases colonic transit time.
- It does not interfere with gastric emptying time.
- It is used in chronic idiopathic constipation in women.

Motilides
- **Macrolide antibiotic:** Erythromycin, clarithromycin.
- **Other motilides:** Mitemcinal.

Macrolide Antibiotics
- Macrolide antibiotic erythromycin stimulates intestinal motilin and promotes intestinal movements.
- By facilitating cholinergic activity, it promotes intestinal motility.
- It can be used in hypomotility associated with diabetic gastroparesis, ileus and scleroderma.

- It can cause bacterial resistance and pseudomembranous colitis.
- Clarithromycin causes minimal stimulation of motilin.

Other Motilides
- Mitemcinal is a macrolide non-antibiotic and stimulates intestinal motility.
- It is used in diabetic gastroparesis.

Miscellaneous Agents

Dexloxiglumide
- It is a cholecystokinin receptor antagonist.
- It promotes gastric emptying.
- It is used in gastroparesis and in constipation dominant IBS.

Sincalide
- It increases intestinal motility.
- It is given intravenously.
- It also stimulates pancreas and gallbladder.
- It is used during diagnostic testing of small intestine, for accelerating transit of barium meal.
- It causes nausea, abdominal pain, dizziness, and gallstones.

DRUGS USED IN PANCREATITIS AND STEATORRHEA
- Chronic pancreatitis causes pain and reduced exocrine secretion of pancreas.
- Functional loss results in steatorrhea or fat malabsorption and protein malabsorption.
- Deficiency of trypsin stimulates cholecystokinin release which causes pain.
- Symptomatic treatment is given for the management of malabsorption and relief of pain.
- Pancreatin and pancrelipase are the two pancreatic enzyme preparations available for treatment.
- They should be given before food.
- Excess administration of pancrelipase causes fibrosing colonopathy.

GALLSTONE DISSOLVING DRUGS
- Bile acids reduce cholesterol synthesis, increase cholesterol excretion and facilitate absorption of lipids and fat soluble vitamins.

- The bile acids chenodeoxycholic acid and ursodeoxycholic acid are used.
- They decrease biliary lipid secretion and reduce cholesterol content of bile.
- They undergo enterohepatic recirculation.
- In addition, ursodeoxycholic acid has cytoprotective effect on liver.
- Chenodeoxycholic acid is more hepatotoxic than ursodeoxycholic acid.

PRIMARY BILIARY CIRRHOSIS
- Primary biliary cirrhosis is a progressive liver disease frequently occurring in women.
- The bile acid ursodeoxycholic acid is used in this condition.
- It reduces the concentration of primary bile acid.
- It is effective in early, primary biliary cirrhosis.
- It also exerts additional cytoprotective effect on hepatocytes.

Anti-Flatulence Agent
Simethicone
- It is an antifoaming agent and forms a layer over bubbles collapsing them.
- It is available as chewable tablets and many other oral formulations.
- It is also combined with many antacid preparations.
- It is nontoxic, insoluble and so not absorbed from GIT.

SECTION X

Respiratory System

- Pharmacotherapy of Bronchial Asthma
- COPD, Mucolytics, Expectorants and Treatment of Cough

CHAPTER 53

Pharmacotherapy of Bronchial Asthma

Bronchial asthma is characterized by hyperresponsiveness and inflammation of airways.

The drugs are classified as:
- β_2 adrenergic agonists
- Methylxanthines
- Corticosteroids
- Leukotriene antagonists
- Anticholinergic drugs
- Monoclonal antibody
- Mast cell stabilizer.

β_2 ADRENERGIC AGONISTS

Actions
- They are the first line drugs in bronchial asthma.
- They are the most effective bronchodilators.
- They are selective agents with minimal side effects.
- They act on β_2 receptors and cause bronchodilatation.
- They also act indirectly by inhibiting histamine release from mast cells.
- They are functional antagonists and reverse the bronchoconstriction.
- They reduce the occurrence of bronchial mucosal edema.
- They enhance the mucociliary clearance.
- Further, they inhibit cholinergic mediated bronchoconstriction.
- They do not inhibit the chronic inflammation of bronchial musculature.

Short-acting β_2 Agonists
They are:
- Albuterol
- Levalbuterol
- Bambuterol.

Actions
- They have rapid onset of action if administered through inhalational route.
- The duration of action is around 3 to 4 hours.
- Inhalational route of administration minimizes the systemic side effects.
- These drugs are indicated 'as required' and not daily.
- They are very effective in severe acute asthma.
- Oral slow release preparations of albuterol and bambuterol are effective in nocturnal asthma.
- Bambuterol is a prodrug of terbutaline.

Long-acting β_2 Agonists (LABA)
They are:
- Salmeterol
- Formoterol
- Arformoterol

Actions
- The duration of action is more than 12 hours.
- The onset of action of formoterol is quick.
- Salmeterol has slow onset of action.
- LABA does not suppress the underlying airway inflammation.
- Hence, LABA should always be combined with inhalational corticosteroids.
- The combination is more effective due to the anti-inflammatory action of corticosteroids.

Adverse Effects
- Tremor, palpitation, tachycardia
- Hypokalemia
- Tolerance

Uses
- Bronchial asthma
- Chronic obstructive pulmonary disease (COPD)

METHYLXANTHINES
The drug are:
- Theophylline
- Aminophylline

- Enprofylline
- Doxofylline

Theophylline

Actions

- It is a second line drug in the treatment of bronchial asthma.
- It is a nonselective phosphodiesterase (PDE) inhibitor.
- Inhibition of PDE increases cellular cyclic adenosine monophospate (cAMP) and cyclic guanosine monophosphate (cGMP) level.
- It causes bronchodilatation, myocardial contraction, diuresis, and central nervous system (CNS) stimulation.
- It inhibits the release of histamine and leukotriene.
- It stimulates apoptosis of eosinophils and neutrophils.
- Further, it exerts anti-inflammatory activity.
- It is a drug of low therapeutic index.
- The sustained release oral preparations are effective in nocturnal asthma.
- Anhydrous theophylline is not administered through intravenous route as it has poor solubility.

Adverse Effects

- Nausea, vomiting
- Headache, seizures, restlessness
- Cardiac arrhythmia

Aminophylline

- Aminophylline (theophylline-ethylenediamine) is water soluble and can be given through intravenous route.
- It is an irritant and cannot be given through intramuscular route.

Doxofylline

Doxofylline is long-acting and is less toxic.

Enprofylline

- It is a derivative of theophylline.
- It inhibits phosphodiesterase enzyme.
- It is more potent and less toxic.

Common Uses of Methylxanthines

- Bronchial asthma
- COPD

CORTICOSTEROIDS

The inhalational steroids are:
- Beclomethasone dipropionate
- Triamcinolone acetonide
- Fluticasone
- Budesonide
- Mometasone
- Ciclesonide

Actions

- Since asthma is a chronic inflammatory condition, corticosteroids are very effective.
- Inhalational corticosteroids are preferred as the incidence of side effects is minimal.
- They inhibit the production of inflammatory cytokines.
- They inhibit the release of granulocyte-macrophage stimulating factor produced by mast cells, lymphocytes and macrophages.
- By inhibiting inflammation and edema, they reduce airway hyperresponsiveness.
- They also improve the lung function.
- Maximum therapeutic benefit occurs only after prolonged administration.
- The symptoms recur on discontinuation of steroids.
- They do not cure the underlying disease.
- They also improve the responsiveness to β_2 adrenergic agonists.
- A fraction of inhaled steroids and the fraction deposited on oropharynx are absorbed into systemic circulation.
- Metered delivery inhaler (MDI) of steroid reduces the systemic absorption.
- Inhaled steroids with β_2 agonist are first line therapy in chronic asthma.
- Inhaled steroids are less effective in COPD.
- However, oral steroids are more effective in acute flares of COPD.
- Intravenous hydrocortisone is effective in acute asthma as it has rapid onset of action.
- Oral prednisolone is equally effective as intravenous hydrocortisone.
- Adverse effects are high after prolonged administration of oral steroid and minimal after inhalational steroid.

- Oral steroid should be withdrawn gradually after prolonged therapy.

Adverse Effects
Inhalational Steroids Cause
- Dermal thinning, impaired growth
- Dysphonia, atrophy of vocal cord
- Cough, increased capillary fragility
- Respiratory infection.

Oral Steroids Cause
- Weight gain, edema
- Hypertension, diabetes mellitus
- Osteoporosis, peptic ulcer
- Cataract and psychosis.

Uses
- Bronchial asthma
- Sarcoidosis
- Pulmonary eosinophilic syndrome
- Interstitial lung disease.

Other details: See Section VIII, Chapter 43

ANTICHOLINERGIC DRUGS
The anticholinergic drugs effective in bronchial asthma are:
- Ipratropium bromide
- Tiotropium bromide.

Actions
- They block muscarinic cholinergic receptors of bronchial smooth muscle.
- They inhibit cholinergic receptor mediated bronchoconstriction.
- They can be administered through inhalational route.
- Tiotropium bromide has longer duration of action.
- These agents are given in addition to β_2 agonist in severe uncontrolled bronchial asthma.
- They are more effective in COPD than in bronchial asthma.

Adverse Effects
- Tiotropium causes dryness of throat and rarely urinary retention
- Inhaled ipratropium bromide causes bitter taste

- Nebulized ipratropium bromide causes glaucoma
- Ipratropium also causes paradoxical bronchoconstriction.

LEUKOTRIENE ANTAGONIST
They are:
- Zileuton
- Zafirlukast
- Montelukast
- Pranlukast.

Actions
- They inhibit leukotriene mediated bronchoconstriction and mucus secretion.
- They suppress bronchoconstriction mediated by allergens, aspirin, cold air or exercise.
- They cause bronchodilatation and improve the lung function.
- They are not the first line therapy.
- They are only 'add on' therapy in bronchial asthma.
- They can be administered through oral route.

Adverse Effects
- Hepatotoxicity
- Churg-Strauss syndrome (vasculitis).

Uses
- Bronchial asthma
- Allergic rhinitis.

MONOCLONAL ANTIBODY
Actions
- Omalizumab is the monoclonal antibody used in bronchial asthma.
- It is a humanized monoclonal antibody.
- It prevents binding of immunoglobulin E (IgE) to mast cells and basophils.
- Thereby it prevents degranulation of mast cells.
- Further, it prevents IgE binding to lymphocytes, macrophages and eosinophils.
- It also reduces the level of circulating IgE.
- It can be given to patients sensitive to allergens.

- It is costly.
- It is given through subcutaneous route.
- It is an additional agent to inhalational corticosteroid in severe asthma.

Adverse Effect
Rare anaphylaxis

Uses
- Bronchial asthma
- Allergic rhinitis.

MAST CELL STABILIZER
They are:
- Cromolyn sodium (sodium cromoglycate)
- Nedocromil sodium.

Actions
- They are mast cell stabilizers.
- They prevent the release of histamine from mast cells.
- They are effective as prophylactic agents.
- They also inhibit chemotaxis of inflammatory cells.
- They are available as metered dose formulation and as nasal spray.

Adverse Effects
- Mild headache
- Bronchospasm
- Throat irritation, nasal congestion, dizziness

Use
Prophylaxis in bronchial asthma.

NURSING RESPONSIBILITIES IN STATUS ASTHMATICUS
- Patients with bronchial asthma should be advised to stop smoking, to avoid pets, to eradicate house dust, mite and molds.
- Since smoke, pollen and household sprays exacerbates asthma, patients should be advised to avoid exposure to these factors.
- They should also be advised to maintain dust free environment at home, to avoid carpets and excessive humidity.

THERAPY OF STATUS ASTHMATICUS
- It is an acute severe exacerbation of asthma.
- Since it is a life-threatening condition, treatment should be started immediately.

Treatment
- High flow oxygen to prevent asphyxia.
- Patient should be advised to inhale β_2 agonists like salbutamol through MDI or nebulizers frequently.
- Intravenous hydrocortisone if the response is inadequate.
- Ipratropium bromide 0.5 mg inhalation or continuous administration.
- Albuterol infusion 5 µg/min and increased up to 10 to 20 µg/min.

Nursing Responsibilities
- Oxygen should be started immediately to prevent asphyxia which is a common cause of death.
- Patient should be hospitalised depending upon the severity of airflow obstruction, duration of asthma, severity of prior exacerbations, and arterial blood gas (ABG) results.

CHAPTER 54: COPD, Mucolytics, Expectorants and Treatment of Cough

CHRONIC OBSTRUCTIVE PULMONARY DISEASE (COPD)
- It is characterized by airflow obstruction due to chronic bronchitis and emphysema.
- The condition is progressive and usually irreversible.
- Pulmonary function test will show reduced midexpiratory flow rate.
- Smoking aggravates the condition.
- Aim of the therapy is to reduce bronchoconstriction and to prevent secondary infection.

Treatment
- Triggering factors such as smoking should be avoided.
- First line drugs are ipratropium bromide or tiotropium bromide
- Short acting or long acting β_2 agonist
- Oral corticosteroid
- Oral theophylline
- Antibiotics
- Mucolytic/expectorant.

MUCOLYTICS
The mucolytics are:
- N-acetylcysteine
- Carbocysteine
- Methylcysteine
- Erdosteine
- Bromhexine
- Dornase alfa

Actions
- They reduce the viscosity of sputum.
- They also have antioxidant property.
- They reduce airway inflammation.

N-acetylcysteine

Actions
- It breaks down the disulfide bridges that bind glycoproteins to secretory immunoglobulin A (IgA).
- Thereby, it makes sputum less viscid.
- It is given as nebulizer.
- Its analog carbocysteine also acts as a mucolytic but should not be given in peptic ulcer patients.

Adverse Effects
- Bronchospasm
- Nausea, vomiting.

Uses
- Cystic fibrosis
- Chronic bronchitis
- Paracetamol poisoning.

Bromhexine

Actions
- It is obtained from the alkaloid vasika.
- It depolymerizes mucopolysaccharides.
- It is a potent mucolytic.
- Its metabolite ambroxol is more effective.

Adverse Effects
- Rhinorrhea, lacrimation
- Nausea, gastric irritation.

Use
Chronic bronchitis.

Dornase-α
- It is a deoxyribonuclease that breaks down the DNA.
- It reduces the viscosity of mucus in cystic fibrosis.

EXPECTORANTS
- They increase the clearance of mucus.
- Guaifenesin increases clearance of mucus through a reflex mechanism.
- Eucalyptus oil and anise oil increase secretion by stimulating bronchial cells directly.
- Ammonium chloride increases bronchial secretion but can cause gastritis and acidosis.

Nursing Responsibilities
- Mucolytics can aggravate cough as they cause bronchospasm. Hence, they should be avoided in patients with bronchial asthma.
- Patient should be informed about the rotten egg smell of N-acetylcysteine.

DRUGS IN THE TREATMENT OF COUGH (ANTITUSSIVES)
Antitussives act either peripherally or centrally. They are not indicated in chronic bronchitis or bronchial asthma.

Centrally Acting Antitussives
- Codeine
- Pholcodine
- Noscapine
- Dextromethorphan.

Actions
- Codeine and pholcodine are opioid antitussives.
- They act by inhibiting cough center by stimulating the central opioid receptors.
- They cause addiction, respiratory suppression and postural hypotension.
- Codeine also causes constipation and drowsiness.
- Pholcodine is long acting and more potent than codeine and causes minimal constipation.
- Dextromethorphan is an antagonist of N-methyl-D-aspartate (NMDA) receptors.
- At high doses it can cause addiction and hallucination.
- Noscapine is an opioid but does not have analgesic activity.
- It is a cough suppressant and does not cause addiction.

Peripherally Acting Antitussives
- Benzonatate
- Moguisteine

Actions
- Benzonatate is a local anaesthetic and inhibits the stretch receptors of lungs, pleura and respiratory passages.
- It suppresses cough reflex by inhibiting the stretch receptors.
- Adverse effects are dizziness, allergy, dysphagia, seizure, and cardiac arrest.
- Moguisteine has moderate antitussive activity.

SECTION XI

Chemotherapy

- Introduction to Chemotherapeutic Agents
- Sulfonamides, Trimethoprim and Co-trimoxazole
- Quinolones
- Beta-Lactam Antibiotics
- Aminoglycosides
- Broad Spectrum Antibiotics
- Macrolides and Ketolides
- Miscellaneous Antibiotics
- Urinary Antiseptics and Chemotherapy of Urinary Tract Infection
- Chemotherapy of Sexually Transmitted Diseases
- Chemotherapy of Tuberculosis
- Chemotherapy of Leprosy
- Chemotherapy of Worm Infestation
- Chemotherapy of Filariasis
- Antimalarial Drugs
- Chemotherapy of Amebiasis
- Chemotherapy of Other Protozoal Infection
- Chemotherapy of Fungal Infection
- Anti Non-retroviral Agents
- HIV Infection and Antiretroviral Agents
- Anticancer Drugs
- Immunosuppressants

CHAPTER 55: Introduction to Chemotherapeutic Agents

- The plasma membrane lies beneath the cell wall in gram positive bacteria.
- In Gram-negative bacteria cell wall, cytoplasmic membrane and outer membrane are present.
- Antimicrobials are classified according to their mechanism of action.
- **Interfering with bacterial cell wall synthesis:** Penicillins, cephalosporins, vancomycin, bacitracin, cycloserine
- **Selective inhibition of bacterial enzymes:** Sulfonamides
- **Inhibition of bacterial protein synthesis:**
  - **Bactericidal inhibitors:** Aminoglycosides
  - **Bacterostatic inhibitors:** Tetracyclines, glycylcyclines, chloramphenicol, macrolides, linezolid, clindamycin
- **Disruption of cell membrane:** Amphotericin B, ketoconazole, daptomycin, polymyxin, colistin, bacitracin
- **Interference with bacterial DNA function:** Metronidazole, rifampin
- **Inhibition of DNA gyrase:** Fluoroquinolones
- **Antimetabolites:** Trimethoprim, sulfonamides, flucytosine
- **Suppression of viral replication:**
  - **Neuraminidase inhibitors:** Oseltamivir, zanamivir
  - **DNA polymerase enzyme inhibitors:** Acyclovir, ganciclovir
  - **Reverse transcriptase enzyme inhibitors:** Zidovudine, lamivudine
  - **Protease inhibitors:** Ritonavir, saquinavir
  - **Fusion inhibitors:** Enfuvirtide.

DEVELOPMENT OF RESISTANCE TO ANTIMICROBIAL DRUGS

- **Excessive synthesis of inactivating enzymes:** Penicillinase producing organism is resistant to penicillin
- **Reduced uptake of drugs:** Tetracyclines
- **Increased exit from cells:** Streptomycin

- **Increased synthesis of substances that antagonize the action of drugs:** Increased para amino benzoic acid (PABA) synthesis inhibits the action of sulfonamides
- **Development of altered target sites:** Fluoroquinolones
- **Genetic modifications:**
    - **Chromosomal mutations:** Methicillin resistant *Staphylococcus aureus* (MRSA)
    - Plasmid mediated mutant transfer through conjugation, transduction, transformation, integrons, and transposon.

Suprainfection
- It develops during the course of treatment of primary infection.
- It is due to suppression of normal protective flora.
- It is resistant to drugs and is difficult to treat.
- Candidiasis following therapy of tetracyclines is a suprainfection.

Prevention of Drug Resistance
- A wiser use of antibiotics which are target specific can prevent drug resistance.
- The culture and sensitivity test helps in the selection of antibiotics.
- Besides, site and type of infection determines the selection of antibiotics.
- Premature discontinuation of antibiotics should be prevented.
- Mixed infection may require more than one antibiotic.

Disadvantages of Antibiotic Combinations
- Higher toxicity
- Allergic reaction
- Suprainfection
- Drug resistance
- Higher cost of therapy

Prophylactic Use of Antimicrobial Drugs
- Prophylactic antibiotics are required in the following conditions:
    - Before an elective surgery to prevent wound infection.
    - Post-exposure prophylaxis in influenza, meningococcal meningitis and exposure to sexually transmitted disease (STD)
    - Febrile neutropenia
    - Patients requiring prosthetic heart valve with high-risk of bacterial endocarditis

- Before dental procedures
- Preemptive therapy to prevent cytomegalovirus infection after stem cell and organ transplantation.

Antibiotic Misuse

Antibiotics misuse in the following conditions results in bacterial resistance:
- Pyrexia of unknown origin
- Untreatable infection
- Inadequate dose and abrupt discontinuation of antibiotics
- Presence of pus or necrotic tissue
- Conditions such as common cold and bronchitis.

Sulfonamides, Trimethoprim and Co-trimoxazole

SULFONAMIDES
- **Short-acting:** Sulfadiazine, sulfisoxazole
- **Intermediate acting:** Sulfamethoxazole
- **Long-acting:** Sulfadoxine
- **Poorly absorbed and locally acting in bowel:** Sulfasalazine
- **Topically used:** Sulfacetamide, silver sulfadiazine, mafenide

Common Properties of Sulfonamides
- They are structural analogs of para-aminobenzoic acid (PABA).
- They are bacterostatic agents.
- They inhibit many Gram-positive and Gram-negative organisms.
- They are competitive inhibitors of the bacterial enzyme dihydropteroate synthase.
- Thus, they inhibit the incorporation of PABA into dihydropteroic acid, the precursor of folic acid.
- Excessive PABA counteracts the action of sulfonamides.
- Spectrum of activity includes *Streptococcus pneumoniae, Streptococcus pyogenes, Haemophilus influenzae, Haemophilus ducreyi, Nocardia, Chlamydia trachomatis* and *Actinomyces*.
- The organisms may develop permanent and irreversible resistance to sulfonamides.
- Gram negative bacilli *Escherichia coli, Neisseria meningitidis* and *Shigella* have developed resistance.
- Cross resistance with other antimicrobial agents does not occur.
- Except those with local action on bowel all other sulfonamides are well absorbed after oral administration.
- Significant absorption occurs from skin and mucous membrane.
- They are well distributed into pleural, peritoneal, ocular, and synovial fluid.
- They accumulate in many tissues and cross the placental barrier.

Adverse Effects
- Crystalluria
- Hematuria

- Hemolytic anemia in glucose-6-phosphate dehydrogenase (G6PD) deficient patients
- Agranulocytosis
- Aplastic anemia
- Hypersensitivity reaction
- Kernicterus in newborn
- Nausea, vomiting, anorexia

Uses
- Urinary tract infection (UTI)
- Acute pyelonephritis
- Nocardiosis
- Toxoplasmosis
- Prophylaxis of streptococcal infection in rheumatic fever.

Short-Acting Sulfonamides
Sulfisoxazole
Actions
- The onset of action is quick but the duration of action is short.
- It is highly soluble and excreted rapidly.
- So, the incidence of hematuria and crystalluria are minimal.
- Its urinary concentration is higher than its plasma concentration.
- Its cerebrospinal fluid (CSF) concentration is one-third of its plasma concentration.
- It is tasteless and easy to administer in children.
- **Other details:** Common properties of sulfonamides.

Sulfadiazine
Actions
- The onset of action is quick but duration is short.
- It attains good CSF concentration.
- It is excreted rapidly initially, followed later by slower rate of excretion.
- Alkalinizing agent sodium bicarbonate facilitates its renal excretion and reduces the risk of crystalluria.
- **Other details:** Common properties of sulfonamides.

Intermediate Acting Sulfonamide
Sulfamethoxazole
Actions
- It has intermediate duration of action.
- It is used in UTI and in systemic infection.

- Its acetylated metabolite is insoluble.
- Hence, the risk of crystalluria is high.
- **Other details:** Common properties of sulfonamides.

Long-Acting Sulfonamide
Sulfadoxine
- It is combined with pyrimethamine for prophylaxis and treatment of malaria.
- It can cause Stevens-Johnson syndrome.
- **Other details:** Common properties of sulfonamides.

Locally Acting Sulfonamides
Sulfasalazine
Actions
- It is poorly absorbed from gastrointestinal tract (GIT).
- It is effective in ulcerative colitis and regional enteritis.
- It is converted by intestinal bacteria into sulfapyridine and mesalamine.
- Mesalamine or 5-aminosalicylic acid (5-ASA) has anti-inflammatory activity.
- Sulfapyridine is responsible for its toxic effects.
- It causes hemolysis in patients with G6PD deficiency.
- Fever, arthralgia, rashes and Heinz-body anemia are the other side effects.
- **Other details:** Common properties of sulfonamides.

Topical Acting Sulfonamides
Sulfacetamide
Actions
- Its aqueous solubility is very high.
- It is available as topical ophthalmic solution.
- This topical ocular preparation is non-irritant to eye.
- The topical solution penetrates into ocular fluid and ocular tissue.
- Hence, it is effective in ocular infection.
- **Other details:** Common properties of sulfonamides.

Silver Sulfadiazine
Actions
- It prevents infection in burns.
- It is not effective in already established infection.

- The silver ion released slowly from the preparation is toxic to the organisms.
- If absorbed, silver can cause rash, itch and burning sensation.
- **Other details:** Common properties of sulfonamides.

Mafenide
Actions
- It is effective in burns.
- It inhibits colonization of burns by gram positive and gram negative organisms.
- Suprainfection is due to *Candida albicans* can occur.
- Systemic absorption can occur during topical application.
- Allergic reactions and intense pain can occur at the site of application.
- Since it inhibits carbonic anhydrase enzyme, it can cause metabolic acidosis and hyperventilation.
- **Other details:** Common properties of sulfonamides.

TRIMETHOPRIM
Actions
- It selectively inhibits the bacterial dihydrofolate reductase enzyme.
- When combined with sulfonamide it causes sequential blockade of tetrahydrofolic acid synthesis.
- Its oral absorption is faster than sulfonamides.
- Its volume of distribution is 9 times higher than sulfonamide.
- It enters CSF and sputum.

Trimethoprim-Sulfamethoxazole (Co-Trimoxazole)
This synergistic combination causes sequential blockade of tetrahydrofolic acid synthesis.

Spectrum of Activity
- Resistant strains of *Streptococcus pyogenes, Streptococcus viridans, Streptococcus pneumoniae, Staphylococcus aureus, Staphylococcus epidermidis, H. influenzae, E. coli, Proteus, Neisseria, Shigella, Salmonella, Pseudomonas, Serratia, Enterobacter, Klebsiella, Brucella, Yersinia enterocolitica, Nocardia, Pasteurella, Chlamydia, Pneumocystis jiroveci* are sensitive.
- Plasma half-life of sulfamethoxazole and trimethoprim is around 10 hours.

- The dose ratio of sulfamethoxazole and trimethoprim is 5:1 (800 mg: 160 mg) since the volume of distribution of trimethoprim is high.
- This ratio provides an optimum minimal inhibitory plasma concentration ratio of 20:1.
- Co-trimoxazole has higher tissue concentration.
- Since it concentrates highly in prostate, it is effective in prostatitis.

Adverse Effects
- Megaloblastic anemia, agranulocytosis, leukopenia, thrombocytopenia
- Stevens-Johnson syndrome
- Exfoliative dermatitis, glossitis, stomatitis
- Toxic epidermal necrolysis, Henoch-Schonlein purpura
- Depression, headache, hallucination.

Uses
- Acute uncomplicated lower UTI due to *E. coli*
- Respiratory tract infection due to *H.influenzae, S.pneumoniae*
- *Pneumocystis jiroveci* infection
- Prostatitis
- Typhoid carrier
- Second line drug in typhoid fever
- Shigellosis
- *Nocardia, Cyclospora* infection
- Prophylaxis in febrile neutropenia.

Nursing Responsibilities
- Advice the patient to always complete a full course of antibiotic.
- Patients on sulfonamide should be advised to consume adequate quantity of fluid.
- Urine output should be maintained at 1.2 L.
- Wound should be cleaned well before applying mafenide cream.
- Periodic monitoring of complete blood count is necessary.

CHAPTER 57

Quinolones

NALIDIXIC ACID

Actions
- Nalidixic acid is a quinolone and all other agents are fluoroquinolones.
- Although it is bactericidal, the development of resistance during therapy is rather rapid.
- It inhibits bacterial DNA gyrase enzyme.
- It acts against *E.coli, Proteus, Shigella, Klebsiella* and *Enterobacter*.
- It is not effective against *Pseudomonas* infection.
- It is well absorbed on oral administration.
- It attains high concentration in urine.

Adverse Effects
- Rash, headache
- Vertigo
- Visual disturbance.

Uses
- Urinary antiseptic.
- Diarrhea due to *Salmonella, Shigella, E.coli, Proteus*.

FLUOROQUINOLONES
- **First generation:** Norfloxacin, ciprofloxacin, ofloxacin, pefloxacin
- **Second generation:** Levofloxacin, lomefloxacin
- **Third generation:** Sparfloxacin, gemifloxacin
- **Fourth generation:** Moxifloxacin, prulifloxacin, trovafloxacin, alatrofloxacin.

Common Mechanism of Action of Fluoroquinolones
- They inhibit DNA gyrase enzyme (topoisomerase II) in Gram-negative organisms.
- They inhibit topoisomerase IV in gram positive organisms.
- DNA gyrase nicks double stranded DNA includes negative supercoils and reseals the nicked ends.

- This prevents excessive positive supercoils or 'overwinding'.
- It inhibit DNA gyrase mediated supercoiling of DNA.
- Quinolones are bactericidal and selectively inhibit bacterial topoisomerase.
- They are contraindicated during pregnancy and in children.

First Generation Fluoroquinolones

Spectrum of activity includes *E. coli, Klebsiella, Salmonella, Shigella Proteus, Haemophilus, Neisseria, Enterobacter, Campylobacter* and *Chlamydia*. They are less active against MRSA, *Pseudomonas, Legionella, Brucella, Mycobacterium* and *Mycoplasma*.

Ciprofloxacin

Details of mechanism of action and spectrum: Common mechanism of action of fluoroquinolones and spectrum of activity of first generation fluoroquinolones.

Actions
- It is well absorbed orally.
- It undergoes first pass metabolism.
- It is also an enzyme inhibitor.
- It has poor efficacy against anerobic organisms.
- It is less effective in peritonitis.
- It attains high concentration in lung, macrophage, bile and prostate but not in cerebrospinal fluid (CSF).
- Its urinary concentration is higher than its plasma concentration.
- It is secreted in milk.

Adverse Effects
- Nausea, anorexia
- Rash, hypersensitivity reaction
- Headache, dizziness
- Tendinitis.

Uses
- Urinary tract infection (UTI)
- Prostatitis
- Gonorrhea
- Typhoid
- Tuberculosis
- Chancroid
- Bacterial gastroenteritis

Quinolones

- Respiratory tract infections due to *H.influenzae, Mycoplasma, Legionella*
- Osteomyelitis
- Meningitis
- Prophylaxis in anthrax
- Shigellosis
- Traveler's diarrhea.

Norfloxacin
Details of mechanism of action and spectrum: Common mechanism of action of fluoroquinolones and spectrum of activity of first generation fluoroquinolones.

Actions
- It is less potent.
- It attains lower concentration in tissues.
- It is used in UTI and gastrointestinal tract (GIT) infection.

Ofloxacin
Details of mechanism of action and spectrum: Common mechanism of action of fluoroquinolones and spectrum of activity of first generation fluoroquinolones.

Actions
- *Chlamydia* and *Mycoplasma* respond well to ofloxacin.
- It is less active than ciprofloxacin against gram negative organisms.
- It is more potent than ciprofloxacin against gram positive organisms.
- It is also effective against anerobic organisms.
- It has high oral bioavailability.
- It attains high concentration in ascitic fluid.
- It is secreted in milk.

Uses
- Cervicitis
- Urethritis
- Prostatitis
- Resistant tuberculosis
- Leprosy
- Ear, nose and throat (ENT) infection
- Respiratory infection
- Single dose in gonorrhea

- Typhoid
- Shigellosis
- Traveler's diarrhea
- Community acquired pneumonia.

Pefloxacin
Details of mechanism of action and spectrum: Common mechanism of action of fluoroquinolones and spectrum of activity of first generation fluoroquinolones.

Actions
- Oral absorption is complete.
- It has adequate tissue concentration.
- It has longer half-life.
- It accumulates in plasma on continued administration.
- It concentrates highly in CSF.
- It is secreted in milk.
- Dose should be reduced in patients with liver dysfunction.

Second Generation Fluoroquinolones
Additional spectrum of activity includes *Mycoplasma, Streptococcus, Legionella* and *Chlamydia*.

Levofloxacin
Details of mechanism of action and spectrum: Common mechanism of action of fluoroquinolones and spectrum of activity of second generation fluoroquinolones.

Actions
- It has 100% oral bioavailability and attains equal plasma concentration after IV and oral administration.
- It has long-duration of action.
- It can be administered once daily.

Uses
- Community acquired pneumonia
- Chronic bronchitis
- Urinary tract infection, skin and soft tissue infection
- Sinusitis, prostatitis, pyelonephritis.

Lomefloxacin
Details of mechanism of action and spectrum: Common mechanism of action of fluoroquinolones and spectrum of activity of second generation fluoroquinolones.

Actions
- It has long-duration of action.
- It can be administered once daily.
- It is concentrated highly in tissues.
- It is very effective than ciprofloxacin in *Chlamydia* and Gram-negative infection.
- It causes QT prolongation and phototoxicity.

Prulifloxacin
Details of mechanism of action and spectrum: Common mechanism of action of fluoroquinolones and spectrum of activity of second generation fluoroquinolones.

Actions
- It is effective against many resistant Gram-positive and Gram-negative organisms.
- It does not prolong QT interval.

Adverse Effects
- Urticaria
- Rarely photosensitivity and blood dyscrasias.

Uses
- Acute uncomplicated UTI
- Complicated lower urinary tract infection
- Chronic bronchitis.

Third Generation Fluoroquinolones
They have higher activity against gram positive organisms such as *Staphylococcus, Streptococcus, Enterococcus, Mycoplasma,* and *Mycobacterium*.

Sparfloxacin
Details of mechanism of action and spectrum: Common mechanism of action of fluoroquinolones and spectrum of activity of third generation fluoroquinolones.

Actions
- It is effective in pneumonia, sinusitis, bronchitis and ENT infection.
- Its efficacy is high in infection due to Gram-positive organisms.
- It can cause severe phototoxicity.
- It can also cause QT prolongation and ventricular arrhythmia.

Gemifloxacin

Details of mechanism of action and spectrum: Common mechanism of action of fluoroquinolones and spectrum of activity of third generation fluoroquinolones.

Actions
- It is rapidly absorbed.
- It is excreted through urine and feces.

Adverse Effects
- Rash
- Nausea, diarrhea
- Headache, dizziness
- QT prolongation.

Uses
- Community acquired pneumonia
- Chronic bronchitis.

Fourth Generation Fluoroquinolones

They show higher activity against Gram-positive organisms and anaerobes.

Moxifloxacin

Details of mechanism of action and spectrum: Common mechanism of action of fluoroquinolones and spectrum of activity of fourth generation fluoroquinolones.

Actions
- It is a 'respiratory fluoroquinolone' and concentrates in lung.
- Hence, it is very effective against *Mycobacterium* species.
- It is metabolized in liver and excreted through bile and feces.
- Since its urinary concentration is low, it is not very suitable for treatment of UTI.
- Moxifloxacin should not be administered in patients with liver dysfunction.

Uses
- Tuberculosis
- Bronchitis
- Pneumonia
- Sinusitis, otitis media.

Nursing Responsibilities
Liver function should be monitored in patients receiving moxifloxacin and gemifloxacin.

CHAPTER 58

Beta-Lactam Antibiotics

Beta-lactam antibiotics are:
- Penicillins
- Cephalosporins
- Carbapenems

COMMON PROPERTIES OF BETA-LACTAM ANTIBIOTICS
- They contain a beta-lactam ring in their structure.
- They are bactericidal in action.
- They bind to penicillin binding proteins (PBP) in bacterial cell wall.
- They inhibit the synthesis of peptidoglycan that forms the basic structure of cell wall.
- By disrupting the synthesis of bacterial cell wall they cause lysis of cells and bacterial death.

COMMON PROPERTIES OF PENICILLINS
- Penicillins are widely used due to their efficacy and safety.
- Their principal adverse effect is hypersensitivity reactions.
- Resistance to penicillins develops due to inability of the bacteria to bind to PBP and inactivation of penicillins by penicillinase or beta-lactamase enzyme produced by organisms.

Adverse Effects
- Hypersensitivity reactions characterized by rash, serum sickness, exfoliative dermatitis, vasculitis, Stevens-Johnson syndrome, angioedema, and anaphylaxis
- Reversible neutropenia
- Tinnitus, headache, dizziness, seizures
- Pain and inflammation at injection site.

Classification
They are classified as:
  A. Narrow spectrum penicillins
  B. Penicillinase resistant penicillins

C. Extended spectrum penicillins
D. Antipseudomonal penicillins

NARROW SPECTRUM PENICILLINS

They are:
- Penicillin G
- Penicillin V

Penicillin G and Penicillin V

Common properties of beta-lactam antibiotics and penicillins to be included.

They are effective against:
- Gram-positive cocci except resistant strains of *Staph. aureus*
- Gram-negative cocci
- Gram-positive bacilli such as *Treponema pallidum* and *Clostridium species* are highly sensitive
- They are not effective against gram negative bacilli.

Actions

- They are well distributed into many tissues.
- They concentrate in cerebrospinal fluid (CSF) only in the presence of meningitis.
- They are excreted through renal tubular secretion.
- Renal excretion is reduced by probenecid.
- In severe infection, penicillin G is more effective than penicillin V.
- Penicillin G is acid labile.
- Parenteral penicillin G is available as procaine penicillin G and benzathine penicillin G.
- Its oral absorption is more in elders, as acidity decreases with age.
- Food reduces its absorption.
- It should be administered either 30 minutes before or 2 hours after food.
- Penicillin V is acid stable and available as potassium penicillin V.
- It is absorbed well after oral administration.
- Intramuscular (IM) preparation of benzathine penicillin is slowly absorbed from the site of administration.
- It has longer duration of action.

Uses
- Infection caused by susceptible strains of *Streptococcus pneumoniae, Streptococcus pyogenes, Streptococcus viridans,* and *Staphylococcus aureus*
- Syphilis
- Diphtheria
- Gas gangrene
- Actinomycosis
- Rat bite fever
- Lyme disease
- Erysipeloid
- Anthrax
- Meningitis caused by susceptible strains of *N. meningitidis*
- Scarlet fever
- Streptococcal toxic shock

Prophylaxis
- Single dose in Streptococcal pharyngitis.
- Once a month in rheumatic fever
- Syphilis after exposure

PENICILLINASE RESISTANT PENICILLINS
They are:
- Methicillin
- Nafcillin
- Cloxacillin
- Oxacillin
- Dicloxacillin

Common properties of beta-lactam antibiotics and penicillins to be included:
- They are effective against penicillinase producing *Staphylococci*.
- They are less active than penicillin G against penicillin sensitive organisms such as non-penicillinase producing *Staphylococci*.
- They are excreted through bile and urine.
- Organisms such as *Staphylococcus aureus* have developed resistance to methicillin.
- Methicillin is destroyed by gastric acid.
- It should be administered parenterally.
- Methicillin causes hematuria and interstitial nephritis.

- Oxacillin, cloxacillin and dicloxacillin are acid resistant and not destroyed by gastric acid.
- Hence, they can be administered through oral route.
- They are not effective against *Listeria* or *Enterococci*.
- Nafcillin is highly resistant to penicillinase enzyme.
- It is more active against penicillin G resistant *Staphylococcus aureus*.
- It attains higher concentration in CSF.
- It is effective in *Staphylococci* meningitis.

EXTENDED SPECTRUM PENICILLINS
They are amino penicillins such as:
- Ampicillin
- Bacampicillin
- Amoxicillin

Common Properties
- They have extended spectrum of activity.
- They are destroyed by β-lactamases produced by Gram-positive and Gram-negative organisms.
- *Enterococci, Listeria* and *H.pylori* are sensitive.
- *Neisseria, Haemophilus, Proteus, E. coli, Shigella* and *Salmonella* are resistant.

Ampicillin
Common properties of beta-lactam antibiotics and aminopenicillins to be included.

Actions
- It is not destroyed by gastric acid.
- It is incompletely absorbed after oral administration.
- This causes gastric irritation and diarrhea.
- Incidence of diarrhea is minimal with its prodrug bacampicillin.
- It undergoes enterohepatic circulation.
- Bacampicillin is absorbed completely from gastrointestinal tract (GIT).

Adverse Effects
- Diarrhea
- Hypersensitivity, rash.

Uses
- Urinary tract infection (UTI)
- Sinusitis
- Bronchitis
- Meningitis
- Otitis media
- Gonorrhea
- Cholecystitis
- Typhoid carrier
- Subacute bacterial endocarditis (SABE)
- Shigellosis

Amoxicillin
Common properties of beta-lactam antibiotics and aminopenicillins to be included.

Actions
- It is not destroyed by gastric acid.
- It has good oral bioavailability.
- Food does not interfere with its absorption.
- Its oral absorption is complete.
- The incidence of diarrhea is minimal.
- It is more effective against penicillin resistant *Streptococcus pneumoniae*.
- It is less effective than ampicillin against shigellosis.

ANTIPSEUDOMONAL PENICILLINS
They are:
- Carbenicillin
- Piperacillin
- Ticarcillin
- Mezlocillin

Common properties of beta-lactam antibiotics to be included:
- They are effective against ampicillin resistant *Pseudomonas* and *Proteus*.
- They are ineffective against *Staphylococcus aureus, Enterococcus, Klebsiella, Listeria* and *Bacteroides*.
- Mezlocillin and piperacillin are more effective against *Pseudomonas* infection.
- Carbenicillin is neither acid resistant nor penicillinase resistant.

- It is given through IM or intravenous (IV) route.
- Carbenicillin indanyl sodium is acid stable and can be administered orally.
- It is effective in UTI and attains high urinary concentration.
- Piperacillin is more effective than carbenicillin against *Klebsiella* and *Bacteroides*.
- It is combined with penicillinase inhibitor tazobactam for better therapeutic benefit.
- It is useful in the treatment of hospital acquired nosocomial infection.
- It is also effective in patients with febrile neutropenia.
- Ticarcillin is more effective than carbenicillin against *Pseudomonas* infection.
- It is combined with clavulanic acid.
- Mezlocillin acts against both *Pseudomonas* and *Klebsiella*.

Nursing Responsibilities

- Procaine and benzathine penicillin G should never be administered through intravenous route.
- Penicillin should never be combined with an aminoglycoside antibiotic in the same syringe.
- Intradermal test dose should be given to determine drug hypersensitivity before administering penicillin injection.
- Even if the intradermal test is negative, adrenaline should be kept ready before first time administration of parenteral penicillin.

CEPHALOSPORINS

- They are bactericidal and disrupt the synthesis of bacterial cell wall by binding to PBP.
- They are highly resistant to penicillinase.
- Patients allergic to penicillins show cross sensitivity to cephalosporins.
- They do not act against *Listeria, Enterococci,* methicillin-resistant *Staphylococcus aureus* (MRSA), *Clostridium difficile, Legionella,* methicillin resistant *Staphylococcus epidermidis, Campylobacter, Acinetobacter, Enterobacteriaceae,* and penicillin-resistant *S. pneumoniae.*
- Probenecid reduces their renal excretion.
- They cross placenta and accumulate in pericardial, ocular as well as synovial fluids.

- They penetrate into aqueous humor but not into vitreous humor of eye.
- Third and fourth generation cephalosporins cross blood-brain barrier (BBB) and are effective in meningitis.

Common Adverse Effects
- Anaphylaxis, hypersensitivity reaction, urticaria, rash
- Fever, bronchospasm
- Diarrhea, thrombocytopenia, nephrotoxicity

They are broadly classified as:
  A. First generation cephalosporins
  B. Second generation cephalosporins
  C. Third generation cephalosporins
  D. Fourth generation cephalosporins

First Generation Cephalosporins
- **Oral:** Cefadroxil, cephalexin, cefradine.
- **Parenteral:** Cefazolin, cefradine.

Common properties of beta-lactam antibiotics to be included.

Actions
- They have good activity against most Gram-positive organisms.
- They have modest activity against Gram-negative organisms.
- Cefazolin has modest activity against *Enterobacter.*
- It is well tolerated through IM or IV route.
- It has long half-life.
- Cefazolin is used in skin and soft tissue infection.
- Cefradine attains equal plasma concentration after oral, IM or IV administration.
- Cephalexin is less active against penicillinase producing *Staphylococcus aureus.*
- It can be administered orally.
- Both cefradine and cephalexin are equally effective.
- Cefadroxil is preferred in UTI as it attains higher concentration in urine.

Second Generation Cephalosporins
- **Oral:** Cefaclor, cefprozil, cefuroxime.
- **Parenteral:** Cefotetan, cefoxitin, cefuroxime axetil, ceforanide.

Common properties of beta-lactam antibiotics to be included.

Actions
- They have broader spectrum of activity than first generation cephalosporins.
- They exert higher activity against Gram-negative organisms than first generation agents.
- Cefoxitin is effective against anaerobe *B. fragilis.*
- It is also effective against mixed aerobic-anaerobic infection.
- Cefaclor is effective against resistant strains of *H.influenzae* and *Moraxella catarrhalis.*
- Cefuroxime crosses blood brain barrier but is less effective than ceftriaxone in meningitis.
- Cefuroxime is less effective against *B. fragilis.*
- Cefoxitin, cefotetan are used in pelvic inflammatory disease, diabetic foot infection.

Third Generation Cephalosporins
- **Oral:** Cefixime, ceftibuten, cefdinir, cefditoren pivoxil, cefpodoxime proxetil.
- **Parenteral:** Cefotaxime, ceftizoxime, ceftazidime, ceftriaxone.

Common properties of beta-lactam antibiotics to be included.

Actions
- Cefotaxime is effective even against resistant strains of many Gram-positive and Gram-negative aerobic bacteria.
- It is highly effective against *Enterobacteriaceae* and less effective against *B. fragilis.*
- It is effective in meningitis as it crosses blood brain barrier.
- Ceftizoxime has long duration of action and effective in UTI.
- It is more effective against *B. fragilis.*
- Ceftriaxone is highly effective in meningitis, gonorrhea and in typhoid fever.
- Cefditoren is effective against susceptible strains of *S.aureus, MRSA, Haemophilus, Moraxella* and *Streptococcus.*
- Ceftazidime has excellent activity against *Pseudomonas.*
- Cefixime is effective in UTI, otitis media, pharyngitis, and uncomplicated gonorrhea.
- Ceftibuten is used in chronic bronchitis, acute bacterial otitis media, tonsillitis, and pharyngitis.
- Cefotaxime, ceftriaxone are used in meningitis due to strains of *H. influenzae, S. pneumoniae* and *N. meningitidis.*
- Ceftazidime is used in meningitis due to *Pseudomonas* organisms.

Fourth Generation Cephalosporins
Parenteral: Cefepime, cefpirome.
Common properties of beta-lactam antibiotics to be included.

Actions
- They are effective against strains of *Enterobacteriaceae* and *Pseudomonas*.
- They are resistant to β-lactamases expressed by many organisms.
- Cefepime is effective in meningitis as it acts against many organisms causing meningitis.
- Besides its concentration in CSF is very high.
- It is not effective in MRSA, penicillin resistant *Pneumococci* or *Enterococci* infection.
- Cefpirome is very effective in the treatment of hospital acquired infection.
- Cefepime is used in nosocomial infection.
- Ceftaroline is a newer cephalosporin active against MRSA.

Nursing Responsibilities
- Cephalosporins are contraindicated in patients with known allergy to penicillins.
- Deep intramuscular injection is preferable as they are very painful.
- Redness, pain and induration at the site of IM injection should be notified to the physician.

CARBAPENEMS

They cause disruption of cell wall by binding to PBP. They have broader spectrum of activity than other beta-lactam antibiotics.
The drugs are:
- Imipenem
- Meropenem
- Doripenem
- Ertapenem

Imipenem
Common properties of beta-lactam antibiotics to be included.

Actions
- It is resistant to many bacterial β-lactamases.
- It is hydrolysed by renal tubular dipeptidase enzyme.

- Hence, it is combined with dipeptidase inhibitor cilastatin.
- It has wide spectrum of activity.
- It is effective against many aerobic and anaerobic microorganisms.
- Spectrum also includes *Listeria, Bacteroides, Pseudomonas, Acinetobacter* and *Enterobacteriaceae*.
- Resistant-strains of *Streptococcus, Staphylococcus* and *Enterococcus* are also susceptible.
- It is administered intravenously as it is not absorbed orally.

Adverse Effects
Nausea, vomiting, seizure, hypersensitivity reactions.

Uses
- Urinary tract infection
- Lower respiratory tract infections
- Intra-abdominal and gynecological infections
- Skin, soft tissue, bone and joint infection.

Meropenem
Common properties of beta-lactam antibiotics to be included.

Actions
- It is not hydrolysed by renal dipeptidase.
- Hence, it need not be combined with cilastatin.
- It is similar to imipenem in efficacy.
- It causes minimal incidence of seizures.
- Doripenem is more active than meropenem on resistant strains of *Pseudomonas*.
- Ertapenem has longer duration of action.
- It is less active against *Pseudomonas* and *Acinetobacter*.

Aztreonam
Common properties of beta-lactam antibiotics to be included.

Actions
- It is a monobactam and inhibits cell wall synthesis.
- It is resistant to β-lactamases produced by Gram-negative bacteria.
- It is also resistant to metallo-β-lactamases expressed by many organisms.
- The incidence of allergic reactions due to aztreonam is minimal.
- Patients allergic to penicillin and all cephalosporins except ceftazidime are not allergic to aztreonam.

- It is effective against Gram-negative but not against Gram-positive or anaerobic bacteria.
- It is administered through IM or IV route.
- Dose adjustment is necessary in renal dysfunction.

β-LACTAMASE INHIBITORS

They are most effective against plasmid encoded β-lactamases. These drugs are not effective against type-I chromosomal, β-lactamases producing strains of *Enterobacter, Citrobacter* and *Acinetobacter*.
The drugs are:
- Clavulanic acid
- Sulbactam
- Tazobactam.

Clavulanic Acid

Actions
- It is a suicide inhibitor of β-lactamases.
- It binds irreversibly to β-lactamases.
- It can be administered both orally and parenterally.
- It is available in combination with amoxicillin as oral preparation.
- It is combined with ticarcillin as parenteral preparation.
- Combination of amoxicillin and clavulanic acid is effective against β-lactamases producing strains of *H. influenzae, Staphylococcus, E. coli* and *Gonococci*.
- Combination of ticarcillin and clavulanic acid is effective against aerobic Gram-negative bacilli and in mixed nosocomial infection.

Uses
Combined with antibiotics and given in the treatment of:
- Cancer chemotherapy induced neutropenia
- Sinusitis, otitis media
- Cellulitis, diabetic foot infection.

Sulbactam

Actions
- It can be administered orally as well as parenterally.
- It is effective against Gram-positive cocci including resistant strains of *Staphylococcus aureus,* susceptible strains of Gram-negative aerobes and anaerobes.
- It is available in combination of ampicillin.

Use

Mixed intra-abdominal and pelvic infection.

Tazobactam

Actions

- It is available in combination with piperacillin. It is available as parenteral preparation.
- It does not increase the activity of piperacillin.

CHAPTER 59

Aminoglycosides

COMMON PROPERTIES
- Aminoglycoside antibiotics are bactericidal in action.
- They inhibit protein synthesis by binding primarily to 30S ribosomal subunit.
- They are effective mainly against aerobic gram negative organisms.
- They are effective only in alkaline pH.
- They are not absorbed orally and should be administered parenterally.
- Tobramycin and amikacin can be administered through inhalational route.
- Aminoglycosides have limited distribution.
- They do not accumulate in ocular fluid.
- They do not cross blood-brain barrier (BBB) adequately and cannot be used in meningitis.
- Their concentration in other secretion and tissues is low.
- Their renal excretion is slow.
- Hence, they can be detected in urine for many days after discontinuation of drug.
- They accumulate in renal cortex, endolymph and perilymph of inner ear.
- Therefore, they cause ototoxicity and nephrotoxicity.
- They also result in neuromuscular blockade.
- Resistance occurs due to reduced entry, inactivation by microbial enzymes and low affinity to target site.

Common Adverse Effects
- Ototoxicity
- Nephrotoxicity
- Neuromuscular blockade

STREPTOMYCIN
Actions
Common properties of aminoglycosides to be included.
- While penicillin G is bacteriostatic to *Enterococci* species, streptomycin is bactericidal.

- Hence, the combination is synergistic in the treatment of *Enterococci* infection.
- They should not be combined in the same syringe to prevent inactivation.
- Many organisms have developed resistance to streptomycin.
- It is given as deep IM injection.
- It is also administered intravenously.
- Streptomycin causes irreversible vestibular toxicity.
- It can also cause scotoma and peripheral neuritis.
- It is used in plague, pulmonary tuberculosis, tularemia and subacute bacterial endocarditis (SABE).

GENTAMICIN

Actions

Common properties of aminoglycosides to be included.
- It is the aminoglycoside of choice due to its low cost and high efficacy.
- It is more effective than streptomycin against *E.coli, Klebsiella, Pseudomonas* and *Serratia*.
- Many organisms have developed resistance to gentamicin.
- It is available as parenteral, topical and ophthalmic preparations.
- It is used topically in burns.
- It is administered with penicillin or vancomycin for *Enterococci* endocarditis.
- It is effective in uncomplicated urinary tract infection (UTI) due to *E.coli* infection.

Uses

Gentamicin is coadministered with other antibiotics in the treatment of:
- Nosocomial pneumonia
- Intrathecal administration in meningitis due to *Pseudomonas* or *Acinetobacter* infection
- Enterococcal endocarditis
- Peritonitis
- Sepsis due to resistant *Pseudomonas, Enterobacter, Serratia,* and *Klebsiella* organisms.

TOBRAMYCIN

Actions

Common properties and adverse effects of aminoglycosides to be included.

- It is more effective than gentamicin in *Pseudomonas* infection.
- It is less effective in *Enterococci* infection.
- It is ineffective against *Mycobacteria*.
- It can be given through inhalational route in cystic fibrosis.
- Tobramycin causes both auditory and vestibular dysfunction.

AMIKACIN
Actions
Common properties and adverse effects of aminoglycosides to be included.
- Among the aminoglycosides, amikacin has a wider spectrum of activity.
- It is effective in infection due to aerobic Gram-negative bacilli.
- It is resistant to aminoglycosidase enzyme expressed by many organisms.
- Hence, it is preferred in the treatment of organisms resistant to gentamicin or tobramycin.
- It is preferred in nosocomial infection.
- It is effective against *M. tuberculosis* and atypical *Mycobacteria*.
- It is less effective against *Enterococci*.
- It causes more auditory toxicity than vestibular dysfunction.

NETILMICIN
Actions
Common properties and adverse effects of aminoglycosides to be included.
- It has wider spectrum of activity against aerobic Gram-negative bacilli.
- It is not inactivated by aminoglycosidase produced by organisms.
- Hence it is effective against many resistant organisms.
- It is effective against severe infections caused by *Enterobacteriaceae*.
- It is less ototoxic.

NEOMYCIN
Actions
Common properties of aminoglycosides to be included.
- It is a broad spectrum aminoglycoside antibiotic.

- It is available as topical application for ocular, skin and ear infection.
- Its oral absorption is poor.
- It is given orally for preoperative preparation of bowel prior to intestinal surgery and in hepatic encephalopathy.
- Oral administration can result in sprue-like syndrome causing diarrhea and steatorrhea.
- It is highly ototoxic and nephrotoxic.
- Hence, it is not administered parenterally.

KANAMYCIN

Actions

Common properties of aminoglycosides to be included.
- It is the most toxic aminoglycoside antibiotic.
- It has limited spectrum of activity.
- The organisms *Pseudomonas* and *Serratia* have developed resistance to kanamycin.
- It is given orally adjunct in hepatic encephalopathy.
- It is also available as parenteral preparation.
- Oral administration can result in malabsorption and suprainfection.
- It is highly ototoxic and nephrotoxic.

PAROMOMYCIN

Actions

- It is not absorbed orally.
- It exerts local action on gastrointestinal tract (GIT).
- It is used as a luminal amebicide in intestinal amebiasis.
- It can cause nausea and abdominal cramps.

Nursing Responsibilities

- High frequency hearing loss, tinnitus, dizziness and vertigo indicate ototoxicity and should be reported to the attending physician.
- All aminoglycosides except amikacin should not be admixed in the same syringe with penicillins as they inactivate the aminoglycosides.

CHAPTER 60

Broad Spectrum Antibiotics

The broad spectrum antibiotics are:
- Tetracyclines and glycylcyclines
- Chloramphenicol.

COMMON PROPERTIES
- They are effective against aerobic and anaerobic Gram-positive and Gram-negative organisms.
- They are also effective against strains of *Mycoplasma, Rickettsia* and *Chlamydia*.
- They are bacterostatic and inhibit protein synthesis.
- They are not effective in fungal or viral infection.

TETRACYCLINES
Actions
Common properties of broad spectrum antibiotics to be included.
- They are more active on Gram-positive than on Gram-negative bacteria.
- In addition, tetracyclines are also effective against *Legionella, Coxiella, Ureaplasma, Borrelia, Treponema, Mycobacteria, atypical Mycobacteria,* and *Plasmodia*.
- Tetracycline, oxytetracycline, demeclocycline, doxycycline and minocycline belong to this group.
- They inhibit protein synthesis by binding to 30S ribosomal subunit.
- Doxycycline and minocycline are commonly used.
- Except doxycycline and minocycline, food interferes with absorption of all other tetracyclines.
- Other tetracyclines form insoluble complexes with iron, calcium, magnesium, aluminum, and zinc.
- Hence, they should be administered on empty stomach.
- They are widely distributed into tissues and body fluids.
- They cross placenta and are secreted in milk.
- In meningitis, they cross the blood-brain barrier (BBB) adequately.

- They accumulate in liver, spleen, bone marrow, bone and teeth.
- Doxycycline is excreted through bile and kidney while minocycline is excreted mainly through bile.
- Both doxycycline and minocycline can be given to patients with renal dysfunction.
- All tetracyclines undergo enterohepatic circulation.
- They also attain high concentration in prostate and urine.
- They are contraindicated during pregnancy and in children between 2 to 8 years of age.

Adverse Effects
- Nausea, vomiting, diarrhea, epigastric burning, esophagitis, pancreatitis
- Brown discoloration of teeth.
- Pseudomembranous colitis due to superinfection by *Clostridium difficile*.
- *Candida albicans* overgrowth in mouth, pharynx, vagina, and bowel
- Vestibulotoxicity by minocycline
- Hepatotoxicity
- Nephrogenic diabetes mellitus by demeclocycline
- Fanconi syndrome due to outdated pills
- Photosensitivity
- Pseudotumor cerebri in infants.

Uses
- Doxycycline and minocycline are preferred.
- Methicillin-resistant *Staphylococcus aureus* (MRSA)
- Respiratory tract infections due to *S. pneumoniae, H. influenzae, Mycoplasma* and *Chlamydia*
- Acne
- Cholera
- Urethritis, salpingitis, endometritis, peritonitis and epididymitis due to *C.trachomatis*
- Rocky mountain spotted fever, typhus
- Anthrax
- Actinomycosis
- Brucellosis
- Tularemia
- Leptospirosis

Broad Spectrum Antibiotics

- Relapsing fever
- Lyme disease
- Yaws.

TIGECYCLINE
Actions
Common properties of broad spectrum antibiotics to be included.
- It is a glycylcycline.
- It is more active against tetracycline resistant Gram-negative organisms.
- It inhibits protein synthesis by binding to 30S ribosomal subunit.
- It is not well absorbed orally.
- So, it is administered only through parenteral route.
- It undergoes extensive and rapid distribution into tissue.
- Due to this, its plasma concentration is low.
- It is excreted through urine.
- It requires dose adjustment in hepatic dysfunction.
- It undergoes enterohepatic circulation.

Adverse Effects
- Photosensitivity reaction
- Brownish discoloration of teeth
- Hepatotoxicity.

Uses
- Complicated skin and soft tissue infection
- Community acquired pneumonia in hospitalized patients
- Complicated intra-abdominal infection is due to *Enterococci* organisms
- Urinary tract infection (UTI) due to *E. coli*.

CHLORAMPHENICOL
Actions
Other details: Common properties of broad spectrum antibiotics to be included.
- It is a reserve drug for life-threatening meningitis or rickettsial infection.
- It inhibits protein synthesis by binding to 50S ribosomal subunit.
- It is well absorbed orally.

- It is also available in the form of prodrug for parenteral administration.
- It is extensively distributed into body fluids such as bile and aqueous humor.
- It accumulates in cerebospinal fluid (CSF).
- It crosses placenta and is secreted in milk.

Adverse Effects
- Irreversible bone marrow depression, pancytopenia and aplastic anemia
- Hypersensitivity reaction
- Nausea, vomiting, diarrhea, unpleasant taste
- Blurring of vision
- Gray baby syndrome in neonate characterized by refusal to suck, abdominal distention, cyanosis, passage of green stools as well as irregular, and rapid respiration.

Uses
- Typhoid fever
- Bacterial meningitis due to *H. influenzae, N. meningitidis* and *S. pneumoniae*
- Rocky Mountain spotted fever
- Typhus
- Q fever

Nursing Responsibilities
- All tetracyclines except doxycycline and minocycline should be taken on empty stomach.
- All tetracyclines except doxycycline and minocycline should not be administered with calcium supplements, milk, iron, antacids or laxatives.

CHAPTER 61

Macrolides and Ketolides

- Erythromycin, clarithromycin, roxithromycin and azithromycin are the macrolides.
- Clarithromycin and roxithromycin are the semisynthetic derivatives of erythromycin.
- Telithromycin is a ketolide and is also a semisynthetic derivative of erythromycin.

COMMON PROPERTIES

- They are bacterostatic at lower concentration and bactericidal at higher concentration.
- They are very effective against aerobic Gram-positive cocci and bacilli.
- Spectrum of activity includes *Streptococci, Staphylococci, Clostridium perfringens, Neisseria, Corynebacterium diphtheriae, Listeria, Pasteurella multocida, Borrelia, Bordetella, Bacteroides, M. pneumoniae, Legionella, Campylobacter, Chlamydia* and some strains *of atypical Mycobacteria.*
- They inhibit protein synthesis by binding to 50S ribosomal subunit.
- Resistance develops due to increased efflux, faster destruction and altered target.

Adverse Effects

- Cholestatic hepatitis
- Hepatotoxicity (severe with telithromycin)
- Epigastric distress, abdominal cramps (more with erythromycin)
- Prolonged QT interval (not seen with azithromycin)
- Visual disturbance (telithromycin)
- Auditory impairment (erythromycin)
- Enzyme inhibition and elevated plasma concentration of coadministered drugs (except azithromycin)
- Skin eruptions, fever, eosinophilia.

Uses

- Community acquired pneumonia
- Pneumonia due to *Mycoplasma, Legionella* or *Chlamydia* organisms
- Cellulitis, erysipelas
- First line drug in Chlamydial urogenital infections
- Diphtheria
- Whooping cough
- Gastroenteritis due to *Campylobacter* infection
- *H.pylori* infection in peptic ulcer (clarithromycin, azithromycin)
- Mycobacterial infection
- As prophylaxis in recurrent rheumatic fever for prevention of bacterial endocarditis.

ERYTHROMYCIN

Actions

Common properties and uses to be included.
- It is effective against aerobic Gram-positive cocci and bacilli.
- It is ineffective against aerobic Gram-negative bacilli.
- It is incompletely but adequately absorbed through oral route.
- It is available as estolate, ethylsuccinate and stearate salts.
- It is given as immediate release or enteric coated delayed release preparations.
- It is well distributed and highly concentrated in prostate.
- It undergoes enterohepatic circulation, excreted in bile and urine.
- It does not accumulate in cerebrospinal fluid (CSF).
- It crosses placenta.
- It is secreted in milk.
- Its concentration in middle ear is inadequate for treatment of otitis media.
- It is an enzyme inhibitor and increases the plasma concentration of coadministered drugs.
- It stimulates motilin receptors resulting in abdominal cramps.
- It prolongs QT interval and causes transient hearing loss.
- It is highly hepatotoxic and causes cholestatic jaundice.
- It causes allergic reactions.
- It is preferred in the treatment of ophthalmia neonatorum and pneumonia due to *Chlamydia*.

Macrolides and Ketolides

CLARITHROMYCIN
Actions
Common properties and uses to be included:
- It has rapid and adequate oral absorption.
- It undergoes first pass metabolism.
- It is available as extended release preparation.
- It concentrates more in tissues than in serum.
- It accumulates in middle ear.
- It has better gastrointestinal tract (GIT) tolerability.
- It can cause hepatotoxicity, QT prolongation and allergic reactions.
- It is an enzyme inhibitor and increases the plasma concentration of coadministered drugs.
- It is excreted in bile and urine.
- It is used in *H. pylori* infection.

ROXITHROMYCIN
Actions
Common properties and uses to be included:
- It has long duration of action.
- It is more effective in *Legionella* infection.
- It is less effective in *B. pertussis* infection.
- It has better gastric tolerability.
- It does not cause abdominal cramps.
- It can prolong QT interval.
- It can cause allergic reactions.
- It is an enzyme inhibitor and increases the plasma concentration of coadministered drugs.
- It is a suitable alternative to erythromycin in skin, soft tissue and ear, nose and throat (ENT) infection.

AZITHROMYCIN
Actions
Common properties and uses to be included:
- It has rapid and adequate oral absorption when given in empty stomach.
- It has very good gastric tolerability.
- It is administered once daily.
- It is widely distributed.

- It concentrates more in tissues than in plasma.
- It accumulates in phagocytes but does not accumulate in CSF.
- Its major route of excretion is bile.
- It does not cause drug interactions.
- It causes hepatotoxicity, allergic reactions and minimal GIT toxicity.
- It does not prolong QT interval.
- It is used in community acquired pneumonia, pharyngitis, otitis media and skin infection.

TELITHROMYCIN

Actions

Common properties and uses to be included:
- It is available only as oral formulation and not as parenteral preparation.
- It has good oral bioavailability.
- It is well distributed into many tissues.
- It concentrates in macrophages and in WBC.
- It is excreted primarily in bile.
- It causes severe hepatotoxicity.
- It prolongs QT interval.
- It causes visual disturbances and allergic reactions.
- It is very effective in community acquired pneumonia.
- It is contraindicated in patients with myasthenia gravis.
- It is an enzyme inhibitor and increases the plasma concentration of coadministered drugs.

Nursing Responsibilities

- ECG should be regularly monitored in patients receiving these drugs.
- Liver function test should be monitored for all patients on these antibiotics.
- Patients taking azithromycin should be told to take it on empty stomach.

CHAPTER 62

Miscellaneous Antibiotics

LINCOSAMIDE (CLINDAMYCIN)

Actions
- It is effective against susceptible strains of anaerobic bacteria.
- It is effective against susceptible strains of *Streptococci, Pneumococci* and methicillin susceptible strains of *S. aureus.*
- It is more effective against anaerobic organisms such as *Bacteroides, Fusobacterium, Peptococcus, Peptostreptococcus, Clostridia, Actinomyces* and *Nocardia.*
- It is not effective against aerobic Gram-negative bacilli.
- It is bacterostatic and inhibits protein synthesis by binding to 50S ribosomal subunit.
- It is completely absorbed orally.
- It is distributed into body fluids, tissues and bone.
- It does not accumulate in CSF.

Adverse Effects
- Pseudomembranous colitis
- Granulocytopenia, thrombocytopenia
- Anaphylaxis, skin rashes
- Stevens-Johnson syndrome.

Uses
- Necrotizing skin and soft tissue infection
- *P. jirovecii* pneumonia in HIV patients
- Lung abscess
- Pleural infection
- *T. gondii* encephalitis.

Nursing Responsibilities
If patients on clindamycin develop frequent watery diarrhea, it should be immediately notified to the attending physician.

STREPTOGRAMINS (QUINUPRISTIN/DALFOPRISTIN)

Actions
- Quinupristin is streptogramin B and dalfopristin is streptogramin A.
- This combination is effective against Gram-positive cocci.
- Quinupristin/dalfopristin combination inhibits protein synthesis by binding to 50S ribosomal subunit.
- It can be administered only by intravenous route.
- It is mainly excreted through bile.
- Hence, it does not require dose reduction in renal insufficiency.
- It is an enzyme inhibitor and increases the plasma concentration of coadministered drugs.

Adverse Effects
- Infusion related events such as pain and phlebitis
- Arthralgia, myalgia.

Uses
- Skin infection
- Vancomycin resistant *E. faecium* infection
- Nosocomial pneumonia due to methicillin-resistant *Staphylococcus aureus* (MRSA).

Nursing Responsibilities
- Administer streptogramin as slow intravenous infusion.
- Never mix streptogramin in saline.
- It should be mixed only with 5% glucose.

OXAZOLIDINONE (LINEZOLID)

Actions
- It is a reserve drug.
- It inhibits protein synthesis by binding to 50S ribosomal subunit.
- It has 100% bioavailability by both oral and IV route of administration.
- It is effective against Gram-positive aerobic and anaerobic cocci and bacilli.
- It is ineffective against most Gram-negative aerobic and anaerobic bacteria.
- It is bacterostatic against *Staphylococci* and *enterococci* organisms.

- It is bactericidal against *Streptococci* organisms.
- It is effective against methicillin resistant *Staphylococcus aureus*.
- It is also effective in vancomycin resistant *Enterococci* infection.

Adverse Effects
- Pancytopenia, peripheral neuropathy
- Optic neuritis, lactic acidosis.

Uses
Reserve drug in:
- Nosocomial and community acquired pneumonia
- Complicated and uncomplicated skin infection.

Nursing Responsibilities
Complete blood count should be monitored in patients on linezolid.

AMINOCYCLITOLS (SPECTINOMYCIN)
Actions
- It is effective against Gram-negative bacteria.
- It inhibits protein synthesis by binding to 30S ribosomal subunit.
- It is administered as intramuscular injection.
- It is effective in uncomplicated gonorrhea resistant to first line drugs.
- It causes urticaria, chills and fever.

POLYMYXIN B AND COLISTIN
Actions
- Polymyxin B is a mixture of polymyxin B_1 and B_2.
- Colistin is polymyxin E.
- They are effective against Gram-negative organisms.
- They are bactericidal.
- They increase bacterial cell permeability.
- They are not absorbed orally.
- They are poorly absorbed from mucous membrane.

Adverse Effects
- Nephrotoxicity
- Vertigo, paresthesia, muscle weakness

Uses

Topically in:
- Skin infection
- Otitis externa, corneal ulcer
- Bladder irrigation.

Systemic administration for:
- Multidrug resistant strains of Gram-negative organisms.

Nursing Responsibilities

Urine output, urea and creatinine level should be monitored closely in patients on polymyxin to rule out renal dysfunction.

GLYCOPEPTIDES

- Vancomycin and teicoplanin are glycopeptides.
- They have broad spectrum of activity against Gram-positive bacteria.
- They are bactericidal and inhibit the cell wall synthesis.

VANCOMYCIN

Actions

- It is bactericidal except against resistant *Enterococci* organisms.
- It is administered only through intravenous route.
- It enters cerebrospinal fluid (CSF) during meningitis.
- It is well distributed to pleural, pericardial, synovial and ascitic fluid.
- It is excreted mainly through kidney.

Adverse Effects

- 'Red man syndrome' characterized by vasodilatation, redness and flushing, urticaria, tachycardia, hypotension. It occurs during rapid IV administration of vancomycin. It is due to histamine release from mast cells
- Nephrotoxicity
- Rash, anaphylaxis, fever, chills
- Ototoxicity.

Uses

- Skin and soft tissue infection
- Bone and joint infection
- Hospital and community acquired pneumonia

- Community acquired bacterial meningitis
- Streptococcal endocarditis
- Pseudomembranous colitis due to *C. difficile.*

TEICOPLANIN

Actions
- It is effective in methicillin resistant and methicillin susceptible *Staphylococcus aureus* infection.
- It is also effective against *Listeria, Clostridium* and *Corynebacterium* organisms.
- It is bactericidal.
- Vancomycin resistant strains of *Enterococci* and *Lactobacillus* are also resistant to teicoplanin.
- It is highly bound to plasma proteins.
- It can be administered through intramuscular and intravenous route.

Adverse Effects
- Nephrotoxicity
- Rash, anaphylaxis
- Chills, fever
- Ototoxicity

Uses
- Skin and soft tissue infection
- Bone and joint infection
- Hospital and community acquired pneumonia
- Community acquired bacterial meningitis
- Streptococcal endocarditis
- Pseudomembranous colitis due to *C. difficile.*

Nursing Responsibilities
- Never administer vancomycin through intramuscular route.
- Give vancomycin infusion slowly to prevent hypotension and 'red man syndrome'.
- Keep a loaded syringe of adrenaline ready before starting vancomycin or teicoplanin infusion as these drugs have the potential to cause anaphylaxis.
- Monitor renal function test periodically in patients receiving vancomycin.

LIPOPEPTIDE (DAPTOMYCIN)

Actions
- It is effective against vancomycin resistant aerobic, facultative and anaerobic Gram-positive organisms.
- It is bactericidal but resistance among susceptible organisms is emerging.
- It is administered only through intravenous route.

Adverse Effects
Myopathy, rhabdomyolysis.

Uses
Skin and soft tissue infection.

BACITRACIN

Actions
- It is bactericidal.
- It inhibits cell wall synthesis.
- It is effective against Gram-positive cocci and bacilli.
- It is used as topical application.
- It is available as skin and eye ointment.
- It is also available as powder.
- Further, it is available in combination with neomycin and polymyxin.

Adverse Effect
Hypersensitivity reaction.

Uses
- Carbuncle, furuncle, impetigo, pyoderma
- Superficial and deep abscess
- Suppurative conjunctivitis, corneal ulcer
- Oral administration for antibiotic associated diarrhea
- Meningeal irrigation during neurosurgical procedure.

MUPIROCIN

Actions
- It is effective against Gram-positive and few Gram-negative organisms.

Miscellaneous Antibiotics

- It inhibits protein synthesis.
- It is available as nasal cream as well as nasal and skin ointment.

Adverse Effects
- Irritation and sensitization at the site of application.
- Systemic absorption of polyethylene glycol present in ointment can cause nephrotoxicity.

Use
Prophylaxis of nosocomial *Staphylococcus aureus* infection in nasal carriers.

Nursing Responsibilities
- Monitor serum creatinine kinase level in patients on daptomycin.
- Do not touch eyes after applying mupirocin as it can cause severe burning sensation, irritation and pain.

Urinary Antiseptics and Chemotherapy of Urinary Tract Infection

- Urinary tract infection (UTI) is mainly caused by Gram-negative organisms.
- *E.coli* is the most common causative organism.
- Antimicrobial agents that attain high concentration in urine are effective in lower urinary tract infection.
- Those that attain high concentration in kidney are effective in pyelonephritis.
- The antimicrobials selected should be effective against the causative organisms and should be safe.

The drugs used in UTI are:
  I. **Sulfonamides:** Sulfamethoxazole-trimethoprim
 II. **Fluoroquinolones:** Ciprofloxacin, ofloxacin, norfloxacin
III. **Cephalosporins:** Cephalexin, cefadroxil, cefixime, ceftizoxime
IV. **Penicillins:** Amoxicillin, cloxacillin, piperacillin, carbenicillin
 V. **Aminoglycosides:** Gentamicin.

SULFAMETHOXAZOLE-TRIMETHOPRIM
- It is effective in alkaline pH.
- It acts against susceptible organisms in uncomplicated upper UTI.
- It is effective in prostatitis as trimethoprim concentrates in prostate.
- It is used prophylactically for recurrent cystitis in women.
- It should not be used during pregnancy.

FLUOROQUINOLONES
- Norfloxacin and ciprofloxacin attain high concentration in urine.
- They are effective in lower UTI and in prostatitis.
- They are effective in alkaline pH.
- They are not indicated during pregnancy.

CEPHALOSPORINS
- They have higher efficacy in alkaline pH.
- They are effective in UTI due to *Pseudomonas* and *Klebsiella* organisms.
- Cephalexin is given as a prophylactic agent in recurrent cystitis.

PENICILLINS
- Amoxicillin and clavulanic acid combination is effective in UTI due to *E.coli*.
- Most *E.coli* organisms have developed resistance to ampicillin.
- Cloxacillin is effective in acidic pH and acts against β-lactamase producing *Staphylococcal* infection.
- Urinary tract infection due to *Pseudomonas* and *Klebsiella* respond to piperacillin and carbenicillin.

AMINOGLYCOSIDES
- Gentamicin is effective in uncomplicated UTI due to *E.coli* organisms.
- Aminoglycosides are coadministered with other antibiotics in pyelonephritis and nosocomial infections.
- They are effective in alkaline pH.

URINARY ANTISEPTICS
They concentrate in renal tubules and are effective in lower UTI.
They are:
- Nitrofurantoin
- Methenamine

Nitrofurantoin
Actions
- It is bacteriostatic at therapeutic concentration and bactericidal at higher concentration.
- It is effective against *E.coli* organisms.
- It is administered orally.
- Its concentration in urine is high.
- Its antibacterial action is high in acidic pH and it colors urine brown.

- Although it is highly soluble in alkaline pH, alkalinization should not be tried as it reduces its therapeutic efficacy.
- It is contraindicated during pregnancy and in neonates.

Adverse Effects
- Nausea, diarrhea, epigastric distress, leukopenia, granulocytopenia
- Polyneuropathy, demyelination of sensory and motor nerves.
- Hemolytic anemia in patients with G6PD deficiency and in neonates
- Pulmonary fibrosis, headache, vertigo, nystagmus.

Use
Uncomplicated UTI.

Methenamine

Actions
- It is prodrug and releases formaldehyde in acidic pH which inhibits the organisms.
- Hence, acidification of urine promotes its activity.
- It is available as enteric coated tablet for oral administration.
- It is effective against *E.coli, S. aureus* and *S. epidermidis* organisms.
- Methenamine mandelate can cause crystalluria.

Adverse Effects
- Hematuria, painful micturition
- Gastrointestinal infection (GI) distress, crystalluria
- Rash.

Use
Only in chronic suppressive therapy of UTI.

URINARY ANALGESIC (PHENAZOPYRIDINE)
- It is a urinary analgesic and not a urinary antiseptic.
- It relieves burning sensation, dysuria and urinary urgency.
- It colors urine orange or red.
- It can cause methemoglobinemia.

Nursing Responsibilities
- Patients should be told not to mistake the reddish orange urine as hematuria.
- Patients on nitrofurantoin should be told that the drug colors urine brown.

CHAPTER 64

Chemotherapy of Sexually Transmitted Diseases

SYPHILIS

- It is caused by the spirochete *Treponema pallidum*.
- The three stages of syphilis are primary, secondary or tertiary syphilis.
- Chancre is characteristic of primary syphilis.
- Flu-like symptoms, joint pain and enlarged lymph nodes occur in secondary syphilis.
- Neurosyphilis or cardiac lesions can occur in tertiary syphilis.
- Penicillin G is the drug of choice in treatment of syphilis.
- Syphilis of less than one year duration can be treated by IM benzathine penicillin G 2.4 MU every week for 3 weeks.
- Benzathine penicillin G 2.4 MU daily for 14 days is given in tertiary syphilis.
- For congenital syphilis aqueous penicillin G 50,000 units/kg in 2 divided doses or 50,000 U/kg of procaine penicillin G as single daily dose for 10 days.
- Doxycycline is given for patients allergic to penicillin.

GONORRHEA

- It is caused by *Neisseria gonorrhoeae*.
- The symptoms are burning micturition and milky discharge in men.
- In women, it can be either asymptomatic or can be symptomatic.
- It varies from mild cervicitis or severe infection of female reproductive tract.
- In patients with *C. trachomatis* coinfection, doxycycline or azithromycin are effective.
- Urethral, cervical and rectal gonorrhea is treated with single dose of cefixime/ceftriaxone/ciprofloxacin/ofloxacin/levofloxacin.
- Single dose of ceftriaxone/ciprofloxacin is effective in oropharyngeal gonococci.
- Ceftriaxone as a single dose is effective in gonococcal conjunctivitis.

- IV ceftriaxone 1g every 24 hours is preferred in disseminated gonococcal infection.
- Single dose of IM or IV ceftriaxone 25 to 50 mg/kg is effective for neonatal gonococcal ocular infection.
- **Nongonococcal urethritis:** Azithromycin/doxycycline.
- **Chancroid:** Azithromycin/ceftriaxone/erythromycin/ciprofloxacin.
- **Trichomoniasis:** Metronidazole/tinidazole.
- **Genital and anal warts:** Podophyllin, trichloroacetic acid and bichlororoacetic acid or podofilox and imiquimod.
- **Chlamydia trachomatis infection:** Azithromycin/doxycycline.
- **Lymphogranuloma venereum:** Doxycycline.
- **Bacterial vaginosis:** Topical metronidazole/topical clindamycin.
- **Genital herpes:** Acyclovir/famciclovir/valacyclovir. Valacyclovir suppresses the transmission of genital herpes infection.

Nursing Responsibilities

- *Chlamydia trachomatis* infection is usually asymptomatic in women. Hence, routine screening can prevent serious complications.
- In trichomoniasis concurrent treatment of asymptomatic male partners of infected women is required.
- Patients with genital herpes should be advised to use condoms permanently or to abstain from sex during active infection.

CHAPTER 65

Chemotherapy of Tuberculosis

FIRST-LINE DRUGS
- Isonicotinic acid hydrazide (INH)
- Rifampin
- Streptomycin
- Ethambutol
- Pyrazinamide

SECOND LINE DRUGS
- Para-aminosalicylic acid (PAS)
- Thiacetazone
- Ethionamide
- Cycloserine
- Fluoroquinolones
- Aminoglycosides
- Terizodine.

ISONICOTINIC ACID HYDRAZIDE (INH)

Actions
- It is a prodrug.
- It is converted to active drug by the enzyme catalase peroxidase.
- It is highly effective against *M. tuberculosis*.
- It has moderate efficacy against some atypical mycobacteria.
- It inhibits synthesis of mycolic acid in mycobacterial cell wall.
- It is tuberculocidal.
- Many organisms have developed resistance to INH.
- It has 100% oral bioavailability.
- It accumulates in pleural, pericardial, pulmonary cavities and in ascitic fluid as well as in tissues.
- It undergoes acetylation, crosses blood-brain barrier (BBB) and accumulates in cerebrospinal fluid (CSF).
- The effective daily dose is 300 mg or 5 mg/kg.
- Pyridoxine 10 mg/day should be coadministered to prevent peripheral neuritis.

Adverse Effects
- Peripheral neuritis, hepatotoxicity
- Optic neuritis, paresthesia, dizziness, ataxia, psychosis
- Vasculitis, arthritis.

RIFAMPIN
Actions
- Rifamycins include rifampin, rifabutin and rifapentine.
- Rifamycins act against *Mycobacterium tuberculosis, M. leprae* and atypical mycobacteria.
- Rifampin also inhibits most Gram-positive bacteria and many Gram-negative bacteria.
- It is also effective against *Proteus, Pseudomonas, Klebsiella, E. coli, Staphylococcus aureus, Haemophilus, N. meningitidis, and Legionella.*
- It is tuberculocidal.
- It inhibits deoxyribonucleic acid (DNA) dependent ribonucleic acid (RNA) polymerase.
- Resistance to rifampin is prevalent among the organisms.
- Food interferes with absorption of rifampin.
- So, it should be given on empty stomach.
- It is an enzyme inducer and causes failure of contraception in women on oral contraceptives.
- It undergoes enterohepatic circulation.
- It accumulates in tissues and in CSF.
- It stains body fluids red.
- Its daily dose is 450 to 600 mg or 10 mg/kg.
- While food does not interfere with absorption of rifabutin, high fat diet increases the absorption of rifapentine.
- The daily dose of rifabutin is 5 mg/kg/day and rifapentine is 10 mg/kg/week.

Adverse Effects
- Fever, rash, flu like syndrome, hepatitis, hypersensitivity, hemolytic anemia
- Red skin, reddish fluid and mucosa
- Interstitial nephritis, thrombocytopenic purpura, myalgia
- Rifabutin also causes polymyalgia, pseudojaundice, anterior uveitis.

Uses
- Tuberculosis (TB), leprosy
- Endocarditis or osteomyelitis by *Staphylococci* organisms
- Prophylaxis for meningitis due to *Meningococcus* and *Haemophilus influenzae*.

PYRAZINAMIDE
Actions
- It is tuberculocidal.
- It is effective in acidic pH.
- It interferes with the synthesis of mycolic acid.
- Resistance is prevalent among strains of *Mycobacterium* that express pyrazinamide.
- It has 90% bioavailability.
- It concentrates in lung.
- It is not safe during pregnancy.
- The effective dose is 15 to 30 mg/kg/day.

Adverse Effects
Hepatotoxicity, hyperuricemia, arthralgia, anorexia, dysuria, fever.

ETHAMBUTOL
Actions
- It inhibits the synthesis of arabinogalactan.
- Thereby, it interferes with the integrity of mycobacterial cell wall.
- It is very effective against typical and atypical Mycobacteria.
- The resistance is prevalent among strains of *Mycobacterium*.
- It has 80% oral bioavailability.
- Its daily dose is 15 to 25 mg/kg/day.

Adverse Effects
- Diminished visual acuity and inability to discriminate red or green color
- Headache, dizziness, mental confusion, pruritus, rash, hyperuricemia

STREPTOMYCIN
Actions
- It is tuberculocidal.
- It acts only on extracellular organisms in alkaline pH.

- Tubercle bacilli develop both streptomycin resistance as well as streptomycin dependence.
- The effective daily dose is 0.75 to 1 g.
- It is not absorbed orally.
- It should be administered as intramuscular injection.
- It causes ototoxicity and nephrotoxicity.

ETHIONAMIDE
Actions
- It is tuberculocidal.
- It interferes with cell wall synthesis.
- It has 100% oral bioavailability.
- Its plasma and tissue concentration are equal.
- The maximum daily dose is 15 to 25 mg/kg.
- Coadministration of pyridoxine prevents its neurological side effects.

Adverse Effects
- Nausea, vomiting, anorexia, gastric irritation, postural hypotension
- Depression, impotence
- Diplopia, dizziness, tremor, blurred vision.

PARA-AMINOSALICYLIC ACID (PAS)
Actions
- It is a structural analog of para-aminobenzoic acid (PABA).
- It inhibits folate synthesis.
- It is tuberculostatic.
- It has more than 90% bioavailability.
- Food increases its bioavailability.
- It is effective only at a high daily dose of 10 to 12 g.

Adverse Effects
Fever, skin eruptions, eosinophilia, blood dyscrasias.

CYCLOSERINE
Actions
- It inhibits mycobacterial cell wall synthesis.
- Organisms have developed resistance to cycloserine.

- It is completely absorbed orally.
- Its CSF concentration is equal to its plasma concentration.
- Its dose is 250 to 500 mg twice daily.

Adverse Effects
- Headache, psychosis (psyche serine), seizure
- Somnolence, suicidal tendencies.

FLUOROQUINOLONES
- Moxifloxacin, ciprofloxacin, ofloxacin, and levofloxacin are used.
- They are effective against *Mycobacterium tuberculosis* and atypical mycobacteria.
- Moxifloxacin is an alternative to ethambutol as first line drug.
- The daily dose of moxifloxacin is 400 mg in pulmonary tuberculosis.

AMINOGLYCOSIDES
- Amikacin, kanamycin and capreomycin are effective against *mycobacteria*.
- Cross resistance can develop between kanamycin and capreomycin.

THIACETAZONE
- It has low efficacy.
- Hence, it is not indicated for the treatment of tuberculosis.

TERIZODINE
- It is similar to cycloserine but less neurotoxic.
- It is a substitute to cycloserine in genitourinary tuberculosis.

REGIMES FOR PULMONARY TUBERCULOSIS
Pyridoxine 10 to 50 mg should be added with INH to minimize the neurotoxicity in elders, diabetics, alcoholics, pregnant women and for HIV infection in malnourished patients.

Directly Observed Treatment Short Course (DOTS)
Very effective with minimal side effects
Intensive phase: INH+R+Z+E thrice weekly for 2 months.
If sputum is positive, than intensive phase is continued for 1 more month.

Continuation phase: INH + R thrice weekly for 4 months.
Total duration 6 months.
INH = Isonicotinic acid hydrazide
R = Rifampin
Z = Pyrazinamide
E = Ethambutol
SM = Streptomycin

Optimal Therapy
- **Intensive phase:** INH+R+Z+E daily for 2 months.
- **Continuation phase:** INH+R daily for 4 months.
Total duration 6 months.

Previously Treated Patients
Intensive phase:
- INH+ R+Z+E+SM daily for 2 months.
- INH+R+Z+E daily for 1 month.

Continuation phase: INH+R+E daily for 8 months.
Total duration 11 months.

MULTIDRUG RESISTANT (MDR) TB REGIME
- **Intensive phase:** Kanamycin, ofloxacin/levofloxacin, cycloserine, ethionamide, pyrazinamide and ethambutol daily for 6 to 9 months are given. Pyridoxine 100 mg/day should be added.
- **Continuation phase:** Ofloxacin/levofloxacin, cycloserine, ethionamide, and ethambutol are given daily for 18 months.

TUBERCULOSIS IN PREGNANCY
- **Intensive phase:** INH+R+E daily for 2 months.
- **Continuation phase**: INH+R daily for 7 months.
Total duration 9 months.

TUBERCULOSIS IN HIV
- **Intensive phase:** INH+R+Z+E daily for 2 months.
- **Continuation phase:** INH+R daily for 7 months.
Total duration 9 months.
- Thrice daily regimen can cause relapse and not recommended.
- In HIV patients on protease inhibitors and non-nucleoside reverse-transcriptase inhibitors (NNRTIs), rifampin is not advised as it causes enzyme induction.
- Rifabutin can be substituted to rifampin in such patients.

CHEMOPROPHYLAXIS
- INH (300 mg or 10 mg/kg) daily for 6 months (or)
- INH (5 mg) +R (10 mg/kg) daily for 3 months.

CORTICOSTEROIDS IN TUBERCULOSIS
- They are used only in seriously ill patients with miliary or severe pulmonary, meningeal, pericardial or renal tuberculosis.
- They are also given to reduce the hypersensitivity reaction to anti-tuberculous drugs.
- They are contraindicated in intestinal tuberculosis.
- They should be withdrawn carefully.

MYCOBACTERIUM AVIUM COMPLEX (MAC) INFECTION
- *Mycobacterium avium* complex causes disseminated tuberculosis.
- The drugs provide only symptomatic relief.

The combinations are:
- (Clarithromycin/azithromycin) + rifabutin+ ethambutol ± fluoroquinolone daily during intensive phase till symptoms subside
- It is followed by maintenance phase with: (Clarithromycin/azithromycin) + (rifabutin/ethambutol/fluoroquinolone).

NURSING RESPONSIBILITIES
- Liver function in patients on anti-tuberculous regimes should be monitored.
- Persistent nausea, vomiting, anorexia, fatigue, jaundice, dark urine and upper abdominal pain are all signs of hepatic dysfunction and patients having such symptoms should be monitored for liver enzymes and referred to the attending physician.
- Since small daily dose (10 mg) of pyridoxine prevents INH induced peripheral neuropathy, patients should be advised to take pyridoxine regularly.
- Patients on rifampin should be informed about its ability to impart red color to urine, tears, saliva, sweat, and other body fluids.

CHAPTER 66

Chemotherapy of Leprosy

Drugs used in leprosy are:
- Dapsone
- Rifampin
- Clofazimine
- Ethionamide
- Clarithromycin
- Ofloxacin
- Moxifloxacin
- Minocycline.

DAPSONE

Actions

- It is a diamino-diphenyl sulfone.
- It inhibits incorporation of para-aminobenzoic acid (PABA) into folic acid.
- Excessive PABA can antagonize its action.
- It is effective against *M. leprae, Toxoplasma gondii, P. falciparum* and *Pneumocystis jirovecii.*
- It is well absorbed and widely distributed.
- Its concentration in red blood cell (RBC) is high but its concentration in cerebrospinal fluid (CSF) is poor.
- It also has an anti-inflammatory property.
- It concentrates in skin, liver, muscle, and kidney.
- It undergoes enterohepatic circulation and metabolized by acetylation.

Adverse Effects

- Hemolytic anemia in patients with glucose-6-phosphate dehydrogenase (G6PD) deficiency, methemoglobinemia
- Nervousness, headache, rash, insomnia
- Sulfone syndrome characterized by fever, lymphadenopathy, anemia, jaundice.

Uses
- Leprosy
- Chloroquine resistant malaria
- Toxoplasmosis
- Pemphigoid, dermatitis herpetiformis
- *P. jirovecii* infection.

CLOFAZIMINE
Actions
- It has antibacterial and anti-inflammatory properties.
- It causes membrane disruption of susceptible organisms.
- It inhibits macrophages, neutrophils and T cells.
- It is absorbed on oral administration and high fat meal increases its absorption.
- Crystal deposition occurs in intestinal mucosa, liver, spleen and abdominal lymph nodes.

Adverse Effects
- Alternate reddish black discoloration of skin and hair.
- Abdominal pain, nausea, vomiting, diarrhea.

Uses
- Leprosy
- Lepra reaction

RIFAMPIN
- The daily required dose of rifampin in leprosy is 600 mg.
- It has rapid action.
- It is included in the therapy of multibacillary leprosy.
- It should be avoided in patients with erythema nodosum leprosum.

Other details: See Section XI, Chapter 65

OFLOXACIN
- It is included in Multi-drug therapy as an alternate drug.
- It is leprocidal and used only in rifampin resistant infection.
- The daily required dose is 400 mg.
- Other fluoroquinolones used in leprosy are pefloxacin, moxifloxacin and sparfloxacin.

MINOCYCLINE
- It concentrates within *M. leprae.*
- It is highly lipophilic and can cause vertigo.

CLARITHROMYCIN
- It causes rapid clinical improvement.
- Its action is synergistic with minocycline.

ETHIONAMIDE
It shows significant activity against *M. leprae* but is highly hepatotoxic.

REGIME FOR PAUCIBACILLARY LEPROSY
Dapsone 100 mg daily and rifampin 600 mg once a month supervised for 6 months.

REGIME FOR MULTIBACILLARY LEPROSY
- Dapsone 100 mg and clofazimine 50 mg daily
- Rifampin 600 mg and clofazimine 300 mg once monthly
- Duration of treatment is 1 year
- This is followed by dapsone 100 mg as monotherapy for 10 years.

Lepra Reaction
- It may be mild or very severe (erythema nodosum leprosum).
- It occurs due to release of antigens from lepra bacilli.
- It has an abrupt onset and necessitates discontinuation of dapsone.
- Clofazimine 200 mg daily and prednisolone 40 to 60 mg/day are effective.
- Thalidomide is also effective as it has an anti-inflammatory action.

Reversal Reaction
- It occurs after a successful completion of full course of therapy.
- It is due to delayed hypersensitivity reaction to *M. leprae* antigens.
- It is characterized by painful, swollen nerves and skin ulcers.
- Thalidomide is not effective in reversal reaction.
- Only corticosteroids and clofazimine are effective.

Nursing Responsibilities
Since dapsone can cause hemolysis in patients with G6PD deficiency, patients on dapsone should be informed to report hematuria.

CHAPTER 67

Chemotherapy of Worm Infestation

NEMATODES
- **Roundworm:** *Ascaris lumbricoides*
- **Hookworm:** *Necator americanus, Ancylostoma duodenale*
- **Threadworm:** *Strongyloides stercoralis*
- **Whipworm:** *Trichuris trichiura, Trichinella spiralis*
- **Pinworm:** *Enterobius vermicularis*
- **Guinea worm:** *Dracunculus medinensis.*

CESTODES
- **Fish tapeworm:** *Diphyllobothrium latum*
- **Beef tapeworm:** *Taenia saginata*
- **Pork tapeworm:** *Taenia solium*
- **Dwarf tapeworm:** *Hymenolepis nana*
- **Hydatid disease:** *Echinococcus granulosus, Echinococcus multilocularis.*

TREMATODES
- **Blood flukes:** *Schistosoma haematobium, Schistosoma mansoni, Schistosoma japonicum*
- **Lung flukes:** *Paragonimus westermani*
- **Liver fluke:** *Fasciola hepatica*
- **Chinese liver fluke:** *Clonorchis sinensis.*

MEBENDAZOLE
- The cure rate is high in roundworm, hookworm, pinworm and whipworm infestation.
- It is less effective in threadworm infestation.
- It reduces the size of hydatid cyst in liver.
- By reducing the glucose uptake, it depletes the glycogen stores of worms.
- Starved worms sometimes migrate from intestine to nose and mouth.

- It is minimally absorbed from gastrointestinal tract (GIT) and acts locally.
- It is contraindicated during pregnancy.

Adverse Effects
- Nausea, vomiting and abdominal pain
- Rarely alopecia, agranulocytosis.

Uses
- 100 mg twice daily for 3 days is effective against roundworm, hookworm and whipworm.
- Second course after 3 weeks if required.
- Single 100 mg dose is adequate in pinworm but should be repeated after 2 weeks to prevent reinfection.

ALBENDAZOLE
Actions
- It is a broad spectrum anthelmintic agent.
- Its efficacy is superior to mebendazole in hookworm, threadworm and whipworm infestation.
- It is also effective in giardiasis and trichomoniasis.
- Unlike mebendazole, it is effective as a single dose in roundworm, hookworm and pinworm infestation.
- It is a second line agent in tapeworm infestation.
- It is more effective than mebendazole in hydatid disease.
- By reducing the glucose uptake, it depletes the glycogen stores of worms.
- Its metabolite albendazole sulfoxide accumulates in tissues including brain.
- Albendazole sulfoxide also has potent anthelmintic action.
- The oral absorption is high after a fatty meal.
- It is contraindicated in pregnancy.

Adverse Effects
- Nausea, vomiting, diarrhea, epigastric pain
- Dizziness, headache.

Uses
- Dose is 400 mg single dose for roundworm, hookworm, whipworm and pinworm infestation.

Chemotherapy of Worm Infestation

- 400 mg daily for 3 days is required in threadworm infestation.
- It is the drug of choice in neurocysticercosis due to larval forms of pork tapeworm.
- Prolonged therapy with twice daily doses of albendazole is required for hydatid disease.
- It is an adjunct to diethylcarbamazine (DEC) or ivermectin in filariasis.

PYRANTEL PAMOATE
Actions
- It is highly effective in roundworm, pinworm and *Ancylostoma duodenale* infestation.
- It is less effective in threadworm and *Necator americanus* infestation.
- It is not effective in whipworm infestation.
- It causes spastic paralysis of worms.
- Purging is not required as the worms are expelled completely.
- It should not be used in children and during pregnancy.

Adverse Effects
- Nausea, vomiting, headache
- Dizziness, rash, fever.

Uses
- 10 mg/kg single dose for roundworm, pinworm and *Ancylostoma duodenale* infestation.
- Dose should be repeated after 2 weeks for pinworm infestation.
- A 3-day course is essential for *Necator americanus* infestation.

PIPERAZINE CITRATE
Actions
- It results in 100% cure rate in roundworm and pinworm infestation.
- It causes flaccid paralysis of worms.
- Hence, purging is necessary to expel the worms.

Adverse Effects
- Nausea, vomiting, urticaria
- Dizziness.

Uses
- 4 g once daily for two days in roundworm infestation.
- 50 mg/kg (maximum 2 g) once daily for 7 days in pinworm infestation.

LEVAMISOLE
Actions
- It causes tonic paralysis of worms.
- It is effective in roundworm infestation and ancylostomiasis.
- It is also an immunomodulator.

Adverse Effects
- Nausea, abdominal pain
- Dizziness, insomnia.

Uses
- Single dose of 150 mg for adults in roundworm infestation
- Two doses of 150 mg at 12 hours interval in ancylostomiasis
- Rheumatoid arthritis
- Aphthous ulcer
- Recurrent herpes infection

NICLOSAMIDE
Actions
- It results in 95% cure rate in beef, fish and dwarf tapeworm infestation.
- It inhibits the adenosine triphosphate (ATP) synthesis in worms.
- Purging is necessary for expulsion of worms.
- Otherwise, ova released from gravid worms develop into larva and cause cysticercosis.
- The scolex should be searched for in stools.

Adverse Effects
Pruritus, dizziness, malaise.

Uses
- Two 500 mg tablets are chewed and swallowed followed by 2 more tablets after 1 hour in pork tapeworm infestation.
- Saline purge should be given 2 hours after last dose
- For dwarf tapeworm a dose of 2 g daily for 5 days.

PRAZIQUANTEL

Actions
- It is effective against most cestodes and trematodes.
- It does not act against nematodes.
- It is the drug of choice in blood fluke infestation.
- It causes spastic paralysis of worms.
- The worms lose grip and are expelled.
- Hence, purging is not necessary for expulsion of worms.
- It causes tegumental damage in worms at high concentration.
- It is not effective against juvenile blood flukes.
- So, it is not effective in early infection.
- It is absorbed after oral administration.
- It undergoes high first pass metabolism.
- It accumulates in cerebrospinal fluid (CSF) as it crosses blood-brain barrier (BBB).
- It is contraindicated in neurocysticercosis and ocular cysticercosis.

Adverse Effects
- Nausea due to bitter taste
- Dizziness, headache, sedation
- Cutaneous reactions such as urticaria and pruritus due to dead worms.

Uses
- 25 mg/kg in dwarf tapeworm infestation
- 10 to 20 mg/kg for fish, beef and pork tapeworm
- Single dose of 40 mg/kg in blood fluke infestation
- 75 mg/kg in 3 divided doses for liver and Chinese liver flukes.

Nursing Responsibilities
- Simultaneous treatment of children with other family members and strict hygienic measures is required to prevent autoinfection in pinworm infestation.
- The scolex of *T. solium* should be searched for in stools to prevent reinfection.

METRIFONATE
- It is effective against blood flukes.
- It is an irreversible anticholinesterase agent.
- It is generally used in veterinary practice.

CHAPTER 68

Chemotherapy of Filariasis

The drugs used in filariasis are:
- Diethylcarbamazine citrate (DEC)
- Ivermectin.

DIETHYLCARBAMAZINE CITRATE (DEC)

Actions
- It is effective against *W. bancrofti* and *B. malayi*.
- It damages the cellular organelles of microfilariae.
- It kills microfilariae in blood but not in transudate (hydrocele) or nodules.
- It is also effective against microfilariae of *L. loa*.
- Rapid destruction of microfilariae of *O. volvulus* can worsen the ocular lesions.
- Hence, it is contraindicated in *O. volvulus*.
- It is well absorbed and acidic urine increases its excretion.
- A dose of 2 mg/kg, 3 times daily results in clinical improvement within 7 days.
- Prolonged therapy is required to kill adult worms.

Adverse Effects
- Nausea, loss of appetite
- Headache, dizziness
- Delayed reaction to adult worms can cause lymphangitis, lymphoid abscess and swelling
- Rapid destruction of worms and larvae can result in Mazzotti reaction causing fever, dizziness, headache, peripheral edema, and hypotension.

Uses
- Filariasis
- Tropical pulmonary eosinophilia

IVERMECTIN
Actions
- It causes rapid and marked reduction in microfilariae of *O. volvulus*.
- It kills microfilariae but not the adult worms of *W. bancrofti, L. loa* and *B. malayi*.
- It is very effective against threadworm, roundworms and cutaneous larva migrans.
- It causes tonic paralysis of worms.
- It suppresses the ocular inflammation due to *O. volvulus*.
- It is well absorbed, has long-duration of action and does not cross blood-brain barrier (BBB).
- It is not indicated in pregnant women or in children.

Adverse Effects
- Nausea, abdominal pain
- Dizziness, pruritus
- Electrocardiogram (ECG) changes
- Rapid destruction of worms and larvae of *O. volvulus* can result in Mazzotti-like reaction causing fever, dizziness, headache, peripheral edema, and hypotension.

Uses
- Single dose of 150 to 200 µg/kg every 6 to 12 months in onchocerciasis
- Single annual dose of 200 µg/kg with 400 mg of albendazole (dual-drug regimen) for eradication of *W. bancrofti* and *B. malayi*
- Single dose of 150 to 200 µg/kg in threadworm infestation.

CHAPTER 69

Antimalarial Drugs

- Of the five *Plasmodium* species, malaria is most frequently caused by *P. vivax* and *P. falciparum*.
- Malaria due to *P. ovale* and *P. malariae* is infrequent but still necessitates treatment.
- The relapse rate is high in malaria due to *P. vivax* and *P. ovale* organisms.
- *P. malariae* organisms can be transmitted during blood transfusion.
- *P. knowlesi* malaria occurs in South-East Asian countries.

The antimalarial agents are classified as:
- **Causal prophylactic agents:** Primaquine, proguanil
- **Suppressive prophylactic agents:** Chloroquine, mefloquine, doxycycline
- **Agents causing clinical cure:** Artemisinin, chloroquine, quinine, amodiaquine, mefloquine, halofantrine, atovaquone, lumefantrine, proguanil, pyrimethamine, sulfonamides, tetracyclines, clindamycin
- **Radical cure:** Primaquine
- **Gametocidal:** Primaquine.

ARTEMISININ AND ITS DERIVATIVES

Actions

- It is obtained from *Qing hao* or sweet worm wood.
- Artesunate, artemether and dihydroartemisinin are its derivatives.
- It is fast acting and causes rapid clearance of *Plasmodium* species.
- It is very effective against severe *P. falciparum* infection and asexual erythrocytic stages of *P. vivax*.
- It inhibits the activity of the heme adduct or hemozoin formed by the *Plasmodium*.
- Further, it promotes lipid peroxidation and lysis of parasitized erythrocytes.
- Artemisinin-based combination therapy (ACT) is preferred to monotherapy of artemisinin.

Antimalarial Drugs

- Since the duration of action of artemisinins is short, they are not suitable for chemoprophylaxis.
- Besides they result in higher relapse rate.
- The drug combinations of ACT are artemether-lumefantrine, artesunate-mefloquine, artesunate-amodiaquine, dihydroartemisinin-piperaquine, and artesunate-sulfadoxine-pyrimethamine.
- Artemisinin derivatives are available for oral, rectal, intramuscular (IM) and intravenous (IV) preparations.
- Fatty meal increases the oral absorption of artemether-lumefantrine combination.
- This is an extensively used combination and effective in *P. falciparum* infection.
- The advantages of ACT are that it is well tolerated, causes high cure rate, low relapse rate and delayed development of resistance.

Adverse Effects
- Nausea, vomiting, drug fever
- Tinnitus, headache
- Bleeding, dark urine
- Prolonged QT.

Use
Uncomplicated and severe complicated falciparum malaria.

ATOVAQUONE
Actions
- It is effective against *P. falciparum, P. vivax, Pneumocystis jirovecii* and *Toxoplasma gondii*.
- It acts against asexual erythrocytic forms of *P. falciparum*.
- It is effective against hepatic stages of *P. falciparum* but not against *P. vivax*.
- It inhibits mitochondrial adenosine triphosphate (ATP) production of malarial parasites.
- Proguanil facilitates its action but resistance develops to this combination.
- Fatty meal increases its absorption and it undergoes enterohepatic circulation.
- It is not preferred in pregnant and lactating women.

Adverse Effects
- Nausea, vomiting, diarrhea
- Rash, abdominal pain

Use
Combined with proguanil in chemoprophylaxis and treatment of uncomplicated *P. falciparum* malaria.

PYRIMETHAMINE
Actions
- It is a slow acting blood schizonticide.
- It inhibits folic acid synthesis in malarial parasites.
- It does not eradicate the hypnozoits or gametocytes of *P. vivax* and hepatic forms of *P. falciparum*.
- It results in synergistic inhibition of folic acid synthesis when combined with sulfadoxine.

Adverse Effects
Sulfadoxine-pyrimethamine combination causes:
- Erythema multiforme
- Stevens-Johnson syndrome
- Toxic epidermal necrolysis.

Use
Intermittent prophylaxis of malaria during pregnancy.

PROGUANIL
Actions
- It inhibits both asexual erythrocytic and hepatic stages of *P. falciparum*.
- It is also effective in acute *P. vivax* infection.
- Relapse is common as it does not suppress the latent stages of *P. vivax*.
- It inhibits the DNA synthesis in *Plasmodium* species.
- Oral absorption is slow but adequate.
- It accumulates in red blood cell (RBC).
- It is safe in pregnancy.

Adverse Effects
- Vomiting, diarrhea, abdominal pain
- Hematuria

Use
Chemoprophylaxis for those traveling to endemic areas in Africa.

CHLOROQUINE
Actions
- It is inexpensive.
- It is an erythrocytic schizonticide of all *Plasmodium* species.
- It has rapid action and clinical cure is evident within 3 days.
- It concentrates within the acidic digestive vacuoles of susceptible *Plasmodium*.
- There, it binds to and inhibits the sequestration of heme causing oxidative damage to the parasites.
- It does not prevent relapse in malaria due to *P. vivax* and *P. ovale* organisms.
- Most strains of *Plasmodium* are resistant to chloroquine.
- Resistance is already prevalent in North-Eastern parts of India, Karnataka and Odisha.
- It is also effective against *Giardia lamblia* and *E. histolytica*.
- Chloroquine has anti-inflammatory action.
- Bioavailability after oral, subcutaneous (SC) and intramuscular administration is good.
- It accumulates in liver, spleen, lungs, and kidney.

Precautions and Contraindications
- Myasthenia gravis
- Epilepsy
- Liver disease, gastrointestinal tract (GIT) disorders
- Glucose-6-phosphate dehydrogenase (G6PD) deficiency
- Exfoliative dermatitis, porphyria
- Psoriasis
- Porphyria cutanea tarda.

Adverse Effects
- Hypotension, arrhythmia
- Convulsion, headache, visual disturbance
- Nausea, vomiting
- Pruritus, skin eruption, bleaching of hair, urticaria
- Retinopathy, hemolysis

Uses
- Malaria due to *P. vivax*, *P. ovale* and *P. malariae*
- Chloroquine sensitive *P. falciparum* malaria
- Chemoprophylaxis of malaria

- Rheumatoid arthritis
- Systemic lupus erythematosus (SLE)
- Lepra reaction
- Extraintestinal amebiasis
- Sarcoidosis.

AMODIAQUINE

- It is a congener of chloroquine.
- It is highly toxic and causes agranulocytosis and hepatotoxicity.
- It is effective in treatment of uncomplicated *P. falciparum* malaria.

QUININE

Actions

- It is an alkaloid obtained from Cinchona bark.
- It acts on asexual erythrocytic forms of *Plasmodium* species.
- Resistance to quinine is highly prevalent in India.
- It binds to heme and prevents its detoxification.
- It causes skeletal muscle relaxation.
- It is well absorbed on oral and IM administration.

Adverse Effects

- Hypoglycemia, postural hypotension.
- Nausea, vomiting, headache, QT prolongation.
- **Cinchonism:** High frequency hearing loss, tinnitus, visual disturbances.
- Hypoglycemia can be life-threatening and may require administration of intravenous (IV) glucose.
- **Black water fever:** Occurs due to hypersensitivity reaction to quinine therapy resulting in hemolysis, hemoglobinemia and hemoglobinuria.

Use

P. falciparum malaria

MEFLOQUINE

Actions

- It inhibits the detoxification of heme.
- It is a blood schizonticide but not effective against hepatic forms and gametocytes of *P. falciparum*.
- It does not inhibit the latent stages of *P. vivax* and does not prevent relapse.

- The oral absorption is good and it undergoes enterohepatic circulation.
- It is extensively bound to plasma proteins.
- Its half-life is long and extends upto 24 days.

Contraindications
- Seizures
- Bipolar disorder
- Depression
- Pregnancy.

Adverse Effects
- Seizure, confusion, psychosis, dizziness
- Nausea, vomiting, headache, disturbed sleep.

Uses
- Reserve drug for drug resistant *P. falciparum* and *P. vivax*
- Chemoprophylaxis for travelers to endemic areas.

PRIMAQUINE
Actions
- It is effective against exoerythrocytic stages of *Plasmodium* species.
- Hence, it prevents relapse.
- It is gametocytocidal but inactive against asexual erythrocytic stages of *Plasmodium* species.
- It generates reactive oxygen species (ROS) that interferes with plasmodial mitochondrial function.
- It has 100% oral bioavailability and extensive tissue distribution.

Adverse Effects
- Hemolysis in patients with G6PD deficiency
- Anemia, methemoglobinemia, leukocytosis
- Rarely granulocytopenia, agranulocytosis.

Use
Chemoprophylaxis and radical cure in *P. vivax* and *P. ovale* infection.

SULFONAMIDES
- It is a para-aminobenzoic acid (PABA) analog.
- It inhibits folic acid synthesis of *Plasmodium*.

- Sulfadoxine, the long-acting sulfonamide is combined with pyrimethamine.
- It is approved for intermittent chemoprophylaxis during 2nd and 3rd trimester of pregnancy but *Plasmodium* species is resistant to this combination.

DOXYCYCLINE
- It is a slow acting blood schizonticide.
- It is used for short-term chemoprophylaxis in areas with chloroquine or mefloquine resistant malaria.
- It inhibits protein synthesis in malarial parasites.
- It is not effective as monotherapy for clinical cure in malaria.
- It is not indicated during pregnancy.

LUMEFANTRINE

Actions
- It is a long-acting erythrocytic schizonticide.
- It inhibits the detoxification of heme.
- It is combined with artemether to prevent the development of resistance by *Plasmodium* species to artemether.
- Fatty food increases its absorption.
- It is contraindicated during pregnancy and in lactating mothers.

Adverse Effects
- Pruritus, myalgia, arthralgia
- Dizziness, rash
- QT prolongation.

Use
Drug resistant *P. falciparum* infection.

Nursing Responsibilities
- Heart rate and ECG should be periodically monitored in patients on chloroquine.
- Visual disturbance in patients on chloroquine may indicate retinopathy and should be reported to the attending physician as it may require discontinuation of drug.
- Visual and auditory disturbance in patients on quinine may indicate cinchonism and should be reported to the attending physician.

Chemotherapy of Amebiasis

- Amebiasis is caused by *E. histolytica*.
- It is common in crowded areas with poor sanitation.
- Patients are either symptomatic with active disease or asymptomatic cyst carriers.
- The trophozoites invade into colonic mucosa and reside there, causing colitis.
- They can also invade through colonic mucosa and enter the portal circulation to form amebic abscess.
  - I. **Tissue amebicides:**
    - a. Effective in intestinal and extraintestinal form of amebiasis: Metronidazole, tinidazole, secnidazole, ornidazole, emetine, dehydroemetine.
    - b. Effective only in extraintestinal amebiasis: Chloroquine.
  - II. **Luminal amebicides:** Nitazoxanide, paromomycin, tetracycline, quiniodochlor, diiodohydroxyquin, diloxanide.

METRONIDAZOLE

Actions

- It is effective against anaerobic protozoal organisms such as *E. histolytica, G. lamblia* and *T. vaginalis*.
- It also acts against anaerobic cocci, anaerobic Gram-negative bacilli and spore-forming anaerobic Gram-positive bacilli.
- *Bacteroides, Clostridia, Helicobacter pylori,* and *Campylobacter* are also susceptible.
- It is a prodrug.
- It is converted to its active nitro moiety which is cytotoxic to parasites.
- It is completely absorbed orally.
- It attains high concentration in saliva, milk, seminal fluid, vaginal secretions, and cerebrospinal fluid (CSF).
- It is available as oral, topical, intravenous, and intravaginal preparations.

- Tinidazole has high cure rate with better tolerability and long-duration of action.
- Ornidazole and secnidazole have long-duration of action.

Adverse Effects
- Metallic taste, vomiting, nausea, diarrhea.
- Headache, dizziness, rashes, urticaria, vertigo
- Disulfiram like reaction, flurry tongue, glossitis, stomatitis
- Stevens-Johnson syndrome.

Contraindication
Central nervous system (CNS) disease.

Uses
- Intestinal and extraintestinal amebiasis
- Giardiasis
- Trichomoniasis
- *H. pylori* infection
- Anaerobic infection
- Pseudomembranous colitis due to *Clostridium difficile.*

EMETINE, DEHYDROEMETINE
Actions
- It is effective in severe, invasive intestinal amebiasis and in extraintestinal amebiasis.
- It kills trophozoites but not the amebic cysts.
- It is rarely used nowadays as it is highly toxic.
- It can be administered only through parenteral route.

Adverse Effects
- Emesis, diarrhea, abdominal pain
- Hypotension

CHLOROQUINE
- It is an amebicide.
- It is totally absorbed from gastrointestinal tract (GIT).
- Hence, it cannot be used as a luminal amebicide in intestinal amebiasis.
- It concentrates in liver.
- So, it is effective in hepatic amebiasis.

- Prolonged therapy is required.
- The relapse rate is high.

For other details: See Section XI, Chapter 69

NITAZOXANIDE

Actions

- It is a broad-spectrum antiparasitic agent.
- It is effective against *E. histolytica, G. lamblia* and *T. vaginalis.*
- It is also effective against *H. pylori, Cyclospora* and *Blastocystis.*
- It has marked activity against roundworm, pinworm, whipworm, hookworm, threadworm, dwarf tapeworm and liver fluke.
- It inhibits the enzymes necessary for anaerobic metabolism of protozoa and bacteria.
- It has excellent oral bioavailability.
- Both the drug and its active metabolite are effective against the protozoa and helminths.

Adverse Effects

- Vomiting, diarrhea, abdominal pain
- Headache, greenish urine

Uses

- Amebiasis
- Giardiasis
- Mixed protozoal and helminth intestinal infestation.

PAROMOMYCIN

Actions

- It is an aminoglycoside antibiotic.
- So, it is not absorbed from GIT.
- Hence, it acts in GIT as a luminal amebicide.
- It inhibits protein synthesis of protozoa.
- It is combined with tissue amebicide in the treatment of amebiasis.
- Topical formulation is effective in cutaneous leishmaniasis.
- Parenteral intramuscular (IM) administration is effective in visceral leishmaniasis.

Adverse Effects

- Epigastric distress, diarrhea
- Nausea, vomiting, abdominal cramps
- Steatorrhea.

Uses
- Amebiasis
- Giardiasis in pregnancy
- Trichomoniasis
- Cutaneous and visceral leishmaniasis
- Cryptosporidiosis.

TETRACYCLINES
- They have modest activity against *E. histolytica*.
- They are useful in chronic amebiasis.
- Tetracycline is added as a third drug in metronidazole, luminal amebicide combination.

DILOXANIDE
- It is useful in chronic amebiasis.
- It eradicates the cysts.
- It is well tolerated.
- It causes flatulence and urticaria.

QUINIODOCHLOR, DIIODOHYDROXYQUIN
- They are effective against *E. histolytica, G. lamblia* and *T. vaginalis*
- They kill the cyst forming trophozoites in intestine.
- They are effective in chronic amebiasis.
- They have variable rate of absorption.
- They can cause 'iodism' and goiter.

Nursing Responsibilities
- Symptoms of dizziness, vertigo and ataxia in patients on metronidazole should be reported to the attending physician as it may require discontinuation of the drug.
- Patients on metronidazole should be cautioned to avoid alcohol as it can cause antabuse like reaction.

CHAPTER 71

Chemotherapy of Other Protozoal Infection

AFRICAN TRYPANOSOMIASIS
- It is caused by *Trypanosoma brucei gambiense* and *Trypanosoma brucei rhodesiense*.
- It is transmitted through bites of tsetse flies.

WEST AFRICAN (GAMBIAN) TRYPANOSOMIASIS
- West African trypanosomiasis is caused by *Trypanosoma brucei gambiense*. It is characterized by hemolymphatic stage that progresses to meningoencephalitic stage.
- Pentamidine and eflornithine are effective against West African trypanosomiasis.

EFLORNITHINE

Actions
- It is an irreversible, suicide inhibitor of ornithine decarboxylase required for cell division and cell differentiation.
- It is a cytostatic agent and causes polyamine depletion in trypanosomes.
- *Trypanosoma brucei gambiense* is highly sensitive while *Trypanosoma brucei rhodesiense* is less sensitive.
- Hence, it is effective in West African (Gambian) trypanosomiasis and not effective in East African trypanosomiasis.
- It is administered intravenously.
- It has limited oral bioavailability.
- It does not bind to plasma proteins.
- Its entry into cerebrospinal fluid (CSF) is increased in *T. brucei* infection.
- Suramin increases the CSF uptake of eflornithine.

Adverse Effects
- Headache, abdominal pain
- Infusion site reactions
- Reversible hearing loss

Use
Late stage West African trypanosomiasis.

PENTAMIDINE
Actions
- It is a trypanocidal and inhibits deoxyribonucleic acid (DNA) and protein synthesis of trypanosomes.
- It is effective in early stage but not in late stage trypanosomiasis.
- It is poorly absorbed orally.
- So, it is administered through intramuscular or intravenous route.
- It is also administered as aerosol preparation for prophylaxis of *Pneumocystis pneumoniae* infection.
- It does not cross blood-brain barrier (BBB).
- It is highly toxic.
- It can cause life-threatening hypoglycemia during intravenous infusion.

Adverse Effects
- Infusion related side effects such as hypotension, headache and tachycardia
- Nephrotoxicity
- Anemia, neutropenia, skin rash
- Hypoglycemia, hyperglycemia, pancreatitis, and insulin dependent diabetes mellitus
- Elevation of liver enzymes.

Uses
- Early stages of West African trypanosomiasis
- Cutaneous leishmaniasis
- Prophylaxis and treatment of *Pneumocystis* pneumonia.

EAST AFRICAN (RHODESIAN) TRYPANOSOMIASIS
- It is caused by *Trypanosoma brucei rhodesiense.*
- Suramin is more effective than eflornithine or pentamidine.
- Melarsoprol is effective in meningoencephalitic stage.

SURAMIN
Actions
- It is a slow acting trypanocide.

- It concentrates within the trypanosomes where it inhibits many glycolytic enzymes.
- It does not accumulate in tissues and does not enter CSF.
- Hence, it is not effective in meningoencephalitic stage.
- It is administered intravenously.
- It should not be administered subcutaneously or intramuscularly

Adverse Effects
- Nausea, vomiting, hypotension
- Renal toxicity and albuminuria
- Metallic taste, headache, peripheral neuropathy.

Use
First-line therapy in early stage East African trypanosomiasis.

MELARSOPROL
Actions
- It is an arsenical compound.
- It is a prodrug.
- Its active metabolite is trypanocidal.
- The development of resistance is high for melarsoprol.
- It is administered intravenously and accumulates in CSF.
- It is highly toxic.
- It should be administered only under supervision in a hospital set up.

Adverse Effects
- Encephalopathy
- Peripheral neuropathy
- Albuminuria, hepatic dysfunction
- Hypertension, myocardial damage.

Use
Late meningoencephalitic stage of East African trypanosomiasis.

AMERICAN TRYPANOSOMIASIS (CHAGAS DISEASE)
- It is caused by the protozoan parasite *Trypanosoma cruzi*.
- The acute stage is characterized by fever, headache, raised tender skin nodule (chagoma), and lymphadenopathy.

- Cardiac and smooth muscle abnormalities are common in chronic stage.
- Benznidazole and nifurtimox are effective in the treatment of Chagas disease.

NIFURTIMOX AND BENZNIDAZOLE

Actions
- They are trypanocidal against trypomastigote and amastigote forms of *T. cruzi*.
- They generate nitro radical ions which are trypanocidal.
- Both drugs are well absorbed on oral administration.
- Nifurtimox undergoes first pass metabolism.

Adverse Effects
- Fever, dermatitis, anaphylaxis, pulmonary infiltrates
- Nausea, vomiting, myalgia, weakness.

Use
- Benznidazole is preferred to nifurtimox in Chagas disease as it is more effective and less toxic.

LEISHMANIASIS
- It is a zoonotic infection transmitted by sand fly bite.
- Visceral leishmaniasis (kala azar) and cutaneous leishmaniasis are the two types.
- Cutaneous leishmaniasis is usually self-limiting and miltefosine and paromomycin are effective
- Miltefosine, amphotericin B, sodium stibogluconate, and paromomycin are effective in visceral leishmaniasis.

SODIUM STIBOGLUCONATE

Actions
- It is a pentavalent antimonial derivative.
- It is given alongwith meglumine antimonate.
- It kills both amastigotes and promastigotes stage of trypanosomes.
- It is not effective orally.
- It is administered through intramuscular or intravenous route.
- Generally well tolerated and causes reversible side effects.

Adverse Effects
- Pancreatitis
- Elevated asparete aminotransferase (AST), Aalanine aminotransferase (ALT) level
- Bone marrow depression, QT prolongation.

Use
Visceral leishmaniasis.

MILTEFOSINE
Actions
- It is effective in both visceral and cutaneous leishmaniasis.
- It has potent antileishmanial activity.
- It induces apoptosis of both amastigotes and promastigotes.
- Ninety eight percent cure rate is achieved with miltefosine in visceral leishmaniasis.
- It has good oral bioavailability.
- It is well distributed and has long half-life of 1 week.
- It is contraindicated in pregnant women.

Adverse Effects
- Vomiting, diarrhea
- Reversible elevation of AST and ALT.

Use
Visceral and cutaneous leishmaniasis.
Paromomycin: Refer Chapter 70

Nursing Responsibilities
- Monitor blood glucose in patients on pentamidine during infusion.
- Monitor liver and kidney function in patients on pentamidine or melarsoprol as they can cause hepatotoxicity and nephrotoxicity.
- Administer melarsoprol slowly and advice the patients to remain in bed and to avoid eating for several hours after infusion as it can induce severe vomiting.
- Monitor liver enzymes, serum amylase and peripheral blood picture in patients on sodium stibogluconate.
- Monitor liver enzymes in patients on miltefosine.

CHAPTER 72

Chemotherapy of Fungal Infection

- Fungal infection is a common occurrence in immunocompromised HIV patients.
- Antifungal agents are classified as systemic and topical agents.
- Some antifungal agents act on both systemic and superficial fungal infection.
- Although less frequent, systemic mycosis is difficult to treat.
- Opportunistic systemic fungal infections are aspergillosis, candidiasis, mucormycosis and cryptococcosis.
- Nonopportunistic systemic fungal infections are histoplasmosis, blastomycosis, sporotrichosis, and coccidioidomycosis.
  - **Antifungal antibiotics:** Amphotericin B, nystatin, hamycin, caspofungin, micafungin, griseofulvin, anidulafungin
  - **Antimetabolites:** Flucytosine
  - **Imidazoles:** Clotrimazole, econazole, miconazole, oxiconazole, ketoconazole
  - **Triazoles:** Itraconazole, voriconazole, fluconazole, posaconazole, isavuconazole
  - **Others:** Terbinafine, tolnaftate, benzoic acid, undecylenic acid, quiniodochlor, ciclopirox olamine, butenafine, naftifine.

AMPHOTERICIN B

Actions

- It is a polyene macrolide antifungal antibiotic.
- It is very effective but highly toxic.
- It is available in four different formulations.
- They are conventional amphotericin B (C-AMB), liposomal amphotericin B (L-AMB), amphotericin B colloidal dispersion (ABCD) and amphotericin B lipid complex (ABLC).
- It is fungicidal.
- It increases the permeability of fungal cell membrane by binding to its ergosterol moiety.

Chemotherapy of Fungal Infection

- It is effective against *Candida species, Cryptococcus neoformans, Histoplasma capsulatum, Blastomyces dermatitidis, sporothrix species, Paracoccidioides, and Coccidioides.*
- It is also effective against the protozoa *Leishmania spp.*
- Amphotericin is not absorbed orally.
- So, all four formulations are given intravenously.
- Conventional amphotericin B (C-AMB) is water insoluble but made soluble by admixing it with bile salt, deoxycholate.
- Liposomal amphotericin B (L-AMB) is preferred as it causes minimal infusion related side effects.
- Amphotericin B colloidal dispersion (ABCD) results in higher incidence of infusion related reactions.
- Amphotericin B lipid complex (ABLC) attains lower blood levels and is highly nephrotoxic.

Adverse Effects
- Infusion related reaction such as chills, fever, nausea, headache, hypotension, and rigor
- Nephrotoxicity
- Anemia, weight loss
- Hypokalemia.

Uses
- Deeply invasive candidiasis, invasive aspergillosis
- Blastomycosis, coccidioidomycosis
- Histoplasmosis, cryptococcosis
- Mucormycosis, sporotrichosis
- Trichosporonosis

FLUCYTOSINE
Actions
- It is converted to 5-fluorouracil within the fungal cells.
- It is an antimetabolite and inhibits deoxyribonucleic acid (DNA) synthesis.
- It is effective against *Candida* species and *Cryptococcus neoformans.*
- It is rapidly and adequately absorbed after oral administration.
- It is widely distributed throughout the body.
- Most fungi have developed resistance to flucytosine.

- The development of secondary resistance during therapy contributes to its therapeutic failure.
- It is given with amphotericin B in cryptococcal meningitis.

Adverse Effects
- Bone marrow depression
- Nausea, vomiting, rash
- Enterocolitis.

Use
Cryptococcal meningitis.

IMIDAZOLES AND TRIAZOLES
- They share similar mechanism of action and antifungal spectrum.
- They inhibit synthesis of ergosterol, the essential component of fungal cell.
- They are effective against *Candida* species, *Cryptococcus neoformans*, *Coccidioides species*, *Blastomyces dermatitidis*, *Histoplasma capsulatum*, *Paracoccidioides brasiliensis*, and dermatophytes (ringworm).
- *Aspergillus* species and *Sporothrix* have intermediate susceptibility.
- *Candida krusei* and agents causing mucormycosis are resistant to azoles.
- Triazoles act more selectively on fungal cells than the imidazoles.
    - **Triazoles:** Itraconazole, fluconazole, posaconazole, voriconazole, isavuconazole, terconazole.
    - **Imidazoles:** Clotrimazole, ketoconazole, miconazole, econazole, oxiconazole, sertaconazole, sulconazole, butoconazole.

Ketoconazole
Actions
- It is a broad spectrum antifungal agent.
- Although it is cheaper, it is largely replaced by itraconazole.
- In addition to its antifungal property, it also inhibits the synthesis of corticosteroids.
- It is an enzyme inhibitor and increases the plasma level of coadministered drugs.
- It is also available as topical solution.

Chemotherapy of Fungal Infection

Adverse Effects
- Nausea and vomiting, headache, hair loss, loss of appetite
- Gynecomastia – displaces testosterone from its binding sites.

Uses
- Dermatophytosis
- Systemic mycosis

Itraconazole

Actions
- A loading dose of itraconazole is necessary in deep mycosis.
- Since it is teratogenic, it should be avoided in pregnancy.
- Oral solution is well absorbed in empty stomach.
- Its concentration in cerebrospinal fluid (CSF) is minimal.
- It is an enzyme inhibitor and increases the plasma level of coadministered drugs.

Adverse Effects
- Nausea, diarrhea, anorexia, abdominal cramps
- Hepatotoxicity, congestive heart failure
- Hypokalemia, hypertriglyceridemia

Uses
- Histoplasmosis, blastomycosis
- Tinea infection
- Sporotrichosis, subungual onychomycosis
- Aspergillosis, oropharyngeal candidiasis

Fluconazole

Actions
- It has excellent oral bioavailability even in the presence of food.
- It attains similar plasma concentration after oral and intravenous (IV) administration.
- It is extensively distributed into body fluids and tissues.
- It concentrates highly in saliva, milk, sputum and CSF.
- It can be administered once daily.
- Twice the maintenance dose is given as loading dose on first day.
- It is an enzyme inhibitor.
- It should not be given to pregnant women.

Adverse Effects
- Reversible alopecia
- Nausea, diarrhea, abdominal pain
- Headache, rash

Uses
- Cryptococcal meningitis, febrile neutropenia
- Coccidioidal meningitis
- Oropharyngeal candidiasis
- Uncomplicated vaginal candidiasis

Voriconazole
Actions
- It has expanded spectrum of activity.
- It has 96% oral bioavailability and is widely distributed.
- It is an enzyme inhibitor.
- It is teratogenic and should not be administered during pregnancy.

Adverse Effects
- Prolonged QT syndrome or Torsades de pointes
- Rash, nausea, flushing, and anaphylaxis during first IV administration
- Hepatotoxicity
- Visual and auditory hallucination during IV infusion.

Uses
- Invasive aspergillosis
- Esophageal candidiasis

Posaconazole
Actions
- It is a broad spectrum antifungal agent.
- Food and acidic beverages increases its absorption.
- It is an enzyme inhibitor and extensively bound to plasma proteins.
- It is teratogenic and should not be given during pregnancy.
- It is not available as intravenous formulation.

Adverse Effects
Nausea, vomiting, diarrhea, headache

Uses
- Oropharyngeal candidiasis
- Febrile neutropenia
- Aspergillosis
- Mucormycosis

Isavuconazole
- It is a prodrug.
- Its efficacy is comparable to voriconazole.
- It is available as both oral and parenteral formulation.

Use
Candida esophagitis

ECHINOCANDINS
- Caspofungin, micafungin and anidulafungin are the echinocandins.
- They inhibit the glucan synthesis damaging the structural integrity of fungal cell wall.
- They are effective in azole resistant Candida infections.
- They are not absorbed orally.
- They are extensively bound to plasma proteins.
- They do not cross blood-brain barrier (BBB).
- They are not excreted through kidney.
- They cause minimal adverse effects that rarely lead to drug discontinuation.
- They belong to pregnancy 'category C'.

Caspofungin
Actions
It is administered as slow intravenous infusion extending for 1 hour.

Adverse Effect
Infusion related phlebitis

Uses
- Deeply invasive candidiasis
- Invasive aspergillosis
- Esophageal and oropharyngeal candidiasis
- Febrile neutropenia
- Anidulafungin and micafungin have similar spectrum of activity.

TERBINAFINE

Actions
- It is available for oral and topical administration.
- Given orally, it undergoes high first pass metabolism.
- It accumulates in skin, fat and nails.
- It should not be used in patients with liver dysfunction.
- Topical terbinafine is effective in *Tinea* infection and nail onychomycosis.
- It is available as spray.

Adverse Effects
- Headache, rash
- Stevens-Johnson syndrome
- Hepatotoxicity.

Uses
- Onychomycosis
- Tinea capitis

GRISEOFULVIN

Actions
- It is effective against dermatophytes such as *Microsporum*, *Epidermophyton* and *Trichophyton*.
- It inhibits microtubular function and suppresses mitosis of fungal cells.
- It is fungistatic and deposited in keratin precursor cells providing long-term protection against fungal infection.
- It concentrates in stratum corneum of skin.
- When the fungal infected keratin sheds, it is replaced with normal tissues.
- Treatment should be continued until infected tissue is replaced by normal skin, hair and nails.
- The microionized and ultra microionized formulations of griseofulvin have better oral bioavailability.
- Fatty meal increases its oral absorption as it is absolutely insoluble in water.

Adverse Effects
- Headache, lethargy, peripheral neuritis
- Syncope, vertigo

- Blurred vision, macular edema
- Vomiting, diarrhea, flatulence
- Urticaria, photosensitivity
- Neutropenia, leukopenia

Use

Dermatophytosis

TOPICAL ANTIFUNGAL AGENTS

Clotrimazole

Actions

- It is a fungicidal agent.
- It is applied on skin and mucous membranes.
- It can be absorbed into systemic circulation when applied in vagina.
- The cure rate is 100% in pharyngeal candidiasis of immunocompetant host.
- It is available as cream, lotion, solution, powder and aerosol solution.

Adverse Effects

- Burning sensation
- Lower abdominal cramp
- Skin rash
- Increased urinary frequency

Uses

- Vulvovaginal candidiasis
- Cutaneous candidiasis
- Oropharyngeal candidiasis

Econazole

- It penetrates into stratum corneum.
- It causes local erythema, itching, burning, and stinging sensation.
- It is used in oral thrush, dermatophytosis and otomycosis.

Miconazole

- After application on skin, it persists for more than 4 days in stratum corneum.
- It is safe in pregnancy for vaginal application but should be avoided during 1st trimester.

- It is available as ointment, powder, lotion, gel, aerosol, powder and aerosol solution.
- It causes itching, burning, irritation, skin rash, and headache.
- It is used for *Tinea* infection.

TERCONAZOLE, BUTOCONAZOLE
- Terconazole is available as vaginal suppository or cream.
- It is usually applied for 3 days.
- Butoconazole is available as vaginal cream.
- Due to slow response during 2nd and 3rd trimester of pregnancy, butoconazole application should be extended for 6 days.

TIOCONAZOLE, OXICONAZOLE, SULCONAZOLE, SERTACONAZOLE
- Tioconazole is effective in vulvovaginal candidiasis.
- Oxiconazole, sulconazole and sertaconazole are effective in dermatophytic infection.

Ciclopirox Olamine
- It is a fungicidal agent with broad spectrum antifungal activity.
- It penetrates through epidermis into dermis.
- It also penetrates into hair follicles and sebaceous glands.
- It is available as cream, gel, suspension, shampoo, and lotion.
- It is used in cutaneous candidiasis, ringworm infection and seborrheic dermatitis.

Haloprogin
- It is a fungicide.
- It is effective in *Epidermophyton, Trichophyton, Candida, Pityrosporum* folliculitus, and *Microsporum* infection.
- It causes irritation, burning sensation, pruritus, and hypersensitization.
- It is used in *Tinea* infection.

Tolnaftate
- It is used in cutaneous mycosis caused by *Tinea, Microsporum* and *Epidermophyton* organisms.
- It is available as cream, gel, powder, and topical solution.
- It can cause pruritus.

Naftifine
- It is a broad spectrum fungicidal agent.
- It is effective in *Tinea* infection.
- It causes allergic contact dermatitis.

Nystatin
- It increases permeability of fungal cell membrane.
- It is a macrolide and not absorbed from skin, vagina or gastrointestinal tract (GIT).
- So, it is available as liposomal formulation of powder, cream and ointment.
- It is used in cutaneous, vaginal and oral candidiasis.

Hamycin
- It is more water soluble.
- It is used in oral thrush, cutaneous candidiasis, trichomonas vaginitis, otomycosis, and monilial vaginitis.

Undecylenic Acid
- It is a yellow color liquid with rancid odor.
- It is available as powder, cream, spray, liquid, and soap.
- It is fungistatic but can be fungicidal on prolonged administration.
- It is effective against ringworm infection and diaper rash.

Whitfield's Ointment
- It contains benzoic acid and salicylic acid.
- Benzoic acid is a fungistatic agent and salicylic acid is a keratolytic agent.
- They are combined in the ratio of 2:1 in Whitfield ointment.
- It is mainly used in *Tinea pedis*.

CHOICE OF DRUGS

Deep Mycosis
- **Invasive aspergillosis:** Voriconazole, amphotericin B
- **Blastomycosis:** Amphotericin B, itraconazole
- **Candidiasis:** Amphotericin B, fluconazole, voriconazole, caspofungin
- **Coccidioidomycosis:** Amphotericin B, fluconazole, itraconazole
- **Cryptococcosis:** Amphotericin B, flucytosine
- **Histoplasmosis:** Amphotericin B, itraconazole
- **Sporotrichosis:** Amphotericin B, itraconazole.

Superficial Mycosis
- **Vulvovaginal candidiasis:** Butoconazole, clotrimazole, miconazole
- **Oropharyngeal candidiasis:** Clotrimazole, fluconazole, itraconazole

- **Cutaneous candidiasis:** Amphotericin B, clotrimazole
- **Ringworm:** Butenafine, ciclopirox olamine, econazole, clotrimazole, griseofulvin.

Nursing Responsibilities
- Monitor renal function once every 4 days in all patients receiving amphotericin B.
- Monitor platelet and leukocyte count once a week for patients on flucytosine.
- Monitor liver function once weekly in patients on flucytosine.
- Monitor liver function in patients on itraconazole, voriconazole or ketoconazole.
- Inform patients to swish the nystatin powder and keep it in mouth as long as possible in oral candidiasis.

CHAPTER 73

Anti Non-Retroviral Agents

- Viruses contain either single stranded or double stranded deoxyribonucleic acid (DNA) or ribonucleic acid (RNA).
- They are encapsulated in a protein coat called capsid.
- Some may contain lipid envelope derived from infected host cell.
- Both capsid and lipid membrane contain antigenic glycoproteins.
- Pox virus, herpes virus, hepadna virus, adeno virus and papilloma virus are DNA viruses.
- After entry into host cells, viral DNA is converted into messenger ribonucleic acid (mRNA) by host cell polymerase.
- Ribonucleic acid (RNA) viruses are rubella virus, picornavirus, rhabdovirus, arenavirus, flavivirus, orthomyxovirus, paramyxovirus, and coronavirus.
- Ribonucleic acid (RNA) virus can synthesize its own mRNA or serves as its own mRNA.
- Retrovirus such as HIV virus are special group of RNA virus.

DRUGS USED IN HERPES VIRUS INFECTION
- Herpes simplex-I (HSV-1) causes infection of face, mouth, skin, brain, and esophagus.
- Herpes simplex-II (HSV-2) causes infection of rectum, genitals, skin, hands, and meninges.

Acyclovir
Actions
- It is very effective in HSV-1 infection.
- It is less effective in HSV-2 infection.
- It is much less effective in Varicella-Zoster virus (VZV) and Epstein-Barr virus (EBV) infection.
- It is least effective against Cytomegalovirus (CMV) infection
- It is phosphorylated to acyclovir triphosphate.
- It inhibits viral DNA polymerase irreversibly.
- It is more specific to viral enzymes and does not inhibit mammalian enzymes.

- Resistance to acyclovir is prevalent among these viruses.
- Acyclovir is widely distributed into body fluids.
- It concentration is high in aqueous humor, seminal vesicular fluid, cerebrospinal fluid (CSF), milk, and amniotic fluid.

Adverse Effects
- Burning, mucosal irritation
- Nausea, diarrhea, rash
- Headache, neutropenia
- Reversible nephrotoxicity, central nervous system (CNS) toxicity.

Uses
- Genital HSV
- Herpetic gingivostomatitis
- Varicella pneumonia
- Localized herpes zoster infection
- Zoster ophthalmicus
- Mucocutaneous HSV
- Herpes simplex virus (HSV) encephalitis.

Valacyclovir

Actions
- Valacyclovir is a prodrug and converted to acyclovir after absorption.
- Hence, it increases the plasma concentration of acyclovir.
- Pain associated with localized herpes zoster is relieved better with valacyclovir and acyclovir.

Adverse Effects
- Nephrotoxicity
- Nausea, diarrhea, headache, hallucination
- Rarely thrombocytopenia.

Uses
- Varicella infection
- Recurrent orolabial herpes
- Localized herpes zoster.

Penciclovir

Actions
- It is phosphorylated to penciclovir triphosphate.
- It inhibits viral DNA synthesis.

- It is as potent as acyclovir against HSV and VZV infection.
- It has low oral bioavailability and administered through intravenous route.
- It is also available for topical application.

Adverse Effects
- Mutagenicity
- Topical formulation can cause irritation at the site of application.

Uses
- Mucocutaneous HSV
- Orolabial HSV.

Famciclovir
Actions
- It is a prodrug of penciclovir.
- It is converted to penciclovir.
- Since it has 75% oral bioavailability, it can increase the plasma concentration of penciclovir after oral administration.

Adverse Effects
- Nausea, diarrhea, headache, urticaria
- Rash, hallucination.

Uses
- Recurrent genital herpes infection
- Zoster associated pain
- Ophthalmic zoster.

Cidofovir
Actions
- It is effective against herpes, papilloma, polyoma, pox, and adeno virus.
- It is phosphorylated to cidofovir diphosphate.
- It acts as an alternate substrate to viral DNA polymerase.
- Thereby, it inhibits viral DNA synthesis.
- It has low oral bioavailability.
- Hence, it is administered through IV route.
- Probenecid increases its plasma concentration.
- It has prolonged intracellular half-life.
- So, it can be given as weekly infusion.
- It is also available as topical gel.

Adverse Effects
- Nephrotoxicity
- Anterior uveitis
- Hypersensitivity reaction, anaphylaxis
- Burning sensation and pruritus at application site.

Uses
- Cytomegalovirus (CMV) retinitis
- Acyclovir resistant mucocutaneous HSV
- Molluscum contagiosum
- Anogenital wart
- Adenovirus infection.

Fomivirsen

Actions
- It inhibits the binding of virus to host cells.
- Thereby, it prevents replication of the virus.
- It is effective against CMV resistant to ganciclovir, cidofovir and foscarnet.
- It is administered as weekly intravitreal injection in CMV retinitis.

Adverse Effects
- Iritis, vitritis
- Cataract
- Increased intraocular pressure.

Use
Resistant CMV retinitis.

Foscarnet

Actions
- It inhibits the synthesis of viral nucleic acid.
- It inhibits DNA polymerase of herpes virus and human immunodeficiency virus (HIV) reverse transcriptase.
- It is effective in the treatment of CMV retinitis in acquired immunodeficiency syndrome (AIDS) patients.
- It is also effective in ganciclovir resistant CMV and acyclovir resistant HSV and VZV.
- It is more specific to viral DNA polymerase than the host enzyme.

Adverse Effects
- Nephrotoxicity, hypocalcemia, hypomagnesemia, hypokalemia, hypophosphatemia

- Tetany, seizures, headache, tremor, nephrogenic diabetes insipidus
- Anemia, leukopenia, liver dysfunction, electrocardiogram (ECG) changes, genital ulceration.

Uses
- Ganciclovir resistant CMV retinitis
- Cytomegalovirus (CMV) retinitis in AIDS patients
- Acyclovir resistant HSV, VZV.

Ganciclovir

Actions
- It is very effective in CMV infection.
- It inhibits viral DNA synthesis.
- It is phosphorylated to ganciclovir di and triphosphates.
- It has low oral bioavailability.
- Hence, it is administered through intravenous route.
- It accumulates in vitreous humor following intravenous (IV) administration.
- Probenecid reduces its excretion.
- It belongs to pregnancy category C.

Adverse Effects
Fatal neutropenia, headache, convulsion.

Uses
- CMV retinitis
- HSV keratitis
- Other CMV syndromes in HIV infected and transplant recipients.

Valganciclovir

Actions
- Food increases the oral bioavailability of valganciclovir.
- It is converted to ganciclovir.
- It inhibits viral DNA synthesis.

Adverse Effects
Headache, nausea, diarrhea, neutropenia.

Uses
- To prevent CMV infection in transplant patients.
- Cytomegalovirus (CMV) retinitis.

Docosanol
- It is available as topical cream for recurrent orolabial herpes infection.
- It inhibits viral replication by inhibiting the fusion of virus with host cell preventing its entry.

Idoxuridine
- It inhibits viral replication by inhibiting viral DNA synthesis.
- It is effective against HSV and pox virus.
- It is not selective to viral DNA and also affects uninfected cells.
- It is used topically in HSV keratitis and herpes genital infection.
- It causes pain, pruritus and edema of eyelids.

Trifluridine
- It is effective in HSV-1, HSV-2 and CMV infection.
- It inhibits viral DNA synthesis.
- It is used in viral keratoconjunctivitis and recurrent epithelial keratitis.
- Hypersensitivity reactions, epithelial keratopathy or irritation can occur.

Nursing Responsibilities
- A state of confusion can be expected in elderly patients on famciclovir.
- Maintain adequate hydration during and after infusion of acyclovir to reduce nephrotoxicity.
- Monitor serum creatinine and blood urea nitrogen in patients on acyclovir.
- Do not administer acyclovir infusion rapidly.
- Monitor blood cell count frequently in patients on ganciclovir and cidofovir.

DRUGS USED FOR INFLUENZA VIRUS INFECTION
Amantadine and Rimantadine
Actions
- They inhibit viral uncoating and viral replication.
- They are effective in influenza-A virus infection.
- Both drugs are well absorbed after oral administration.
- Rimantadine is more effective and better tolerated than amantadine.

Adverse Effects
- Nausea, anorexia
- Dizziness, insomnia
- Cardiac arrhythmia.

Uses
- Prophylaxis and treatment of influenza-A infection.
- Amantadine is used in Parkinsonism.

Oseltamivir
Actions
- It is a neuraminidase inhibitor of influenza-A virus and inhibits viral spread.
- It is rapidly absorbed after oral administration.
- Seasonal influenza-A of H_1N_1 strain has become totally resistant to oseltamivir.
- Swine influenza (H_1N_1) is still susceptible.

Adverse Effects
- Nausea, vomiting, abdominal pain
- Headache.

Use
Prophylaxis and treatment of influenza-A and B infection.

Zanamivir
Actions
- It inhibits neuraminidase enzyme of influenza-A and B viruses.
- It is available as dry powder for oral inhalation.

Adverse Effects
Wheeze, bronchospasm.

Use
Prevention and treatment of influenza-A and B virus infection.

DRUGS USED IN VIRAL HEPATITIS
- Hepatitis C virus (HCV) causes chronic viral infection of liver.
- It can result in hepatocellular carcinoma.

Interferons (IFNs)
Actions
- Interferons are cytokines and have antiviral, immunomodulatory and antiproliferative actions.

- Interferons (IFN)-α, β and γ are the major form with significant antiviral activity.
- Interferons -α and IFN -β have anti viral and antiproliferative actions.
- Interferons-γ has higher immunomodulatory activity than antiviral activity.
- Pegylated α interferons (peg interferon α2a, peg interferon α2b) are available for therapy.
- Ribonucleic acid (RNA) viruses are more sensitive to interferons than DNA viruses.
- They act by inhibiting protein synthesis.
- They are administered parenterally.
- Conventional interferon preparations have short-duration of action.
- Long-acting polyethylene (PEG) interferon preparation can be administered once weekly.

Adverse Effects
- Nausea, vomiting, diarrhea
- Myalgia, arthralgia
- Headache
- Myelosuppression, neurotoxicity, behavioral disturbance, hypothyroidism.

Uses
- Chronic HCV infection, chronic HBV infection
- Condyloma acuminatum
- Kaposi's sarcoma, idiopathic pulmonary fibrosis
- Multiple sclerosis, juvenile rheumatoid arthritis.

Ribavirin

Actions
- It is effective against orthomyxovirus, paramyxovirus, flavivirus, bunyavirus, and arenavirus.
- It is also effective against influenza virus, parainfluenza virus and respiratory syncytial virus.
- It is phosphorylated to its active form ribavirin triphosphate in both infected and noninfected host cells.
- It inhibits synthesis of viral mRNA.
- It enhances viral mutagenesis and inhibits its replication.
- So far, the development of resistance is minimal.
- Food increases its oral bioavailability.

- It accumulates in plasma and in red blood cells (RBC).
- It exits from RBC gradually.
- It is administered orally and intravenously.
- It is also available as aerosolized formulation.
- It is teratogenic and not safe in pregnancy.

Adverse Effects
- Aerosolized formulation causes rash, conjunctival irritation, and wheeze.
- Systemic administration causes anemia, fatigue, pruritus, dyspnea and increase in serum iron, uric acid as well as bilirubin level.

Uses
- Hepatitis C virus
- Respiratory syntytial virus (RSV) bronchiolitis and pneumonia
- Severe influenza.

DRUGS USED IN HEPATITIS B VIRUS (HBV)
- Hepatitis B virus can cause lifelong infection.
- It can cause hepatitis, cirrhosis and fibrosis.

Adefovir
Actions
- It is used mainly for HBV infection although it can inhibit many DNA and RNA viruses.
- It is phosphorylated to adefovir diphosphate and inhibits viral DNA polymerase as well as reverse transcriptase enzymes.
- Food does not inhibit the oral bioavailability of adefovir.

Adverse effects
- Nephrotoxicity
- Headache, asthenia
- Hepatotoxicity.

Use
Chronic HBV infections.

Entecavir
Actions
- It is phosphorylated to entecavir triphosphate and inhibits HBV polymerase.
- It should be administered in empty stomach.

Adverse Effects
Headache, dizziness, fatigue

Uses
Chronic HBV infection

Lamivudine

Actions
- Lamivudine triphosphate inhibits DNA polymerase of HBV and HIV reverse transcriptase.
- It is combined with penciclovir or adefovir in the treatment of HBV infection.
- Its duration of action is long.
- So, it is given once daily.

Adverse Effects
Increase in serum aminotransferase level.

Uses
Chronic HBV hepatitis
Other details: See Section XI, Chapter 74

Telbivudine

Actions
- It is phosphorylated to its triphosphate form that inhibits HBV DNA polymerase.
- It is well absorbed orally and widely distributed.
- It has long half-life.
- Hence, it is given once daily.

Adverse Effects
- Nausea, diarrhea
- Fatigue, myalgia, myopathy.

Uses
Chronic HBV infection

Tenofovir
- It is effective against HIV and HBV viruses.
- It is safer, more effective with very minimal resistance profile.
- It is preferred to adefovir in treatment of HBV infection.

For other details: See Section XI, Chapter 74

Imiquimod

Actions
- It is a topical immunomodulatory agent.
- It is effective in skin infection due to *Molluscum contagiosum, Condylomata acuminata* and other DNA viruses.
- It induces immunomodulatory activity of cytokines.
- It reduces the viral load and wart size at the site of application.

Adverse Effects
Erythema, burning, itching at the site of application.

Uses
- Genital wart
- Perianal wart.

Nursing Responsibilities
- Monitor valves of the mechanical ventilators for blocks when ribavirin aerosolized formulation is given.
- Avoid exposure to ribavirin during administration of aerosolized formulation.
- Monitor hematuria and anemia during therapy of ribavirin.
- Pegylated interferons are more tolerable than conventional preparations.
- Patients and their attendants should be warned about the capacity of interferons in causing depression and behavioral disturbances.
- Monitor renal function in patients on adefovir.
- Prophylaxis of oseltamivir is necessary for the family members of patients with swine flu.
- Monitor liver function and thyroid function in patients receiving interferon.

HIV Infection and Antiretroviral Agents

- Human immunodeficiency virus (HIV) is a retrovirus with a small RNA genome.
- Nucleocapsid core contains two copies of genome.
- It is surrounded by a lipid bilayer or envelope.
- The viral genome codes for *gag, pol* and *env* genomes.
- While *gag* and *pol* genes code for reverse transcriptase, *env* gene codes for envelope.
- These surface glycoproteins on envelope are antigenic and promote attachment to $CD4^+$ receptors of lymphocytes and macrophages as well as chemokine receptors on macrophages.
- After fusion with host cells, the virus uncoats and viral RNA synthesizes DNA by reverse transcriptase enzyme.
- This viral DNA integrates into host DNA by viral integrase forming provirus.
- Activated provirus forms mRNA and viral proteins, which form nucleocapsid around genomic RNA.
- Reverse transcriptase is incorporated into new, enveloped HIV particles that contain two single stranded RNA.
- Replication begins as soon as virus enters the new cell.
- *Viral load* depends upon host immunity and infecting virus.
- $CD4^+$ T lymphocytes decline as the concentration of plasma HIV RNA increases.

The antiretroviral drugs are classified as:
  A. Nucleoside reverse transcriptase inhibitors (NRTIs)
  B. Non-nucleoside reverse transcriptase inhibitors (NNRTIs)
  C. Nucleotide reverse transcriptase inhibitors (NtRTIs)
  D. Protease inhibitors (PIs)
  E. Fusion inhibitors
  F. Integrase inhibitors

NUCLEOSIDE REVERSE TRANSCRIPTASE INHIBITORS
They are:
- Zidovudine
- Stavudine

- Lamivudine
- Didanosine
- Abacavir
- Emtricitabine.

Common Mechanism of NRTIs
- Zidovudine, stavudine and didanosine inhibit human DNA polymerase.
- So, they cause anemia, granulocytopenia, myopathy, peripheral neuropathy, pancreatitis, and lactic acidosis.
- NRTIs are phosphorylated to their active triphosphate form.
- They incorporate into reverse transcriptase enzyme and inhibit the conversion of viral RNA into proviral RNA.
- This inhibits the viral replication.

Zidovudine
Actions
- It is the oldest drug but still used widely.
- It has good efficacy, tolerability with well known toxicity profile.
- It is effective in HIV-1, HIV-2 and human T lymphocyte viruses I and II.
- It has rapid oral absorption but undergoes very high first pass metabolism.
- It attains high concentration in milk, semen and fetal tissue.
- It concentrates highly in male genital tract.
- Its fetal plasma concentration is equal to its maternal concentration.
- Hence, it reduces the incidence of neonatal HIV infection.
- It is given in HIV infected mother.
- Stavudine should never be coadministered with zidovudine as it inhibits the clinical outcome of zidovudine.

Adverse Effects
- Nausea, malaise, anorexia
- Headache, fatigue, insomnia
- Bone marrow depression in advanced HIV infection.

Uses
- HIV infection during pregnancy
- HIV infection in adults and children.

Nursing Responsibilities
Monitor blood count periodically in patients on zidovudine.

Stavudine

Actions
- Due to its toxicity, it is less frequently used now.
- Its active form is stavudine triphosphate.
- It is well absorbed and food does not interfere with its absorption.
- It crosses placenta and blood-brain barrier.
- If combined with didanosine, it increases the incidence of pancreatitis.
- Further, it should not be combined with zidovudine.

Adverse Effects
- Peripheral neuropathy
- Lactic acidosis
- Lipoatrophy.

Uses
HIV infection in neonates, children and adults.

Lamivudine

Actions
- It is one of the least toxic antiretroviral drugs.
- Its oral bioavailability exceeds 80% and food does not interfere with its absorption.
- It concentrates more in male genital tract.
- It crosses placenta freely and enters fetal circulation.
- It is more effective when combined with zidovudine.

Adverse Effects
- Neutropenia
- Headache, nausea.

Uses
- HIV infection in adults and in children above 3 months
- Chronic hepatitis B infection.

Abacavir

Actions
- Its active form is carbovir triphosphate.
- Its oral bioavailability exceeds 80% irrespective of food intake.

Adverse Effects
- Fatal hypersensitivity syndrome
- Increased risk of myocardial infarction.

Uses
Combination therapy in HIV infection.

Nursing Responsibilities
Before administering abacavir to patients, history of previous hypersensitivity reaction should be enquired as it should not be given in patients who have experienced hypersensitivity reaction.

Didanosine
Actions
- It should be administered either 30 minutes before or 2 hours after food.
- It has long-duration of action so can be administered once daily.
- Tenofovir increases toxicity of didanosine.
- Combination with stavudine increases the likelihood of peripheral neuropathy and pancreatitis.

Adverse Effects
- Peripheral neuropathy
- Pancreatitis
- Optic neuritis
- Hyperuricemia
- Hypertriglyceridemia
- Hypertension
- Diarrhea.

Use
Combination therapy in HIV infection in adults and children.

Emtricitabine
Actions
- It is one of the least toxic antiretroviral drug.
- The prevalence of resistance is very high for emtricitabine.
- Its oral bioavailability is around 93%.
- It has long-duration of action.
- So, it can be administered once daily.

Adverse Effects
- Hyperpigmentation
- Hepatitis
- Pancreatitis.

Use
Combination therapy in HIV infection in adults.

NON-NUCLEOSIDE REVERSE TRANSCRIPTASE INHIBITORS (NNRTIs)
They are:
- Efavirenz
- Delavirdine
- Nevirapine
- Etravirine.

Common Properties
- NNRTIs do not require intracellular phosphorylation for clinical action.
- They are noncompetitive inhibitors of reverse transcriptase enzyme.
- They are effective in HIV-1 and not against HIV-2 infection.
- Except etravirine, HIV virus has developed resistance to all other NNRTIs.

Efavirenz
Actions
- Fatty meal increases the bioavailability of efavirenz.
- Still, the initial dose should be given in empty stomach at bed time to reduce the side effects.
- Although its CSF concentration is minimal, it causes CNS toxicity.
- It is administered once daily and is a moderate enzyme inducer.
- It is effective and preferred due to its convenient once daily dosage schedule.
- Hence, it is widely used for combination therapy in HIV infections.
- It is highly teratogenic and should be avoided in pregnancy.

Adverse Effects
- Dysphoria, vivid dreams, frank psychosis
- Dizziness, insomnia.

Use
HIV infection of adults and children above 3 years.

Nevirapine
Actions
- It is well absorbed and food does not interfere with its absorption.
- It crosses placenta.
- It is secreted in milk.

HIV Infection and Antiretroviral Agents **483**

- Hence, it is used to prevent transmission of HIV infection to fetus during pregnancy.
- It is an enzyme inducer.
- Although it is started initially as once daily dose, it is administered twice daily after 2 weeks.
- Development of resistance and treatment failure can occur during nevirapine therapy.
- Cross resistance with efavirenz and delavirdine can also occur.

Adverse Effects
- Rash, pruritus
- Stevens-Johnson syndrome
- Fatal hepatitis, more common in women.

Uses
- Combination therapy in HIV infection of adults and children
- Single dose in HIV infection during pregnancy.

Etravirine

Actions
- It inhibits reverse transcriptase enzyme, resistant to other NNRTIs.
- It is rapidly absorbed after oral administration.
- Food improves its oral absorption.
- It is highly plasma protein bound.
- It is suitable for once daily dosage.

Adverse Effects
- Rash
- Epidermal necrolysis
- Stevens-Johnson syndrome.

Use
HIV infection in adults.

Delavirdine

Actions
- Resistance emerges rapidly if delavirdine is used alone.
- Besides, its short half-life necessitates thrice daily administration.
- Hence, it is a not preferred drug in therapy of HIV infection.
- It is well absorbed after oral administration even in the presence of food.
- As an enzyme inhibitor, it increases the plasma concentration of coadministered protease inhibitors.

Adverse Effects
- Rash, erythema multiforme
- Stevens-Johnson syndrome.

Use
Combination therapy in HIV infection.

NUCLEOTIDE REVERSE TRANSCRIPTASE INHIBITORS (NtRTIs)
Tenofovir is the NtRTI used in treatment of HIV infection.

Tenofovir
Actions
- It is nucleotide reverse transcriptase inhibitor used in HIV infection.
- It is used in HIV-1, HIV-2 and HBV infection.
- It is available as tenofovir disoproxil, a prodrug with better oral bioavailability.
- Its active metabolite tenofovir diphosphate inhibits reverse transcriptase enzyme.
- It should not be coadministered with didanosine.
- It reduces the clinical efficacy of atazanavir.

Adverse effects
Flatulence.

Use
Combination therapy in HIV infection in adults.

PROTEASE INHIBITORS
They are:
- Saquinavir
- Nelfinavir
- Indinavir
- Ritonavir
- Fosamprenavir
- Atazanavir
- Lopinavir
- Darunavir
- Tipranavir.

Common Properties
- Protease inhibitors inhibit viral protease enzyme competitively.
- They are enzyme inhibitors and effective in HIV infection.
- Pharmacokinetic inter-individual variation occurs among protease inhibitors.
- Unlike NNRTIs and NRTIs they attain minimal concentration in semen.
- They are highly protein bound and attain low CSF concentration.
- Low dose ritonavir increases the bioavailability and duration of action of other protease inhibitors.
- Hence, therapy with dual protease inhibitors are combined with ritonavir in HIV infection.
- The initial GIT side effects such as nausea, vomiting and diarrhea are short lived and resolve on continuation of therapy.

Saquinavir
Actions
- Given alone, it has poor oral bioavailability as it undergoes high first pass metabolism.
- Hence, it should be combined with low dose ritonavir.

Adverse Effects
- Nausea, vomiting, diarrhea that are short lived
- Lipodystrophy on prolonged therapy.

Ritonavir
Actions
- At a low dose, it is a pharmacokinetic enhancer, in dual protease inhibitor combinations.
- Nelfinavir does not require ritonavir as pharmacokinetic enhancer.
- Food increases the oral bioavailability of capsule formulation.
- Bioavailability of oral solution is less in the presence of food.
- It is highly protein bound.

Adverse Effects
- Nausea, vomiting, diarrhea that are short lived
- Lipodystrophy, atherosclerosis.

Use
Pharmacokinetic enhancer for all protease inhibitors except nelfinavir.

Fosamprenavir

Actions
- It is a prodrug of amprenavir with better oral bioavailability.
- It is dephosphorylated to amprenavir.
- It is well tolerated and more effective than amprenavir.
- It is highly protein bound.
- A low dose ritonavir increases its plasma concentration.

Adverse Effects
- Nausea, vomiting, diarrhea that are short lived
- Hyperglycemia, headache, fatigue, paresthesia.

Use
HIV infection in adults and pediatric patients above 2 years of age.

Lopinavir

Actions
- It is effective even in patients who do not benefit with other protease inhibitors.
- Since food does not interfere with its oral absorption, it can be taken with or without food.
- Given alone, it undergoes very high first pass metabolism.
- So, it is given as combination with low dose ritonavir to increase its plasma concentration.

Adverse Effects
- Nausea, vomiting, diarrhea that are short lived
- Hypercholestrolemia
- Hypertriglyceridemia.

Use
Resistant HIV infection in adults and children.

Atazanavir

Actions
- Fatty meal increases its oral absorption.
- It is highly protein bound.
- It attains higher concentration in seminal fluid.
- It is combined with low dose ritonavir which increases its plasma concentration.

Adverse Effects
- Nausea, vomiting, diarrhea that are short lived
- Hyperbilirubinemia, cholecystitis, cholelithiasis.

Use
HIV infection in adults.

Darunavir

Actions
- Food increases its oral absorption.
- Coadministration of low dose ritonavir increases its bioavailability.
- It is highly protein bound.
- It is administered twice daily.
- Efavirenz reduces plasma concentration of darunavir.

Adverse Effects
- Nausea, vomiting, diarrhea that are short lived
- Rash, hypertriglyceridemia.

Use
HIV infection in adults and children above 6 months.

Indinavir

Actions
- It differs from other protease inhibitors in its pharmacokinetics.
- Unlike other protease inhibitors, fatty food reduces its oral absorption.
- Hence, it is given on empty stomach in combination with ritonavir.
- It is minimally protein bound.
- It attains significant concentration in CSF.
- It has short-duration of action.
- Hence, it is given three times daily when given as monotherapy.
- Twice daily administration is effective when combined with low dose ritonavir.
- It is not widely preferred due to its moderate efficacy and high toxicity.

Adverse Effects
- Nephrolithiasis, crystalluria
- Hyperglycemia, hair loss, dry skin, ingrown toe nails.

Use
HIV infection.

Nelfinavir
Actions
- It is the only protease inhibitor whose plasma concentration is not increased by ritonavir.
- Its oral absorption is highly sensitive to fatty meal which increases its oral absorption.
- This causes high inter-individual variation.
- Although it is not teratogenic, it is carcinogenic so not used in pregnant women.

Adverse Effects
- Secretory diarrhea
- Glucose intolerance
- Hypercholesterolemia, hypertriglyceridemia.

Use
Combination therapy in HIV infection in adults and children.

Tipranavir
Actions
- It is combined with high dose ritonavir to enhance its bioavailability.
- This combination should not be coadministered with other protease inhibitors as they reduce the plasma concentration of these drugs.
- Food reduces its GIT side effects and it is highly protein bound.

Adverse Effects
- Fatal hepatotoxicity
- Intracranial hemorrhage
- Hypertriglyceridemia.

Use
Resistant HIV infection in adults and children.

ENTRY INHIBITORS
They are:
- Maraviroc
- Enfuvirtide.

Maraviroc

Actions
- It inhibits fusion of HIV outer envelope to CCR5 chemokine receptor.
- It is effective in resistant HIV infection.
- Its oral bioavailability depends on its dose.
- Food reduces its absorption.

Adverse effects
Hepatotoxicity.

Use
HIV infection in adults.

Enfuvirtide

Actions
- It is a reserve drug.
- It is the only antiretroviral drug that should be administered parenterally.
- It inhibits viral fusion with $CD4^+$ receptors.
- It is a costly drug.
- It causes cutaneous toxicity.
- It should be administered either through subcutaneous or through IV route.
- These factors limit its use in HIV infection.
- It is highly bound to plasma proteins.
- It should be administered twice daily.
- It does not undergo drug interaction with other coadministered drugs.

Adverse Effects
- Pain, erythema at site of injection
- Nodules, cysts
- Lymphadenopathy, pneumonia.

Use
Reserve drug for resistant HIV infection in adults.

INTEGRASE INHIBITORS
Raltegravir is an integrase inhibitor.

Raltegravir

Actions
- It blocks the activity of the viral integrase enzyme.
- It prevents the integration of viral DNA into host chromosome.
- Fatty meal increases its oral bioavailability.
- Inter-individual variation occurs during its therapy.
- It is highly protein bound.
- Atazanavir and tenofovir increase the plasma concentration of raltegravir.

Adverse Effects
Fatigue, asthenia, myopathy, rhabdomyolysis.

Use
Multidrug resistant HIV infection in adults.

PREFERRED DRUG COMBINATIONS

Two drug regimen for low risk persons and three drug regimen for high-risk persons.
- Lamivudine + zidovudine + nevirapine
- Lamivudine + zidovudine + efavirenz
- Lamivudine + stavudine + nevirapine
- Lamivudine + stavudine + efavirenz
- Lamivudine + tenofovir + efavirenz
- Lamivudine + zidovudine + tenofovir
- Lamivudine + nevirapine + tenofovir.

HIGHLY ACTIVE ANTIRETROVIRAL THERAPY (HAART)

The principles of HAART therapy are:
- Lifelong treatment is required and drug holidays are not indicated.
- Three drugs belonging to different classes of antiretroviral drugs are preferred.
- The regimen should have 1 NNRTI and 2 NRTI.
- 3 NRTI can be used only if an NNRTI cannot be given.
- Commonly used NRTI is lamivudine.
- Stavudine or zidovudine can also be used.
- Nevirapine or efavirenz are the preferred NNRTI.
- Efavirenz should be avoided in pregnancy and in patients with hepatic dysfunction.
- Regimen with PI should be reserved for resistant/treatment failure patients.

- Low dose ritonavir is the preferred PI in any dual PI combination except in combination with nelfinavir.
- Development of adverse effects necessitates discontinuation of that particular regimen or the concerned drug.

THERAPY OF HIV INFECTION DURING PREGNANCY
The preferred combination is:
Lamivudine + zidovudine + nevirapine.

Nursing Responsibilities
- Motivate the patient to adhere to therapy of antiretroviral agents.
- Monitor treatment adherence continuously for better clinical outcome.
- Monitor liver enzymes in women patients on nevirapine.
- Patients on indinavir should be advised to drink more water to avoid crystalluria.
- Accidental needle prick, sharing contaminated needle used by infected patients and contact with infected blood and body fluids of the patients may increase the risk of developing HIV infection in health personnel.
- Monitor blood sugar periodically in patients on protease inhibitors as they cause diabetes mellitus.

CHAPTER 75

Anticancer Drugs

- Cancer cells undergo rapid proliferation and are unresponsive to normal feedback mechanism that control growth cycle.
- The unique property of cancer cells is its rapid spread resulting in metastasis to distant sites from primary tumor.
- The four main stages of cell cycle are G_1 or presynthetic phase, S or synthetic phase, G_2 or pre-mitotic interval and M or mitotic phase.
- G_0 is the quiescent stage where cells remain in dormant stage.
- Anticancer drugs are not selective and are toxic to normal cells too.
- Besides, at any given dose, they kill a constant fraction or percentage of cancer cells and it is difficult to achieve a complete cell kill.
- Drug resistance is the major problem interfering with successful treatment of cancer.
- So combination chemotherapy is more effective in the management of cancer as it prevents development of resistance and reduces the toxicity of anticancer drugs.
- The common side effects of anticancer drugs are gastrointestinal (GIT) toxicity, bone marrow depression, alopecia, and toxicity to reproductive organs.
- **Bone marrow:** Aplastic anemia, granulocytopenia, thrombocytopenia, agranulocytosis, leukopenia.
- **GIT:** Stomatitis, nausea, vomiting, mucosal ulceration, hemorrhage.
- **Skin:** Alopecia, dermatitis.
- **Gonads:** Oligozoospermia, impotence, amenorrhea, inhibition of ovulation.
- **Fetus:** Abortion, teratogenicity, fetal death.
- **Carcinogenicity:** Lymphoma, leukemia.
- They also cause hyperuricemia, neuropathy, cardiotoxicity, hemorrhagic cystitis.

The anticancer agents are broadly classified as:
   I. Alkylating agents
  II. Antimetabolites

III. Natural compounds
IV. Miscellaneous agents
V. Hormones.

ALKYLATING AGENTS

- They are either bifunctional or monofunctional cytotoxic agents.
- They alkylate the DNA, cause mispairing and interfere with DNA function and induce cell death.
- They are cytotoxic, non cell-cycle specific and act on rapidly multiplying cells.
- Resistance to alkylating agents develops rapidly if used alone.
- They cause bone marrow depression, GIT toxicity, alopecia, and toxicity to reproductive organs.

The alkylating agents are:
  A. **Nitrogen mustards:** Mechlorethamine, cyclophosphamide, ifosfamide, melphalan, chlorambucil.
  B. **Alkyl sulfonate:** Busulfan.
  C. **Ethyleneimines:** Thiotepa, altretamine.
  D. **Nitrosoureas:** Carmustine, semustine, bendamustine, streptozotocin.
  E. **Triazenes:** Dacarbazine, temozolomide.
  F. **Methyl hydrazine:** Procarbazine.
  G. **Platinum complexes:** Cisplatin, carboplatin, oxaliplatin.

Nitrogen Mustards

Mechlorethamine

- It is rarely used now as it causes severe local reactions at the site of injection.
- It was formerly used in mechlorethamine, oncovin (vincristine), procarbazine, prednisone (MOPP) regime for Hodgkin's disease.

Cyclophosphamide

Actions
- It is a prodrug.
- It is metabolized to phosphoramide mustard and acrolein.
- Phosphoramide mustard has antitumor activity.
- Acrolein causes hemorrhagic cystitis.
- It can be administered by oral and intravenous route.

Adverse Effects
- Hemorrhagic cystitis. MESNA (2-mercaptoethane sulfonate) reduces this toxicity

- Alopecia, syndrome of inappropriate ADH secretion (SIADH)
- Myelosuppression
- Nausea, vomiting, mucosal ulceration
- Pulmonary fibrosis
- Renal, hepatic and cardiac toxicity.

Uses
- Chronic lymphocytic leukemia (CLL)
- Hodgkin's lymphoma, non-Hodgkin's lymphoma, Burkitt's lymphoma
- Carcinoma of cervix, breast, ovary, lung
- Neuroblastoma
- Immunosuppressant in rheumatoid arthritis, Wegener's granulomatosis, nephrotic syndrome.

Ifosfamide
Actions
- It is a derivative of cyclophosphamide.
- Its metabolite chloracetaldehyde causes CNS toxicity.

Adverse Effects
- Hemorrhagic cystitis. MESNA (2-mercaptoethane sulfonate) reduces this toxicity.
- Seizure, confusion, hallucination.
- Nausea, vomiting, leukopenia, thrombocytopenia.

Uses
- Germ cell testicular cancer relapse
- Pediatric and adult sarcoma.

Melphalan
Actions
- It is a bifunctional alkylating agent.
- It is not a vesicant.
- Its oral absorption is incomplete.
- So, it is given intravenously.

Adverse Effect
Severe bone marrow depression.

Use
Multiple myeloma.

Chlorambucil
Actions
- It is well tolerated.
- It is given for months to years in treatment of CLL.
- Even after prolonged administration, it does not cause significant toxicity.
- It is adequately absorbed through oral administration.

Adverse Effects
- Moderate and reversible myelosuppression
- Gastrointestinal (GI) discomfort
- Pulmonary fibrosis
- Hepatotoxicity
- Azoospermia, amenorrhea.

Use
Chronic lymphocytic leukemia.

Busulfan
Actions
- It is well absorbed orally.
- It is also available as IV formulation.
- It results in 90% remission in chronic myeloid leukemia.
- It is the first line drug in Hodgkin's lymphoma.

Adverse Effects
- Bone marrow depression
- Pulmonary fibrosis
- Nausea, vomiting, veno-occlusive disease of liver
- Alopecia, azoospermia, amenorrhea.

Uses
- Chronic myelogenous leukemia (CML)
- Allogenic bone marrow transplantation
- Hodgkin's lymphoma.

Thiotepa
- Thiotepa is used in high dose chemotherapy regimes.
- It causes bone marrow depression, mucositis and neurotoxicity.

Altretamine
Actions
- It is also known as hexamethylmelamine.
- Its absorption is adequate through oral route.

Adverse Effects
- Myelosuppression
- Nausea, vomiting, rash
- Neurotoxicity, alopecia, hepatotoxicity.

Use
Ovarian cancer.

Nitrosoureas

- Carmustine and lomustine are bifunctional alkylating agents.
- They are highly lipophilic and attain high concentration in CSF.
- Hence, they are used in malignant gliomas.
- They cause delayed myelosuppression, severe nausea and vomiting.
- Long-term therapy of semustine results in renal failure.
- Carmustine is used in Hodgkin's and non-Hodgkin's lymphoma.
- Bendamustine is used in chronic lymphocytic leukemia and non-Hodgkin's lymphoma.
- Carmustine causes veno-occlusive disease of liver, pulmonary fibrosis and secondary leukemia.
- Bendamustine causes mucositis and myelosuppression.
- Streptozotocin is selectively taken up by pancreatic islet cells.
- Hence, it is used in islet cell carcinoma and in malignant carcinoid tumors.
- It is also used to induce diabetes mellitus in experimental animals.
- It causes severe nausea, anemia, leukopenia, thrombocytopenia, renal, and hepatic toxicity.

Triazenes

Actions

- Dacarbazine is used in regime for Hodgkin's lymphoma.
- It is also used in malignant melanoma and soft tissue sarcoma.
- Temozolomide is converted to its active metabolite which has anticancer activity.
- It has 100% oral bioavailability.
- It is used in the treatment of malignant gliomas and astrocytoma.
- Dacarbazine is administered intravenously while temozolomide can be given orally and intravenously.

Adverse Effect

Both drugs cause nausea, vomiting, bone marrow depression, and flu-like syndrome.

Platinum Complexes
Actions
- On entry into cancer cells, platinum complexes get aquated
- This aquated moiety cross links with DNA, inhibits its replication and cause apoptosis.

Cisplatin
- Cisplatin is given only as intravenous infusion.
- It is highly emetogenic and causes severe nausea and vomiting.
- Neurokinin inhibitors such as aprepitant or fosaprepitant and serotonin antagonist ondansetron or palonosetron with high dose corticosteroids are effective in reducing the emesis induced by cisplatin.
- Its concentration in CSF is poor.
- It concentrates in liver, kidney, intestine, and testes.
- 'Chloride diuresis' or administration of 1 to 2 L of normal saline prior to cisplatin administration reduces its renal toxicity.

Adverse Effects
- Nephrotoxicity
- Marked nausea and vomiting
- Ototoxicity
- Peripheral motor and sensory neuropathy
- Severe electrolyte disturbance (hypokalemia, hypomagnesemia, hypocalcemia)
- Myelosuppression, predominantly anemia
- Hyperuricemia
- Anaphylaxis-like reaction.

Uses
- Advanced testicular and ovarian cancer
- Carcinoma of head and neck
- Carcinoma of bladder and endometrium
- All types of lung cancer
- Childhood cancer
- Anal and rectal cancer.

Carboplatin
- It is better tolerated than cisplatin.
- The incidence of neurotoxicity, nephrotoxicity and ototoxicity are minimal.
- It causes myelosuppression, primarily thrombocytopenia.

- It has similar efficacy to cisplatin in ovary and lung cancer.
- It is less effective than cisplatin in cancer of esophagus, head and neck.
- The incidence of nausea and vomiting is less severe with carboplatin.
- It is preferred in patients who develop refractory nausea and vomiting to cisplatin.

Oxaliplatin
- Oxaliplatin is mainly used in colorectal cancer and causes peripheral neuropathy
- It can cause pulmonary fibrosis.

Procarbazine
Actions
- Procarbazine methylates DNA and causes cytotoxicity.
- It undergoes extensive first pass metabolism.
- It is highly carcinogenic, mutagenic and teratogenic substance.
- Hence, it is rarely used in Hodgkin's regime nowadays.

Adverse Effects
- Leukopenia, thrombocytopenia
- Nausea, vomiting, diarrhea, rash
- Behavioral disturbance
- Antabuse-like action.

Use
Malignant brain tumors.

ANTIMETABOLITES
- Being structural analogs of metabolites, they undergo incorporation into DNA and interfere with its function and replication.
- Some antimetabolites inhibit the enzymes necessary for synthesis of essential cellular constituents.

The antimetabolites are:
- Folic acid analogs
- Pyrimidine analogs
- Purine analogs.

Folic Acid Analogs
They are:
- Methotrexate
- Pemetrexed

Anticancer Drugs

- Raltitrexed
- Trimetrexate.

Actions
- They inhibit dihydrofolate reductase, an enzyme that converts dihydrofolic acid into tetrahydrofolic acid.
- Folic acid analogs inhibit synthesis of folic acid necessary for synthesis of DNA.
- Leucovorin/folinic acid/citrovorum factor is given as 'rescue' of host cells from the toxic actions of folic acid analogs.
- Leucovorin repletes the folate cofactors.
- This selectively permits the normal cells to synthesize thymidylate required for DNA synthesis.

Methotrexate
Actions
- It is converted to polyglutamates which block dihydrofolate reductase and thymidylate synthase.
- This inhibits the synthesis of thymidylate and purines.
- It can be administered through oral, IM and IV route.
- Since it does not effectively cross Blood-brain barrier (BBB), it is given through intrathecal or intraventricular route in brain tumor.
- Polyglutamates accumulate in tissues and prolong its action.
- Prolonged accumulation of methotrexate as polyglutamates in chorionic epithelium is responsible for its abortifacient action as well as its therapeutic efficacy in choriocarcinoma.
- It is given with misoprostol to induce abortion in first trimester.
- It accumulates in liver and kidney as polyglutamates causing hepatotoxicity and nephrotoxicity.

Adverse Effects
- Severe myelosuppression
- Nausea, vomiting, diarrhea
- Alopecia, dermatitis, interstitial pneumonitis
- Nephrotoxicity
- Hepatic fibrosis
- Seizure
- Meningismus on intrathecal administration.

Uses
- Acute lymphoblastic leukemia in children
- Choriocarcinoma

- Burkitt's and other non-Hodgkin's lymphoma.
- Cancer of breast, ovary, bladder, head, and neck
- Rheumatoid arthritis, psoriasis.

Pemetrexed
Actions
- It inhibits not only DHFRase but also thymidylate synthase and other enzymes necessary for synthesis of DNA.
- It acts on S phase of growth cycle.
- It has greater capacity to enter into cells where it is stored as polyglutamates.

Adverse Effects
- Erythematous and pruritic rash
- Nausea, diarrhea, mucosal ulceration
- Myelosuppression.

Uses
- Mesothelioma
- Ovarian cancer
- Adenocarcinoma of lung.

Raltitrexed
Its primary action is inhibition of thymidylate synthase.

Trimetrexate
- It is highly lipid soluble and crosses BBB.
- It has modest antitumor activity.
- It is effective in the treatment of *Pneumocystis jirovecii* infection.

Pyrimidine Analogs
They are:
- Fluorouracil
- Floxuridine
- Cytosine arabinoside
- Gemcitabine
- Azacitidine
- Capecitabine.

Actions
- Pyrimidines are required in the biosynthesis of DNA and RNA.
- Pyrimidine analogs have structural similarity to pyrimidine and incorporate into nucleic acids and inhibit their function.

5-Fluorouracil (5-FU)
Actions
- It is converted to its active form floxuridine which incorporates into nucleic acids and inhibits their function and exerts cytotoxicity.
- Its oral absorption is unpredictable and incomplete.
- Hence, it is administered parenterally.
- Its duration of action is short.
- It is rarely used as single agent and combined with other anticancer drugs for treatment of cancer.

Adverse Effects
- Bone marrow depression
- Alopecia, hyperpigmentation
- Diarrhea, stomatitis
- Neuropathy and hand-foot syndrome.

Uses
- Metastatic colon cancer with oxaliplatin and leucovorin
- Breast cancer
- Upper GIT cancer.

Floxuridine
It is given as continuous infusion into hepatic artery for metastatic colon cancer.

Cytosine Arabinoside (Cytarabine)
Actions
- The conventional cytosine arabinoside should be administered through IV route.
- Liposomal cytosine arabinoside is available for intrathecal administration.
- If given orally, its bioavailability is reduced by cytidine deaminase present in GIT and liver.
- Children can tolerate higher dose of cytosine arabinoside better than adults.
- It has a very short half-life of 10 minutes.

Adverse Effects
- Myelosuppression
- Nausea, vomiting, stomatitis
- Pulmonary edema
- Arachnoiditis, delirium, seizure, and cerebellar toxicity

- Dermatitis, conjunctivitis
- Reversible elevation of liver enzymes.

Uses
- Acute and chronic myeloid leukemia
- Acute lymphocytic leukemia
- Meningeal and lymphomatous leukemia.

Capecitabine
- It is a prodrug of 5-fluorouracil.
- It can be administered orally.
- It is used in metastatic breast cancer and metastatic colon cancer.
- It can cause nausea, anorexia, diarrhea, stomatitis, alopecia, and myelosuppression.
- Hand-foot syndrome occurs more frequently with capecitabine than with 5-fluorouracil.

Gemcitabine
Actions
- It acts on S phase and inhibits DNA synthesis.
- It is administered through intravenous route.
- It increases the severity of cisplatin adverse effects.

Adverse Effects
- Myelosuppression
- Hepatotoxicity
- Posterior leukoencephalopathy syndrome
- Flu-like syndrome
- Asthenia.

Uses
- Metastatic pancreatic cancer
- Non-small cell cancer lung
- Bladder cancer
- Ovarian cancer.

Azacitidine
- It is used in the treatment of myelodysplasia.
- It causes severe nausea and vomiting.
- It also causes bone marrow depression.

Purine Analogs
The drugs are:
- 6-Mercaptopurine
- 6-Thioguanine

- Azathioprine
- Pentostatin
- Fludarabine
- Clofarabine
- Nelarabine
- Cladribine.

Actions
- They act as analogs for guanine and hypoxanthine.
- So, they incorporate into nucleic acids and inhibit purine synthesis.

6-Mercaptopurine (6-MP)
Actions
- 6-mercaptopurine and 6-thioguanine are both 6-thiopurine analogs.
- They interfere with the synthesis of DNA.
- The oral absorption is incomplete.
- They undergo first pass metabolism.
- 6-MP attains high concentration in WBC and bone marrow.
- They are metabolized by xanthine oxidase.
- Prolonged therapy can cause acute myeloid leukemia.

Adverse Effects
- Bone marrow depression
- Anorexia, nausea, vomiting
- Hepatic dysfunction.

Use
Acute lymphocytic leukemia (ALL).

Fludarabine
Actions
- It can be administered both orally and parenterally.
- It is also an immunosuppressant.

Adverse Effects
- Thrombocytopenia, lymphopenia
- Tumor lysis syndrome
- Anorexia, peripheral neuropathy.

Use
Chronic lymphocytic leukemia (CLL).

Cladribine

Actions
- It is given intravenously.
- It crosses BBB and its CSF concentration is higher than its plasma concentration.

Adverse Effects
- Cumulative thrombocytopenia
- Fever, headache, rash.

Uses
- Hairy cell leukemia
- CLL
- Waldenstrom macroglobinemia.

Clofarabine

Actions
- It is given intravenously.
- It has long intracellular half-life.

Adverse Effects
- Myelosuppression
- Capillary leak syndrome
- Hepatic dysfunction.

Uses
- Pediatric and adult acute myeloid leukemia (AML)
- Pediatric acute lymphocytic leukemia (ALL)
- Myelodysplasia.

Nelarabine

Actions
- It is given as IV infusion.
- It has long half-life.

Adverse Effects
- Myelosuppression
- Liver dysfunction
- Guillain-Barre syndrome
- Neurotoxicity.

Use

T-cell leukemia.

Pentostatin
Actions
It is given as intravenous infusion as single bolus dose.
Adverse Effects
- Myelosuppression
- Nausea, vomiting, fever, rash
- Opportunistic infection.

Use
Hairy cell leukemia.

NATURAL PRODUCTS
They are:
  I. **Vinca alkaloids:** Vincristine, vinblastine, vinorelbine.
 II. **Taxanes:** Paclitaxel, docetaxel.
III. **Epipodophyllotoxins:** Etoposide, teniposide.
IV. **Camptothecin:** Topotecan, irinotecan.
 V. **Epothilone:** Ixabepilone.
VI. **Antibiotics:** Dactinomycin (actinomycin), doxorubicin, daunorubicin, epirubicin, idarubicin.
VII. **Anthracenediones:** Mitoxantrone, mitomycin, bleomycin.
VIII. **Echinocandin:** Yondelis (trabectedin).
IX. **Enzyme:** L-Asparaginase.

Vinca Alkaloids
- They are isolated from Madagascar periwinkle plant *Vinca rosea*, a species of myrtle.
- They are cell cycle specific and act on M phase.
- They inhibit mitosis by preventing the formation of microtubules.
- Cross resistance occurs among the vinca alkaloids.
- They are mainly excreted in bile.

Vincristine
Actions
- It is tolerated better by children than by adults.
- Hence, it is mainly used in childhood leukemia
- It causes minimal bone marrow toxicity but can cause severe neurotoxicity.

Adverse Effects
- Peripheral neuropathy, alopecia

- Paresthesia, sensory loss, urinary hesitancy
- Severe constipation.

Uses
- Hodgkin's and non-Hodgkin's lymphoma
- Acute lymphocytic leukemia
- Neuroblastoma, rhabdomyosarcoma
- Wilms' tumor.

Vinblastine
- It is given with bleomycin and cisplatin in metastatic testicular cancer.
- It is also used in Hodgkin's disease and bladder cancer.
- It causes minimal neurotoxicity and its main adverse effect is myelosuppression.

Vinorelbine
- It is mainly indicated in non-small cell cancer of lung.
- It has intermediate toxicity profile.
- It causes mild neurotoxicity but profound bone marrow depression.

Taxanes

Actions
- They are isolated from the bark of Western yew tree.
- They inhibit mitosis by forming stable microtubules that fail to divide.
- Nab-paclitaxel is more water soluble formulation than paclitaxel.
- Docetaxel is more water soluble than paclitaxel.
- They are used with other drugs in advanced metastatic cancer.

Adverse Effects
- Bone marrow depression
- Peripheral neuropathy with Nab-paclitaxel
- Hypersensitivity reaction with paclitaxel and not with Nab-paclitaxel
- Docetaxel causes higher incidence of neutropenia but minimal asthenia and peripheral neuropathy
- Peripheral edema, pulmonary edema, interstitial pneumonitis are other side effects of docetaxel.

Use
Metastatic ovarian, breast, lung, GIT, genitourinary, head, and neck cancer.

Anticancer Drugs

Epothilones
- They are obtained from myxobacterium found in river bank soil.
- They stabilize the microtubules and inhibit cell division.
- They are used in metastatic breast cancer.
- The solvent used in intravenous formulation causes infusion related reactions.
- Bone marrow depression, peripheral neuropathy, diarrhea, asthenia, and fatigue are the other side effects.

Camptothecins
- They are obtained from the Chinese tree *Camptotheca acuminata*.
- They inhibit the function of DNA topoisomerase I enzyme.
- While topotecan is active as such irinotecan should be converted into its active metabolite SN-38.
- Topotecan is used in ovarian and small-cell cancer of lung.
- Both drugs are given as intravenous infusion.
- The main toxicity of topotecan is neutropenia.
- Irinotecan causes life-threatening diarrhea and severe neutropenia.
- Irinotecan with 5-FU or oxaliplatin is given as first-line therapy in colorectal cancer.

Epipodophyllotoxins
- They are isolated from May apple or mandrake plant.
- They inhibit the function of DNA topoisomerase II enzyme.
- They are used as adjuncts with other agents in the treatment of cancer.
- Etoposide is used in testicular cancer and in ALL.
- Teniposide is used in refractory ALL.
- Etoposide causes leukopenia, reversible alopecia, nausea, vomiting, and stomatitis.
- Long-term complication of etoposide in children with ALL is acute nonlymphocytic leukemia.
- Teniposide causes bone marrow depression, nausea and vomiting.

Antibiotics

Dactinomycin
Actions
- Dactinomycin inhibits DNA dependent RNA polymerase.
- It is the most potent anticancer drug.

- It does not enter CSF after IV administration.
- It is excreted through bile and urine.

Adverse Effects
GIT toxicity, pancytopenia, alopecia.

Uses
- Rhabdomyosarcoma
- Wilm's tumor
- Choriocarcinoma.

Daunorubicin, Doxorubicin, Epirubicin, Idarubicin
- They inhibit the function of DNA by complexing with topoisomerase II enzyme.
- These drugs accumulate in heart, kidneys, lungs, spleen, and liver.
- These drugs are cardiotoxic except idarubicin which is less cardiotoxic.
- They cause tachycardia, hypotension, arrhythmia, and pericardial effusion.
- They also cause bone marrow depression and GIT toxicity
- Doxorubicin causes myelosuppression and 'adriamycin flare' or erythematous streak at the site of infusion.
- Daunorubicin and idarubicin are used in the treatment of AML.
- Doxorubicin and epirubicin are used in solid tumors.

Anthracenediones
- Mitoxantrone inhibits DNA function.
- It causes less cardiotoxicity.
- It is mainly indicated in prostate cancer and acute lymphocytic leukemia.
- It causes nausea, vomiting, alopecia and bone marrow depression.
- Bleomycin causes DNA damage.
- It causes minimal bone marrow toxicity but causes severe pulmonary fibrosis and cutaneous lesions.
- It is indicated in testicular tumor, ovarian cancer and in Hodgkin's lymphoma.
- It is included in first-line ABVD (Adriamycin, Bleomycin, Vinblatine and Dacarbazine) regimen in Hodgkin's lymphoma.
- Mitomycin inhibits DNA synthesis.
- It is indicated for bladder and anal cancer.
- It causes bone marrow depression, GIT toxicity and hemolytic-uremic syndrome.

Yondelis (Trabectedin)
- It is an alkylating agent.
- It is derived from a sea animal.
- It is a drug with 'orphan' status.
- It is indicated in ovarian cancer, pancreatic cancer and in sarcoma.
- Severe hepatic dysfunction, myelosuppression and rhabdomyolysis are its important side effects.

L-Asparaginase
- It deprives the aminoacid asparagine to malignant cells and causes cell death.
- It is mainly administered through IM or IV route.
- Anaphylaxis, urticaria, hypersensitivity reaction, pancreatitis, hyperglycemia, and deficiency of clotting factors are its main side effects.
- It is mainly used in the treatment of ALL.

MISCELLANEOUS AGENTS
They are:
- A. **DDT like compound:** Mitotane
- B. **Substituted urea:** Hydroxyurea
- C. **Differentiating agents:** Retinoids, arsenic trioxide, histone deacetylase inhibitors.

Mitotane
- Mitotane causes destruction of adrenocortical cells.
- It is used in adrenal cortex tumor.
- It causes nausea, anorexia, somnolence and lethargy.

Hydroxyurea
Actions
- It inhibits ribonucleoside reductase, an enzyme necessary for DNA synthesis.
- It has almost 100% oral bioavailability.

Adverse Effects
- Anemia, leukopenia
- Stomatitis, interstitial pneumonitis, alopecia.

Uses
- Chronic myeloid leukemia (CML)

- Myeloid metaplasia
- Polycythemia vera.

Differentiating Agents
- They induce differentiation of undifferentiated tumors.
- Retinoids such as tretinoin cause complete remission in acute promyelocytic leukemia.
- It can cause pseudotumor cerebri, dry skin, liver dysfunction, and bone tenderness.
- Arsenic trioxide is indicated for CML and for acute promyelocytic leukemia relapse.
- Liver dysfunction, hyperglycemia, fatigue, and dizziness are some of the side effects.
- Vorinostat is a histone deacetylase inhibitor.
- It is an epigenetic modifier and inhibits histone function.
- It is indicated in refractory cutaneous T-cell lymphoma.
- Thrombocytopenia, fatigue, nausea, and diarrhea are the main side effects.

HORMONES
- **Tamoxifen:** SERM used in premenopausal and postmenopausal breast cancer.
- **Toremifene:** SERM used in postmenopausal breast cancer.
- **Fulvestrant:** SERD used in postmenopausal metastatic breast cancer.
- **Anastrozole, letrozole, exemestane:** Inhibitors of estrogen synthesis used in postmenopausal breast cancer.
- **Leuprolide, goserelin:** GnRH agonists used in prostate cancer.
- **Flutamide, nilutamide, bicalutamide:** Androgen antagonists used in prostate cancer.
    - **SERM:** Selective estrogen receptor modulator
    - **SERD:** Selective estrogen receptor down regulator
    - **GnRH agonist:** Gonadotropin release hormone agonist.

Nursing Responsibilities
- Monitor complete blood count periodically for all patients on anticancer agents.
- Patients on cyclophosphamide and ifosfamide should receive vigorous intravenous hydration to reduce the incidence of hemorrhagic cystitis.

Anticancer Drugs

- If patients on oral therapy of cyclophosphamide and ifosfamide develop hematuria, it should be immediately reported to the attending physician.
- Tingling, burning or redness of hand and foot of patients on 5-fluorouracil requires to be reported to the attending physician.
- Renal function should be closely monitored in patients on nelarabine.

TARGETED THERAPY IN CANCER

Protein Tyrosine Kinase Inhibitors
- Protein tyrosine kinase is essential for DNA synthesis.
- Protein tyrosine kinase inhibitors inhibit DNA synthesis.
- Imatinib, nilotinib and dasatinib are used in CML.
- They cause mild GIT toxicity.
- They also cause dependent edema and periorbital swelling.
- While nilotinib prolongs QT interval, dasatinib causes pleural effusion.
- Lapatinib inhibits tyrosine kinase activity of human epidermal growth factor receptor 2 (HER2)/neu glycoprotein and used in refractory breast cancer.
- It causes cardiac failure.
- Geftinib and erlotinib are epidermal growth factor receptor (EGFR) tyrosine kinase inhibitors.
- Both drugs are indicated in non-small cell cancer of lung.
- They cause severe diarrhea, anorexia, fatigue and rash.
- Although rare, they can cause fatal interstitial lung disease.

MONOCLONAL ANTIBODIES IN CANCER
They are:
- Rituximab
- Cetuximab
- Alemtuzumab
- Trastuzumab
- Bevacizumab
- Panitumumab
- Gemtuzumab.

Nomenclature
- **Ximab:** Chimeric antibody.
- **Umab:** Humanized antibody.

- They target the antigens expressed by cancer cells.
- They kill cancer cells either by antibody-dependent cellular toxicity (ADC) or by complement-dependent cytotoxicity (CDC).
- They cause infusion related reaction, rash and bone marrow suppression.
- **Cetuximab:** Cytotoxic EGFR blocker used in metastatic colon as well as head and neck cancer.
- **Panitumumab:** EGFR inhibitor used in metastatic colorectal cancer.
- Both cetuximab and panitumumab can also cause acne, pruritus, diarrhea, fatigue, pulmonary fibrosis, and electrolyte imbalance.
- Trastuzumab inhibits HER2/neu glycoprotein and used in metastatic breast cancer. It can cause cardiotoxicity.
- Rituximab inhibits CD20 B-cell antigen. It is used in B-cell lymphoma. It causes late-onset neutropenia.
- Ofatumumab inhibits CD20 B-cell antigen. It causes antibody dependent and complement dependent cytotoxicity. It is used in CLL. It causes hypersensitivity reaction and immunosuppression.
- Alemtuzumab causes antibody dependent and complement dependent cytotoxicity. It is used in B and T- cell lymphomas. It causes pancytopenia and opportunistic infection.
- Geftuzumab-ozogamicin induces apoptosis and used in AML. It causes myelosuppression and liver dysfunction.
- Tositumomab and ibritumomab are radioimmunoconjugates used in lymphoma. They can cause bone marrow depression, hypersensitivity reactions and secondary leukemias.

ANGIOGENESIS INHIBITORS
- Bevacizumab, sunitinib and sorafenib inhibit vascular endothelial growth factor (VEGF).
- Bevacizumab is indicated as monotherapy in the treatment of renal-cell cancer.
- It is combined with other drugs in the treatment of colorectal, lung and breast cancer.
- Sunitinib is used in metastatic renal cell cancer and sorafenib is used in hepatocellular cancer.
- All these drugs can result in vessel injury, bleeding, hypertension, and proteinuria.
- Thalidomide and lenalidomide have additional immunomodulatory action.

Anticancer Drugs

- They induce tumor cell apoptosis and inhibit production of tumor necrosis factor α and interleukin-6.
- They are used in refractory multiple myeloma.
- In addition, lenalidomide is also used in myelodysplastic syndrome and in CLL.
- Severe neurological manifestation can occur during thalidomide therapy.
- Carpal tunnel syndrome and pyramidal tract involvement occur frequently.
- Painful paresthesia, sensory loss, numbness of toes and feet, weakness and muscle cramps can occur.
- Thalidomide is teratogenic and should be avoided during pregnancy.
- Lenalidomide is not teratogenic and is well tolerated but can cause significant leukopenia.
- It causes mild sedation, neuropathy and constipation.

PROTEASOME INHIBITORS
- Bortezomib, the proteasome inhibitor is used in multiple myeloma.
- It is also used in mantle cell lymphoma.
- It causes thrombocytopenia and peripheral neuropathy.

mTOR INHIBITORS
- Rapamycin analogs inhibit mammalian target of rapamycin (mTOR) and promote apoptosis.
- Everolimus and temsirolimus are the rapamycin analogs.
- They are indicated in renal cell and hepatocellular cancer.
- They cause rash, mucositis, anemia, leukopenia and fatigue.
- **Other details:** See Section XI, Chapter 76

Interleukin-2
- It stimulates proliferation of T-cells.
- It causes capillary leak syndrome, hypotension, myelosuppression, pruritus, liver dysfunction and hypothyroidism.
- It is used in metastatic renal cell cancer and melanoma.

Denileukin Diftitox
- It is an immunotoxin obtained from interleukin-2.
- It inhibits protein synthesis and used in cutaneous T-cell lymphoma.

- It causes vascular leak syndrome and hypersensitivity reactions.

Nursing Responsibilities
- Patients on erlotinib and geftinib should be closely watched for symptoms of lung disease such as cough and dyspnea. If present, they should be reported to the attending physician.
- Liver function should be monitored in patients on erlotinib and geftinib.

CHAPTER 76

Immunosuppressants

CALCINEURIN INHIBITORS

Cyclosporine
- Cyclosporine inhibits calcineurin.
- It suppresses T-cell activation.
- It inhibits graft rejection during transplantation.
- It is indicated in kidney, liver, heart, and other organ transplantation.
- As an immunosuppressive agent, it is used in rheumatoid arthritis and psoriasis.
- It is also used in inflammatory bowel disease and in atopic dermatitis resistant to standard therapy.
- Nephrotoxicity, hirsutism, hyperuricemia, hypertension, and gingival hyperplasia are its side effects.

Tacrolimus
- It also inhibits calcineurin.
- It inhibits activation of T cell.
- It is more effective than cyclosporine.
- Hence, it is preferred during organ transplantation.
- It is also used for Crohn's disease and applied topically for atopic dermatitis.
- It causes neurotoxicity, nephrotoxicity, hyperglycemia, diarrhea, and alopecia.

mTOR Inhibitors
- Sirolimus and everolimus are the rapamycin analogs.
- Rapamycin analogs inhibit mammalian target of rapamycin (mTOR).
- They inhibit activation of T-cells.
- They are used as prophylaxis during organ transplantation with calcineurin inhibitors.
- They help to reduce the dose of calcineurin inhibitors.
- They also reduce calcineurin inhibitors induced renal toxicity.
- They increase serum cholesterol and triglycerides.

- They also cause anemia, leukopenia, thrombocytopenia, mouth ulcer, and delayed wound healing.

Antiproliferative Agents
- Azathioprine is used to prevent graft versus host reaction during renal transplantation.
- It causes bone marrow suppression, hepatotoxicity and increased susceptibility to infection.
- Methotrexate and cyclophosphamide are also used as immunosuppressants during transplantation.
- Mycophenolate mofetil inhibits T and B cell synthesis.
- It is used during renal transplantation.
- It can cause leukopenia, vomiting and diarrhea.

Antithymocyte Globulin
- It is a combination of purified γ globulin from rabbit serum immunized with human thymocytes.
- It is used to prevent acute rejection after renal transplantation.
- Hypotension, leukopenia, thrombocytopenia, increased risk of infection, and serum sickness can occur.

Monoclonal Antibodies
- Muromonab, daclizumab, alemtuzumab, etanercept, and infliximab are useful as immunosuppressants.
- Muromonab is used only in acute organ transplantation rejection reaction.
- Daclizumab is used as prophylaxis in acute organ transplantation rejection reaction.
- Alemtuzumab is used in CLL and in renal transplantation.
- Infliximab is used to suppress TNF in rheumatoid arthritis, Crohn's disease, ulcerative colitis and psoriasis.
- Etanercept and adalimumab also suppress TNF and are used in rheumatoid arthritis.
- Other indications are plaque psoriasis, juvenile arthritis, psoriatic arthritis and ankylosing spondylitis.
- Efalizumab is indicated in renal transplantation and in psoriasis.
- Alefacept is used to prevent transplantation reaction after cardiac transplant.

Nursing Responsibilities
Renal function should be monitored for a long time in patients on sirolimus and everolimus.

SECTION XII

Miscellaneous Topics

- Nonsteroidal Anti-inflammatory Drugs (NSAIDs)
- Pharmacotherapy of Rheumatoid Arthritis
- Pharmacotherapy of Gout
- Chelating Agents
- Antiseptics, Disinfectants and Ectoparasiticides
- Drugs Acting on Skin and Mucous Membrane

Nonsteroidal Anti-Inflammatory Drugs (NSAIDs)

They reduce the synthesis of prostaglandins by inhibiting cyclooxygenase enzyme. They are analgesic, antipyretic and anti-inflammatory drugs. Most of the traditional nonsteroidal anti-inflammatory drugs (NSAIDs) are reversible competitive inhibitors of cyclooxygenase. COX-2 inhibitors are selective agents.

ASPIRIN (ACETYL SALICYLIC ACID)
Actions
- Aspirin, the acetyl salicylic acid is an irreversible inhibitor of cyclooxygenase enzyme.
- It is used in pain of low and moderate intensity such as toothache.
- It is also an antipyretic and anti-inflammatory agent.
- At a low dose of 100 mg/day, aspirin inhibits platelet aggregation.
- This action of aspirin is permanent and lasts till the lifetime of platelets.
- A small dose of 1 to 2 g/day of aspirin decreases uric acid excretion, increasing its plasma level.
- Large dose of >5 g/day is uricosuric and promotes uric acid excretion.
- At high dose, it causes sodium and water retention, increase in cardiac output and noncardiogenic pulmonary edema.
- It is well absorbed orally and is extensively bound to plasma proteins.
- It is widely distributed and crosses placental barrier.

Adverse Effects
- Nausea, vomiting, anorexia, erosive gastritis and heart burn
- Hypoprothrombinemia, vitamin K deficiency
- Respiratory alkalosis
- Nephrotoxicity
- Hepatotoxicity
- Tinnitus

Contraindications
- Peptic ulcer
- Influenza and other viral infection in children and young adults due to the possibility of Reye's syndrome.

Uses
- Inflammation
- Mild pain
- Cardioprotection
- Acute rheumatic fever
- Chemoprevention of colon cancer
- Systemic mastocytosis
- Niacin induced flushing

OTHER SALICYLATES
Actions
- Salicylates are mild analgesic agents and inhibit cyclooxygenase enzyme.
- At higher doses, they exert anti-inflammatory action.
- Their antipyretic action is centrally mediated.
- They cause compensatory respiratory alkalosis initially.
- At toxic dose, they result in compensatory renal acidosis.
- Food delays their absorption.
- They are widely distributed into most body fluids and cross the placental barrier.
- They prolong gestation, reduce birth weight and increase perinatal mortality.
- Their excretion is high in alkaline urine.

Adverse Effects
- Respiratory alkalosis
- Nephrotoxicity
- Noncardiogenic pulmonary edema
- Nausea, vomiting, gastric bleeding and gastritis
- Hepatotoxicity
- Vertigo, tinnitus

Uses
- Diflunisal is used in rheumatoid arthritis, osteoarthritis and musculoskeletal sprain.

- Mesalamine and sulfasalazine are used in inflammatory bowel disease, ulcerative colitis and proctitis.
- Salicylic acid is keratolytic and used in wart, corn and fungal infection.
- Methyl salicylate (oil of wintergreen) is used in musculoskeletal pain.

Salicylate Intoxication

Headache, tinnitus, difficulty in hearing and vision, convulsion, psychosis, stupor, respiratory depression, respiratory alkalosis, renal acidosis, vasomotor depression, and ketonuria.

Treatment
- Activated charcoal
- Intravenous (IV) fluids for dehydration
- Correction of hypokalemia and hyperpyrexia
- Maintenance of acid-base balance
- Blood transfusion and vitamin K in case of blood loss.

PARACETAMOL

Actions
- It is an analgesic and antipyretic agent.
- Its anti-inflammatory action is minimal due to high level of peroxide in the inflammatory fluid.
- It has excellent oral bioavailability.
- It causes minimal gastrointestinal tract (GIT) irritation.
- It is metabolized to N- acetyl-para-benzoquinone imine (NAPQI) that causes hepatotoxicity.
- It is the first-line drug in osteoarthritis.
- It occasionally causes rash and other allergic reactions.
- It can cause neutropenia, thrombocytopenia, pancytopenia, methemoglobinemia, and hemolytic anemia.

Paracetamol Toxicity
- It is a medical emergency.
- The symptoms in first 2 days are mainly anorexia, nausea and abdominal pain.
- Abnormality of liver enzymes occurs 2 to 4 days after ingestion and peaks after 96 hours.
- Ninety percent of patients suffer from fatal hepatic necrosis involving centrilobular area.

- Hypoglycemic coma and renal tubular necrosis can occur.
- Hepatic necrosis occurs due to accumulation of NAPQI.
- NAPQI depletes hepatic glutathione level.
- If mild, hepatic lesion can reverse within few weeks.
- Hepatic encephalopathy indicates poor prognosis.

Treatment
- Activated charcoal within 4 hours of ingestion to reduce paracetamol absorption.
- N-acetylcysteine, the precursor of glutathione to detoxify NAPQI.
- Supportive care.
- Maintenance of renal function and treatment of hypoglycemia.

Nursing Responsibilities
- Since hepatotoxicity is delayed and occurs after 2 days, it should not be missed.
- Plasma glucose levels should be monitored as hypoglycemia occurs in liver failure.
- Gastric lavage is not recommended in paracetamol overdose.

INDOMETHACIN

Actions
- It is a nonselective COX inhibitor.
- It is 20 times more potent than aspirin.
- It is a good anti-inflammatory, analgesic and antipyretic agent.
- It has excellent oral bioavailability.
- It attains low CSF concentration but concentrates highly in synovial fluid.

Adverse Effects
- Frontal headache
- Light headedness, vertigo, tinnitus
- Gastric ulceration, diarrhea
- Hepatitis
- Rarely pancreatitis
- Depression, psychosis, suicidal tendency

Uses
- Rheumatoid arthritis, osteoarthritis, ankylosing spondylitis, gouty arthritis
- Parenteral formulation is available for therapy of patent ductus arteriosus (PDA).

- Refractory fever of Hodgkin's lymphoma.
- Bartter syndrome

Sulindac
- It is a nonselective COX inhibitor.
- Since it is a congener of indomethacin, it was expected to cause minimal GIT toxicity than indomethacin.
- Because as a prodrug, the gastric mucosa is not directly exposed to the drug.
- Still, it causes GIT toxicity due to exposure of gastric mucosa to the drug in systemic circulation.
- It is used in cancer chemoprophylaxis to prevent colon cancer in patients with familial adeno polyposis (FAP).

Etodolac
- It causes minimal gastric irritation and is well tolerated.
- It has uricosuric action.
- It is an excellent analgesic agent and given for postoperative pain.
- It is also used in osteoarthritis and rheumatoid arthritis.
- It is available as sustained release preparation.

Tolmetin
- It accumulates in synovial fluid.
- It is used in osteoarthritis, rheumatoid arthritis and ankylosing spondylitis.
- It is also effective in juvenile rheumatoid arthritis.
- It causes gastric irritation and CNS side effects.

Ketorolac
Actions
- Its analgesic activity is comparable to opioids.
- It has only moderate anti-inflammatory activity.
- It has quick onset of action.
- Its duration of action is short.

Adverse Effects
- Somnolence
- Headache
- Dizziness
- Nausea, dyspepsia

Uses
- Postoperative pain
- Topical application is used for preventing ocular inflammation after cataract surgery and in seasonal allergic conjunctivitis.

Nabumetone
- It is an anti-inflammatory agent.
- It is effective in rheumatoid arthritis and osteoarthritis.
- It can cause abdominal cramp, diarrhea and gastric ulceration.
- Its off label use is for short-term therapy of soft tissue injury.

Diclofenac
Actions
- It has analgesic, anti-inflammatory and antipyretic actions.
- It is more potent than other NSAIDs.
- It is absorbed rapidly and is extensively bound to plasma proteins.
- Its duration of action is short.
- It undergoes vey high first pass metabolism.
- It accumulates in synovial fluid thereby prolonging its therapeutic benefit in joint inflammation.
- It is available as gel and transdermal patch for topical application.
- It is available as immediate release, extended release and sustained release formulation for oral use.
- Diclofenac carries a 'black box' warning for cardiovascular side effects.

Adverse Effects
- Gastrointestinal tract side effect
- Nephrotoxicity, fluid retention and edema
- Hypersensitivity
- Reversible elevation of liver enzymes
- Thrombosis and other cardiovascular events.

Uses
- Rheumatoid arthritis, ankylosing spondylitis, osteoarthritis
- Acute migraine
- Primary dysmenorrhea
- Postoperative inflammation after ocular surgery.

PROPIONIC ACID DERIVATIVES
The drugs are ibuprofen, naproxen, fenoprofen, flurbiprofen, oxaprozin, ketoprofen.

Ibuprofen
Actions
- It is a nonselective cyclooxygenase inhibitor.
- It is absorbed rapidly and extensively bound to plasma proteins.

- Since it accumulates slowly in the synovial fluid, its action persists even after a fall in its plasma concentration.

Adverse Effects
- Gastric irritation
- Headache, dizziness
- Thrombocytopenia, rash
- Toxic ambylopia, blurring of vision
- Fluid retention, edema

Uses
- Rheumatoid arthritis
- Osteoarthritis
- Dysmenorrhea
- Patent ductus arteriosus

Naproxen

Actions
- It is a nonselective NSAID with antiplatelet action.
- Its duration of action is prolonged in elderly patients due to their compromised renal function.
- It is 99% bound to plasma proteins, crosses placenta and is secreted in milk.
- It can be administered rectally in children.
- It is very effective in reducing morning stiffness of joints.

Adverse Effects
- Drowsiness, dizziness, headache, fatigue
- Ototoxicity, depression
- Pruritus

Uses
- Rheumatoid arthritis
- Osteoarthritis, ankylosing spondylitis, tendonitis, bursitis
- Acute gout
- Dysmenorrhea

Mefenamic Acid
- It is used in dysmenorrhea, soft tissue injury, rheumatoid arthritis and osteoarthritis.
- It causes reversible elevation of liver enzymes.

Piroxicam

- It is an anti-inflammatory agent with multiple mechanisms.
- In addition to its inhibitory action on cyclooxygenase enzyme, it also inhibits neutrophils activation.
- Further, it inhibits collagenase and proteoglycanase in the cartilage.
- Its absorption is complete and it undergoes enterohepatic circulation.
- It is extensively bound to plasma proteins.
- After 7 to 12 days, its plasma concentration is equal to its concentration in synovial fluid.
- Since its onset of action is slow, it is not suited for the management of acute pain conditions.
- When compared to other NSAIDs, it causes severe GIT and skin reaction.
- It is useful in rheumatoid arthritis and osteoarthritis.

Selective COX-2 Inhibitors

- Celecoxib, parecoxib, etoricoxib belong to this group.
- Since their action is selective, they cause minimal GIT side effects.

Celecoxib

- It is used in acute pain, dysmenorrhea, juvenile rheumatoid arthritis, adult rheumatoid arthritis, osteoarthritis, and ankylosing spondylitis.
- It is also approved in chemoprevention of familial adeno polyposis.
- It can cause thrombosis and result in myocardial infarction and stroke.
- Inhibition of prostaglandin synthesis in kidney causes edema and hypotension.

Parecoxib

- It is effective in postoperative pain.
- It is the only COX-2 inhibitor available as a parenteral formulation.
- It can cause life-threatening toxic epidermal necrolysis, erythema multiforme and Stevens-Johnson syndrome.
- It results in high incidence of cardiovascular problems and hypersensitivity reactions.

Etoricoxib
- It results in minimal GIT toxicity but increases the risk of stroke and heart attack.
- It can be given once daily in gouty arthritis, rheumatoid arthritis and osteoarthritis.
- It can be given safely in renal dysfunction but requires dose reduction in hepatic dysfunction.

Apazone
- In addition to its analgesic, antipyretic and anti-inflammatory action, it is also a potent uricosuric agent.
- It inhibits neutrophil migration and production of superoxide radicals.
- It is effective in rheumatoid arthritis, gout, osteoarthritis, and ankylosing spondylitis.
- Although well tolerated with minimal GIT side effects it can cause mild CNS toxicity.

Nursing Responsibilities In NSAIDs Therapy
- Dyspepsia, nausea and heart burn occur during the first week of therapy but gastritis occurs later.
- Hypersensitivity reaction such as skin rash and difficulty in breathing should be watched for.
- Twenty four hours urine output, blood urea, serum creatinine should be monitored to rule out nephrotoxicity.
- Do not give ibuprofen within 30 minutes of administration of low dose aspirin.
- Do not give more than the recommended dose of ketorolac as it is highly toxic with FDA black box warning for nephrotoxicity, bleeding, hypersensitivity and GIT side effects.
- Persons with known hypersensitivity to aspirin should not be given ketorolac.

CHAPTER 78

Pharmacotherapy of Rheumatoid Arthritis

The drugs used are:
  I. Nonsteriodal anti-inflammatory drugs (NSAIDs)
 II. Disease-modifying antirheumatoid drugs (DMARDs)
    – **Biological DMARDs:** Adalimumab, golimumab, infliximab, etanercept, certolizumab, abatacept, rituximab, anakinra
    – **Nonbiological DMARDs:** Methotrexate, leflunomide, cyclosporine, cyclophosphamide, chloroquine, minocycline, azathioprine, sulfasalazine.

NONBIOLOGICAL DMARDs

They suppress the progression of disease by reducing the disease activity.

Methotrexate

- Methotrexate is a dihydrofolate reductase inhibitor.
- Low dose methotrexate is generally combined with other nonbiological DMARDs.
- This combination is effective in mild to moderate disease.
- Such a combination is suitable for long-term therapy.
- **Other details:** See Section XI, Chapter 75

Azathioprine

- It is converted to 6-mercaptopurine.
- It suppresses cell mediated immunity.
- It is combined with glucocorticoids in rheumatoid arthritis.
- **Other details:** See Section XI, Chapter 75

Sulfasalazine

- It contains sulfapyridine and 5-amino salicylic acid.
- It has moderate efficacy in rheumatoid arthritis.
- **Other details:** See Section XI, Chapter 56

Chloroquine

- It is an antimalarial drug.

- It inhibits the function of interleukin and monocytes.
- Long-term therapy of chloroquine is required in rheumatoid arthritis.
- **Other details:** See Section XI, Chapter 69

Leflunomide
- It inhibits proliferation of lymphocytes.
- It is an alternative to methotrexate.
- The onset of therapeutic benefit is rapid.
- Its metabolite is active with long half-life.
- Leflunomide causes nausea, rash, headache, alopecia, leukopenia, and thrombocytopenia.

Gold
- It arrests the progression of disease.
- It is given through intramuscular route.
- It causes dermatitis, stomatitis, hypertension, and organ damage.
- Auranofin is an orally acting gold preparation.
- It is less effective and less toxic.

Cyclosporine
- It is an immunosuppressant.
- It is rarely used now.
- It is a reserve drug.

Cyclophosphamide
- It is an alkylating agent and an immunosuppressant.
- It is very toxic and rarely used in rheumatoid arthritis.

Biological DMARDs
- They are reserved for those with persistent symptoms due to bony erosion.
- Such patients are positive for rheumatoid factor and they suffer from fuctional disability.
- Although effective as monotherapy, they are generally combined with methotrexate.
- They are tumor necrosis factor (TNF-α) inhibitors and suppress T-cell function.
- Hence, they are effective in autoimmune condition such as rheumatoid arthritis.
- They cause opportunistic infection such as tuberculosis.

Glucocorticoids
- They are indicated for acute flare-up of the condition.
- They are generally not suited for long-term therapy due to their side effects.

NSAIDs
- They provide only symptomatic relief and do not modify the course of the disease.
- They act as anti-inflammatory agents and do not suppress the progression of the disease.

CHAPTER 79

Pharmacotherapy of Gout

The drugs are:
- Colchicine
- Febuxostat
- Rasburicase
- Allopurinol
- Probenecid
- Benzbromarone

COLCHICINE

Actions

- It is a drug with narrow therapeutic index.
- It results in high side effects.
- It is a second-line drug.
- It arrests the cell division of rapidly dividing cells.
- It interferes with microtubule spindle formation and inhibits mitosis.
- It also suppresses the formation of superoxide anion.
- It inhibits secretion of chemotactic factors and neutrophils adhesion.
- It prevents mast cell degranulation.
- It inhibits insulin secretion and movement of melanin granules into melanophores.
- It inhibits respiratory center and lowers body temperature.
- It increases blood pressure.
- The oral absorption is rapid but variable.
- It is distributed widely and undergoes enterohepatic circulation.
- It accumulates in body causing cumulative toxicity.

Adverse Effects

- Nausea, vomiting, diarrhea, abdominal pain
- Myelosuppression, leukopenia, granulocytopenia, thrombocytopenia, aplastic anemia.

Uses

- Offers dramatic improvement in acute gout if given within 24 hours of attack. Complete remission of symptoms occurs within 72 hours.
- Prevention of amyloidosis.
- Familial mediterranean fever.

Off Label Use

Prevention of recurrent gout.

Nursing Responsibilities

- Minimum gap of 3 days and maximum gap of 14 days is required between subsequent courses of colchicine.
- The earliest sign for discontinuation of colchicine is its gastrointestinal tract (GIT) side effects.
- Delaying the administration of the second dose reduces the GIT toxicity.
- Overdose of colchicine can result in hemorrhagic gastropathy. Hence only the prescribed dose should be taken.
- Intravenous (IV) formulation obviates GIT toxicity but it is banned as it increases the risk of systemic toxicity.
- Blood count to be monitored regularly as it can cause aplastic anemia.

ALLOPURINOL

Actions

- It is used to treat hyperuricemia in gout.
- It reduces urate production through inhibition of the enzyme xanthine oxidase.
- It increases the excretion of xanthine and hypoxanthine.
- Both allopurinol and its metabolite oxypurinol are effective.
- Allopurinol facilitates dissolution of tophi.
- It delays further progression of the disease.
- It prevents development of nephropathy but does not alter the course of preexisting nephropathy.
- Since it mobilizes uric acid from tissue stores, it can precipitate an acute attack immediately after its administration.
- Hence, colchicine is always coadministered to prevent such attacks.
- It is rapidly absorbed and distributed widely.

- It increases the uricosuric effect of probenecid.
- Probenecid increases the clearance of oxypurinol thereby increasing the dose requirement of allopurinol.

Adverse Effects
- Hypersensitivity reaction
- Drowsiness
- Pruritus, urticaria
- Stevens-Johnson syndrome
- Fever, malaise, myalgia

Uses
- Primary and secondary gout.
- Hyperuricemia secondary to malignancy or cancer chemotherapy.
- Post transplantation hyperuricemia.
- Renal calculi with calcium oxalate crystals.
- Hyperuricemia in Lesch-Nyhan syndrome.

Drug Interactions
- Azathioprine and 6-mercaptopurine require dose modification if coadministered with allopurinol.
- It increases plasma concentration of theophylline.

Nursing Responsibilities
- Hypersensitivity reactions are common when it is coadministered with thiazide diuretic.
- It should not be combined with ampicillin as this combination can cause rash.

FEBUXOSTAT
- It is a non-purine xanthine oxidase inhibitor.
- It is more potent than allopurinol.
- It is effective only in patients with gouty hyperuricemia.
- It is not effective in asymptomatic hyperuricemia.
- Food slightly interferes with its oral absorption.
- It increases the plasma level of theophylline, azathioprine and 6-mercaptopurine.

Adverse Effects
- Joint pain, nausea, rash
- Stroke, myocardial infarction (MI)

Nursing Responsibilities
Liver function should be monitored periodically.

RASBURICASE
- It converts uric acid into its inactive metabolite.
- It is more effective than allopurinol in reducing uric acid level.
- It is used for initial therapy of leukemia, lymphoma and solid tumors in children.

Adverse Effects
- Hemolysis in patients with glucose 6-phosphate dehydrogenase (G6PD) deficiency
- Anaphylaxis
- Nausea, vomiting, diarrhea, constipation, abdominal pain, mucositis
- Methemoglobinemia, fever, headache

Nursing Responsibilities
Patient should be watched for signs of anaphylaxis during infusion of rasburicase.

PROBENECID
Actions
- It is a uricosuric agent.
- It inhibits tubular reabsorption of uric acid.
- It is absorbed completely in oral route.
- It is extensively bound to plasma proteins.
- It should not be used in gouty patients with nephrolithiasis.
- Coadministration of colchicine and non-steroidal anti-inflammatory drugs (NSAIDs) is essential during early therapy to prevent acute gouty attack.
- It prolongs the duration of action of penicillin by inhibiting its excretion.
- It is ineffective in patients with renal dysfunction.

Adverse Effects
- Gastritis
- Hypersensitivity reaction

Nursing Responsibilities
Patient should be advised to drink plenty of fluid to prevent the occurrence of renal calculi.

BENZBROMARONE
- It is a potent uricosuric agent.
- It increases the excretion of uric acid.
- Since the drug is excreted through bile, it can be safely administered in patients with renal dysfunction.
- It is more effective when combined with allopurinol.
- It can cause hepatotoxicity.

Nursing Responsibilities
Monitor liver function as benzbromarone can cause hepatic dysfunction.

NSAIDs
- They are used in acute gouty arthritis.
- Naproxen, indomethacin, sulindac, celecoxib, and etoricoxib are commonly used.
- Aspirin should not be given as it increases uric acid level at low doses and increases the risk of renal calculi at higher doses.

CHAPTER 80

Chelating Agents

- They form stable nontoxic complex with metals and promote their excretion.
- An ideal metal chelator should be highly water soluble, not metabolized and should be able to form stable, nontoxic complex with metals.
- It should have wide distribution into tissues and cerebrospinal fluid (CSF) and promote excretion of metal complex.
- It should have low affinity for essential metals in the body such as zinc and calcium.

DIMERCAPROL

Actions
- It is also known as British anti lewisite (BAL).
- Its sulfhydryl groups form chelation complex with heavy metals.
- It binds with the metal in the ratio of 2:1.
- Two molecules of dimercaprol bind with one molecule of the metal.
- It dissociates quickly in acidic urine potentiating metal induced renal toxicity.
- Alkalinization of urine prevents its rapid dissociation from the metal.
- It is lipophilic and crosses blood-brain barrier (BBB).
- Hence, it can mobilize the metals from other tissues to brain.
- It is given as deep intramuscular injection.

Adverse Effects
- Hypertension, tachycardia
- Conjunctivitis, salivation, vomiting, headache
- Anxiety, burning sensation in mouth.

Uses
- Arsenic, mercury, gold poisoning

- Combined with calcium disodium ethylenediamene-tetracetic acid (EDTA) for lead poisoning.

SUCCIMER
- It is less toxic than dimercaprol as it is more water soluble.
- It has good oral bioavailability.
- It does not cross BBB.
- So, it does not mobilize the metals from other tissues to brain.
- It does not chelate essential metals such as zinc, copper and iron.
- It is used in lead, arsenic and mercury poisoning.
- It causes anorexia, diarrhea and rash.

CALCIUM DISODIUM EDTA
Actions
- It is effective in acute but not in chronic lead poisoning.
- It is distributed extracellularly.
- It is rapidly excreted through kidney.
- It has high affinity for metals and acts by exchange of calcium with metals.
- Since it is not absorbed orally, it is given parenterally.
- Intramuscular (IM) injection is very painful so, it is available in combination with a local anesthetic for IM injection.
- Intravenous (IV) is the preferred route of administration.
- It mobilizes endogenous metals such as zinc, manganese and iron.

Adverse Effects
- Renal toxicity, hypocalcemic, tetany
- Frontal headache
- Chills, fever, malaise

Use
Acute lead poisoning

PENICILLAMINE
Actions
- It is inexpensive, orally effective but more toxic.
- It chelates copper, zinc, lead and mercury selectively.
- It is given as low dose following therapy with dimercaprol/calcium disodium EDTA.

Adverse Effects
- Urticaria, fever, pruritus, dry skin
- Renal toxicity
- Myasthenia gravis, lupus erythematosus, dermatomyositis.

Contraindications
- Pregnancy
- Renal insufficiency
- Previous history of penicillamine induced aplastic anemia or agranulocytosis.

Uses
- Wilsons disease
- Lead, zinc and mercury poisoning.

TRIENTINE
- It is less toxic but less potent than penicillamine.
- It is used in Wilson's disease.
- It is effective orally.
- It can cause iron deficiency.

DEFEROXAMINE
Actions
- It has high affinity for ferric ion.
- Hence, it does not remove the iron in cytochrome or hemoglobin.
- It is not absorbed orally.
- It is given through subcutaneous (SC), IM and IV routes.

Adverse Effects
- Rash, pruritus, anaphylaxis
- Diarrhea, tachycardia, leg cramp
- Neurotoxicity, cataract.

Contraindications
- Pregnancy
- Renal insufficiency.

Uses
- Iron poisoning
- Thalassemia.

DEFERASIROX
- It is an orally effective iron chelator.
- It is used to treat chronic iron overload in patients on repeated blood transfusion.

Nursing Responsibilities
- IV infusion of calcium disodium EDTA should be given slowly.
- History of peanut allergy should be asked in patients before parenteral administration of dimercaprol.
- Complete blood count should be monitored in patients on chronic therapy of penicillamine.

CHAPTER 81

Antiseptics, Disinfectants and Ectoparasiticides

- They inhibit or kill microbial organisms.
- The agents used on living tissues are antiseptics.
- Those used on inanimate objects are disinfectants.
- They cause oxidation of bacterial protoplasm, denaturation of proteins and increased cellular permeability.

PHENOL
- It is a weak antiseptic.
- It causes skin burns at higher concentration.
- It is cheap.
- It is used in disinfection of urine, feces and sputum.

CHLOROXYLENOL
- It is noncorrosive and nonirritant to intact skin.
- The commercial preparation of dettol is used as surgical antiseptic.
- It loses activity when kept for long-time after diluting in water.

HEXACHLOROPHENE
- It is usually included in the preparation of soap and other antiseptics.
- It is effective against Gram-positive but not against Gram-negative organisms.
- When used as 3% solution for baby bath it resulted in brain damage.

POTASSIUM PERMANGANATE
- It is an oxidizing agent and damages bacteria by liberating oxygen.
- At the concentration of 1:10,000 it is used for gargling and for irrigation of urethra and wound.
- It is also used in disinfection of water.

HYDROGEN PEROXIDE
- It liberates oxygen which acts against the microorganisms.

Antiseptics, Disinfectants and Ectoparasiticides | 541

- It promotes the decomposition of necrotic tissues resulting in foaming.
- It is used to remove slough and ear wax.

IODINE
- It acts against bacteria, fungi and viruses.
- It kills even the bacterial spores.
- It is available as tincture iodine, Mandel's paint and as ointment.
- Povidone iodine (polyvinyl pyrrolidone iodine) is a nontoxic, nonirritant preparation with germicidal activity.

CHLORINE
- It is a rapidly acting germicide.
- It is used to disinfect water.
- It is more active in neutral and acidic pH.
- Bleaching powder decomposes to release chlorine.
- It is used to disinfect drinking water and swimming pool.
- Sodium hypochlorite is used to disinfect milk cans.
- It is also used as antiseptic for root canal therapy in dentistry.

CHLORHEXIDINE
- It is more active against gram positive organisms.
- It is used as surgical scrub, mouthwash, skin antiseptic and for neonatal bath.
- It can stain teeth if used as mouthwash.

CETRIMIDE
- It is used as a cleansing agent for removing dirt, grease, dried blood, and tar.
- It is used as an antiseptic for surgical instruments.

ALCOHOL
- Ethyl alcohol is effective as antiseptic at 90% concentration.
- It precipitates bacterial proteins.
- As a solvent it enhances the antiseptic activity of chlorhexidine and iodine.
- Since it is an irritant, it should not be applied to mucous membrane.
- It does not kill spores and promotes rusting of metals.
- So, it is not used as antiseptic for instruments.

ALDEHYDE
- Formaldehyde is used in fumigation.
- Formalin is used to preserve dead tissues.
- It is slow acting and has pungent odor.
- It can cause eczema in those who handle it.

ACID
- Boric acid is used for douche, mouthwash and for irrigating eyes.
- It is used as paint in stomatitis and glossitis.

SALTS OF METALS
- Silver nitrate releases silver slowly and used as topical application for aphthous ulcer and in tonsillitis.
- It stains tissues black.
- Zinc sulfate is used in eyewash and to reduce skin perspiration.

DYES
- Gentian violet acts against gram positive bacteria.
- It is applied topically in chronic ulcer, furunculosis, oral thrush, eczema and in bedsore.
- Acriflavine is effective against Gram-positive organisms and gonococci.
- Unlike other agents, its activity is not hindered in the presence of organic matter.
- It is used in chronic ulcer and for cleaning wound.

ECTOPARASITICIDES
Drugs in Scabies and Pediculosis
Permethrin
- It causes paralysis of mites and lice.
- It is effective in both scabies and pediculosis.
- Single application can result in complete cure.
- Burning, itching and rash are the side effects.

Lindane
- It is less effective than permethrin.
- It is effective against scabies and head lice.
- It causes paralysis of mites and lice which develop resistance to lindane.

- It is highly lipid soluble so, can be absorbed from skin.
- It causes vertigo, cardiac arrhythmia and convulsion.

Benzyl Benzoate
- The cure rate in scabies is almost 100%.
- It should be applied twice within 24 hours for an effective cure.
- It causes contact dermatitis.
- It is less effective in pediculosis.

Crotamiton
- It is a second-line drug in both scabies and pediculosis.
- It is also an antipruritic agent.
- It should be applied daily for 5 days for effective treatment of scabies.
- It is preferred in children.

Ivermectin
- It is administered orally for treatment of ectoparasites.
- A single oral dose causes complete cure in scabies.
- It is also effective in the treatment of head lice.
- It is not indicated during pregnancy and in children less than 5 years.

Nursing Responsibilities
- Acriflavine solution should be stored in amber colored bottles away from sunlight otherwise it will lose its efficacy.
- While treating scabies, all other members in patient's family should also be treated concurrently.
- Cloths worn by scabies patients and family members should be washed in hot water and dried in sun to prevent reinfection.
- Care should be taken not to contaminate the eyes while applying ectoparasiticides in pediculosis as they are toxic to eyes.

CHAPTER 82

Drugs Acting on Skin and Mucous Membrane

TREATMENT OF ACNE VULGARIS
- Acne vulgaris is due to excessive production of sebum and colonization of bacteria and yeast.
- The fatty acid produced by bacterial lipase cause retention of secretion forming comedones.
- Both topical and systemic agents are used in the treatment of acne.

Topical Agents
- Benzoyl peroxide is an oxidizing agent and acts as keratolytic, comedolytic and bactericidal agent.
- It removes the comedone caps but causes burning sensation during topical application.
- Its side effects are dry skin, edema and dermatitis.
- Topical retinoids are first-line therapy in acne.
- All-trans retinoic acid (tretinoin) is a comedolytic agent and causes peeling of comedones.
- It has delayed onset of action and can cause skin irritation.
- Edema, erythema and burning sensation are its side effects.
- Tretinoin prevents photoaging of cells.
- Adapalene exerts anti-inflammatory action and suppresses comedone formation.
- It causes minimal irritation.
- It can be combined with benzoyl peroxide.
- Tazarotene is used for topical application in acne.
- Another topical agent azelaic acid inhibits aerobic and anaerobic microorganisms.
- It has delayed action and it also reduces melasma.
- Topical antibiotics used are clindamycin and erythromycin.
- Topical corticosteroid preparations such as clobetasol betamethasone, desonide, fluocinolone dexamethasone and triamcinolone are effective.

Systemic Agents
- Doxycycline, minocycline and erythromycin are preferred.
- Oral isotretinoin reduces sebum production.
- It can cause dry skin, conjunctivitis, pruritus and epistaxis.
- Besides, it is highly teratogenic and should be reserved for resistant acne.

Treatment of Psoriasis
- Psoralen ultraviolet A (PUVA) therapy is effective in severe psoriasis.
- Psoralen interferes with epithelial cell proliferation.
- They induce antiproliferative, anti-inflammatory and immunosuppressive effects.
- Oral methoxsalen is followed by UVA radiation after 1 to 2 hours on alternate days.
- It can cause skin cancer and cataract.
- Topical tazarotene is moderately effective in psoriasis.
- It acts as anti-inflammatory and antiproliferative agent.
- It may cause dermatitis and is also teratogenic.
- Oral acitretin inhibits cutaneous manifestations of psoriasis.
- It can cause erythema, alopecia, arthralgia, dry skin and dry eyes.
- It is mainly useful in pustular psoriasis.
- It is reserved for severe psoriasis as it is teratogenic.
- Hence, women patients on acitretin should avoid pregnancy for a minimum period of 3 years after stopping acitretin.

Demelanizing Agents
- Hydroquinone inhibits melanin forming enzymes.
- Thereby, it inhibits the production of melanocytes.
- It also promotes degradation of melanocytes.
- Its action is incomplete and pigmentation recurs on discontinuation of the drug.
- It can cause irritation and allergy.
- Monobenzone destroys melanocytes and causes permanent depigmentation.
- The treated area should be protected from sunlight by sunscreen.
- It can cause erythema, eczema and permanent hypopigmentation.
- It should not be used in hormonal induced or post inflammatory hyperpigmentation.
- Azelaic acid is a weak demelanizing agent and inhibits melanin synthesis.

ANDROGENIC ALOPECIA
Minoxidil
- Topical solution of minoxidil increases thickness, length and amount of hair.
- The growth of hair stops after discontinuation of minoxidil application.
- Contact dermatitis is its main side effect.

Finasteride
- It inhibits type II 5α-reductase enzyme in hair follicles.
- It is given orally.
- It increases hair growth over frontal scalp and in vertex.
- It is approved for use only in men.
- It can cause decreased libido and erectile dysfunction.

Nursing Responsibilities
Patients should be advised to wash their hands after application of minoxidil solution to prevent hair growth in unwanted areas.

SECTION XIII

Alternative Systems of Medicine

✦ Ayurveda, Siddha, Homeopathy and Unani Medicine

CHAPTER 83

Ayurveda, Siddha, Homeopathy and Unani Medicine

AYURVEDA

- Ayurveda originated in India
- The word ayurveda is derived from the Sanskrit words **ayu**- life and **veda**- knowledge
- The three main fundamental energies of ayurveda are movement, transformation and structure
- They are *vata* (wind), *pitta* (fire) and *kapha* (earth)
- Balance of these three energies results in health, while imbalance leads to disease
- The seven basic tissues mentioned in ayurveda are blood (*rakta*), plasma (*rasa*), bone (*asthi*), marrow (*majja*), muscles (*mamsa*) and semen (*shukra*)
- Earth, fire, water, air and akash (ether) are the five elements (panchabhuta) named in ayurveda
- It also mentions ten pairs of twenty *gunas* (two *gunas* in each pair)
- As per ayurveda, Parinama (effects of climate, cosmic rays and time), Asatmyendriyartha samyoga (improper use of sense organs), and Prajnaparadha (improper diet and behavior) can cause disease
- Diagnosis is based on Nidana (cause), Rupa (symptoms and signs), Purvarupa (prodromal symptoms), Samprapti (pathology) and Upashaya (factors against cause of the disease)
- Chaya (accumulation), Prakopa (aggravation), Prasara (overflowing), Sthanasamsraya (localization), Vyakti (manifestation) and Bheda (dissolution) are the six stages of a disease
- Maintenance of equilibrium is the main concept of therapy in ayurvedic medicine which helps to maintain health in normal individuals and also to treat people with diseases
- Dhanvantari, Charaka and Sushruta are the three important names associated with ayurveda
- The origin of ayurveda is credited to Dhanvantari, physician of the Gods
- Charaka compiled 'Charaka Samhita' that gives details of potential uses of substances as drugs

- Sushruta describes the surgical procedures in his book 'Sushruta Samhita'
- Whole plants, parts of plants, animal parts and minerals are used for therapy in ayurveda
- Cardamom, cinnamon, milk, bones, lead, copper sulfate, gold, sulfur and arsenic are some of the substances prescribed in ayurvedic medicine
- Ayurveda also focuses on diet, exercise, yoga, meditation and hygiene.

SIDDHA
- Siddha originated in India
- Siddhars with *'ashta siddhis'* (eight special powers) developed siddha
- Sage Agastya is the *guru* of these *siddhars*
- 'Siddha medicine' means 'the perfect medicine'
- 'Healthy soul through healthy body' is the concept of siddha
- It also deals with meditation that strengthens body and the soul
- Similar to ayurveda, the three main fundamental energies of siddha are also *vata* (wind), *pitta* (fire) and *kapha* (earth)
- Ratio between these three energies should be maintained at 4:2:1 for perfect health
- As per siddha, plasma (saram) is responsible for growth, blood (chenneer) for nourishment, muscle (ooun) for shape, fat (kozhuppu) for lubrication, bone (elumbu) for structure/posture, brain (moolai) for strength and semen (sukila) for reproduction
- Clinical examination of color (*varna*), voice (swara), eyes (*kan*), tongue (na), touch (sparisam), stool (mala), urine (*neer*) and pulse (*nadi*) help in diagnosis of the disease
- Thavara (herbs), thadhu (inorganic substances) and jangamam (animal products) are mentioned as drugs in siddha
- *Guna* (character), *suvai* (taste), *veerya* (strength), *pirivu* (class) and *mahimai* (action) are the five ways by which the drugs are classified
- They are also classified into 'internal medicine' and 'external medicine' according to their route of administration.

HOMEOPATHY
- Homeopathy was developed by the German physician 'Samuel Hahnemann'

- The seven principles in homeopathy are based on doctrine of 'drugs evaluation' and 'drugs dynamization', theory of 'chronic diseases' and 'vital force' as well as laws of 'similia', 'simplex' and 'minimum dose'
- Doctrine of drugs evaluation (drug proving) deals with investigating the capacity of a substance in inducing a disease while doctrine of drug dynamization deals with potentiating the latent medicinal properties of a substance to be used in therapy
- Theory of chronic diseases states that 'miasm' or disease producing agents cause disease
- As per the theory of vital force, an invisible vital energy or vital force maintains the health of an individual
- Law of similia means administration of substances capable of producing similar symptoms of a disease as the form of therapy to a diseased person
- Law of simplex states that only a single drug can be administered to the patient at any given time
- Law of minimum dose states that only a minute quantity of the drug should be administered to stimulate the dynamically deranged vital force/energy.

UNANI SYSTEM

- The word 'Unani' has originated from the Greek word 'Ionia', a place with thick population of Greeks in the coastal region of Anatolia
- It is a traditional medicine widely practiced in South Asia and means 'Greek medicine' in Hindi
- 'Canon of medicine', the encyclopedia written by Hakim Ibn Sina provides the basic information of unani medicine
- Concept of unani medicine is based on four humors namely phlegm (*balgham*), blood (dam), yellow bile (*safra*) and black bile (*sauda*)
- According to unani system, disequilibrium of these four humors (akhlat) can cause disease
- This can occur due to failure of the body to oppose any factor that disturbs Quwwat-e-Mudabbira-e-Badan (power of body to maintain health)
- Therapy (Usoole ilaj) deals with eradication of cause (Izalae Sabab), restoration of the four humors (Tadeele Akhlat), normalization of tissues/organs (Tadeele Aza), pharmacotherapy with unani drugs (Ilaj-Bil-Advia) and surgery (Ilaj-Bil-Yad).

YOGA
- 'Yoga' means 'to join mind, spirit and body'
- It is derived from the Sanskrit word 'Yuj'
- It results in physical, mental, emotional and spiritual balance of the body
- It helps to live a stress free, healthy and balanced life
- Breathing exercises can reinstate the healthy status of the body from the diseased state
- It helps to maintain equilibrium between all physiological systems of the body
- It improves cardiac respiratory, endocrine, gastrointestinal, autonomic, musculoskeletal and genitourinary functions
- Yoga sutra by sage Patanjali defines 195 sutras and eight-fold path
- The eight fold paths mentioned in yoga sutra are Yama (ethics), niyama (tolerance), asana (postures), pranayama (breath control), pratyahara (sense of withdrawal), dharana (concentration), dhyana (meditation) and samadhi (ecstasy).

NATUROPATHY
- Naturopathy insists that nature is the healer of all diseases
- According to naturopathy, harmony with nature results in perfect health of an individual
- It says that human body has self-healing power and can prevent itself from diseases
- Water therapy, light (photo) therapy and mud therapy are followed in naturopathy
- Balanced diet and prayers also form an important aspect of naturopathy.

AYUSH
- Department of AYUSH (Ayurveda, Unani, Siddha and Homeopathy) has been established under Ministry of Health and Family Welfare
- It deals with the improvement of quality and standards of drugs available under these systems of medicine
- It is also responsible for developing an awareness and improvement of education system of these fields
- It is also concerned with the research and development of these alternative systems of medicine

- The 'essential drug list' of these systems is available under the drug control cell of AYUSH
- Ayurvedic, Siddha and Unani drug technical advisory board (ASUDTAB) stipulates the shelf-life/expiry period of Ayurvedic, Siddha and Unani drugs.

Nursing Responsibilities
- Mode of administration of AYUSH medicines may be different to allopathic system. So, read instructions carefully before administering the drugs
- The AYUSH medicines are prepared by mixing with milk, honey, jaggery or ginger extract in addition to water unlike allopathic medicines which are usually mixed with water or saline
- A basic knowledge of the 'essential drug list', their indications and contraindications is essential before administering these drugs.

Index

A

Abacavir 479, 480
Abarelix 308
Abciximab 238, 240
Abortion 96
Acamprosate 103
Acebutolol 69
Acetyl salicylic acid 519
Acetylcholine 33
Acid 542
   neutralizing capacity 327
   peptic disease 325
Acinetobacter 392, 397
   infection 400
Acne vulgaris 544
   treatment of 544
Acquired immunodeficiency
   syndrome 305
Acting adrenergic agonists 46
Actinomyces 376, 411
Acyclovir 467
Addison's disease 282
Adefovir 475
Adenoma 264, 347
Adenosine 209
   triphosphate 436
Administer melarsoprol 455
Adrenal glands, tumor of 282
Adrenal insufficiency, acute 282
Adrenaline 46
Adrenergic agonists 46
   therapeutic uses of 58
Adrenergic drugs
   directly acting 46
   in hypertension, centrally acting
      203
   indirectly acting 46
Adrenergic neuron blockers 202
Adrenochrome 224

Adriamycin 508
Adverse drug reactions 20
African trypanosomiasis 451
Agents, miscellaneous 153, 509
Agonists-antagonists 145
Albendazole 434, 439
Albuterol 51, 359
   actions 51
Alcohol 541
   addiction, treatment of 102
Aldehyde 542
Aldosterone antagonists 189
Alemtuzumab 511, 516
Alfentanil 144
Alfuzosin 60, 310
Aliskiren 205
Alkyl sulfonate 493
Alkylating agents 493
Allopurinol 531, 532
All-trans retinoic acid 544
Alosetron 350
Alpha blockers 59
Alpha methyl dopa 56
Alteplase 235, 236
Altretamine 495
Aluminum hydroxide 327
Alvimopan 342, 343
Alzheimer's disease, therapy of 137
Amantadine 136, 472
Ambenonium 38
Amebiasis, chemotherapy of 447
American trypanosomiasis 453
Amikacin 399, 401, 427
Amiloride 185
Aminocaproic acid 237
Aminocyclitols 413
Aminoglycosides 399, 418, 419, 427
Aminophylline 360, 361
Aminosalicylates 351
Amiodarone 216

Amlodipine 174
Amodiaquine 440, 444
Amoxicillin 391
Amphetamine 56
Amphotericin B 373, 456
  colloidal dispersion 457
  lipid complex 457
Ampicillin 390
Amylin analog 289
Amyotrophic lateral sclerosis,
  therapy of 138
Anabolic steroids 306
Analgesic 115
  agents, mild 520
Anaphylactic reaction, type I 21
Anastrozole 295, 296, 510
Ancylostoma duodenale infestation 435
Androgen 305
  receptor antagonists 307
Androgenic alopecia 546
Anesthetic
  adjuvants 114
  general 105
  local 81
Angina 178
  combinations in 176
  pharmacotherapy of 178
Angiogenesis inhibitors 512
Angioneurotic edema 279
Angiotensin converting enzyme
  inhibitors 197
Angiotensin II receptor blockers 199
Antacids 327
Antagonism 19
  chemical 19
  competitive 19
  functional 19
  noncompetitive 19
  nonequilibrium 19
  physical 19
  physiological 19
  receptor 19
Anthracenediones 505, 508
Anthraquinone laxatives 340

Antiandrogens 307
Antianginal drugs 169
Antiarrhythmic agent 209, 212, 218
Antibiotic 505, 507
  broad spectrum 403
  combinations, disadvantages of 374
  miscellaneous 411
  misuse 375
Anticholinergics, uses of 44
Anticholinesterases 35, 137
  irreversible 39
Anticoagulants 227
  effective
    in vitro 227
    in vivo 227
Antidepressants, atypical 153
Antidiarrheal agents 344, 346
Antidiuretics 186
Antiemetic drugs 333
Anti-flatulence agent 356
Antifungal agents 456
  topical 463
Antifungal antibiotics 456
Anti-*Helicobacter pylori* drugs 330
Antihistamines 89, 335
Antimetabolites 373, 456, 498
Antimicrobial drugs, development
  of resistance to 373
Anti-nonretroviral agents 467
Antiplatelet agents 238
Antiprogestins 298
Antiproliferative agents 516
Antipseudomonal penicillins 391
Antipsychotic
  agents, nursing responsibilities
    in 163
  atypical 93, 159
  drugs
    common uses of 157
    typical 157
  in depression, atypical 156
Antiretroviral agents 478
Antiretroviral therapy, highly active 490

Index

Antirheumatoid drugs, disease-modifying 528
Antiseptics 540
Antithymocyte globulin 516
Antitussives 369
 centrally acting 369
Anxiolytics 156
Apazone 527
Aplastic anemia 492
Apomorphine 135
Apraclonidine 55
Ardeparin 229
Arformoterol 53, 360
Argatroban 231
Aripiprazole 159, 162
Aromatase inhibitors 295
Arrhythmia, treatment of 209
Artemisinin 440
Arterial blood gas 366
Arteriolar dilator 205
Arteriolar venular dilator 205
Arthrus reaction, type III 22
Articaine 81, 83
Asatmyendriyartha samyoga 549
Asenapine 159
Ashta siddhis 550
Aspirin 238, 519
Atazanavir 484, 486
Atenolol 68
Atomoxetine 153
Atorvastatin 244
Atosiban 319
Atovaquone 440, 441
Atropine 40, 41
 actions 41
 adverse effects 41
 overdose 45
 treatment 45
Attapulgite 344
Autacoids 87
Ayurveda 549
AYUSH 552
Azacitidine 502
Azathioprine 528
Azelaic acid 545
Azelastine 90
Azithromycin 407-409, 429
Aztreonam 396

B

Bacitracin 416
Bacterial cell wall synthesis 373
Bacterial diarrhea 349
Bacterial DNA function 373
Bacterial enzymes 373
Bacterial vaginosis 422
Bactericidal inhibitors 373
Bacteroides 391, 392, 407, 411, 447
 fragilis 394
Bacterostatic inhibitors 373
Balsalazide 352
Bambuterol 359
Barbiturate 119, 123
 poisoning, therapy of 120
Beclomethasone dipropionate 362
Beef tapeworm 433
Benazepril 197, 198
Bendamustine 496
Benzamides 334
Benzbromarone 531, 535
Benznidazole 454
Benzocaine 81, 85
Benzodiazepines 114, 116, 126, 156, 337
Benzoic acid 456
Benzonatate 369
Benzothiazepine 171
Benzyl benzoate 543
Beta blockers 64, 72
 adverse effects of nonselective 64
 common properties of nonselective 64
 in angina 176
Beta receptor blockers in hypertension 200
Beta-adrenergic agonists 319
Beta-lactam antibiotics 387, 389, 393, 395

Betamethasone 281
Betaxolol 70
Bethanechol 34
Bevacizumab 511
Bezafibrate 246
Bicalutamide 307, 510
Biguanides 287
Bile acid sequestrants 242, 244, 345
Biliary cirrhosis, primary 356
Biotransformation 12
Biperiden 44
Bipolar disorder, drugs in 164
Bisacodyl 340
Bisoprolol 69
Bisphosphonates 315
Bivalirudin 231
Black water fever 444
Blastocystis 449
Blastomyces dermatitidis 457, 458
Blastomycosis 465
Bleeding peptic ulcer 331
　management of 331
Bleomycin 508
Blood 221
　flukes 433
　loss 254
Blood-brain barrier 55, 350, 399, 423, 437, 452, 536
Bolus intravenous 236
Bone
　marrow 492
　mineral density 317
　turnover, agents in 311
Bordetella 407
Borrelia 403, 407
Bradycardia 272
Brimonidine 55
Bromhexine 368
Bromocriptine 265
Bronchial asthma,
　pharmacotherapy of 359
Brucella 379, 382
Brugia malayi 438, 439
Buccal mucosa 79

Bucindolol 71
Budesonide 362
Bupivacaine 81, 82
Buprenorphine 145
Bupropion 154
Buspirone 95, 156
Busulfan 495
Butenafine 456
Butoconazole 464
Butorphanol 145
Butyrophenones 334

C

Cabergoline 266
Calcineurin inhibitors 515
Calcitonin 311, 314
Calcium 311
　carbonate 328
　channel blockers 171, 175
　　in hypertension 199
　current, inhibition of T type 121
　polycarbophil 344
Camptothecin 505, 507
Campylobacter 382, 392, 407, 447
　jejuni 349
Cancer
　cells 492
　chemotherapy 264
　therapy of 337
　targeted therapy in 511
Candida 464
Candida albicans 379, 404
Candida species 457, 458
Candidiasis 465
Cangrelor 238, 241
Cannabinoid 166, 333, 336
Capecitabine 502
Captopril 197, 198
Carbachol 34
Carbamazepine 123
Carbapenems 387, 395
Carbimazole 275
Carbonic anhydrase inhibitors 73, 180

Carboplatin 497
Carboprost 322
Carboxymethyl cellulose 344
Carcinogenicity 24, 492
Carcinoid tumor 347
Carcinoma prostate 308
Cardiac glycosides 191
Cardiac impulse 209
Cardiac lesion 421
Cardiovascular system 141, 167
Carmoterol 53
Carvedilol 70
Cascara 340
Caspofungin 461
Castor oil 340
Catechol-o-methyl transferase inhibitors 135
Cefaclor 393
Cefepime 395
Cefprozil 393
Ceftizoxime 394
Cefuroxime 393
Celecoxib 526
Celiprolol 71
Cell membrane, disruption of 373
Central nervous system 41, 99, 101, 119, 140, 166, 361
 actions 140
Cephalosporins 387, 392, 418, 419
 first generation 393
 fourth generation 395
 second generation 393
 third generation 394
Cerebrospinal fluid 124, 408, 430, 437, 447, 536
Cervical priming 96
Cestodes 433
Cetirizine 90
Cetrimide 541
Cetrorelix 270
Cetuximab 511, 512
Chagas disease 453
Chagoma 453
Chancroid 422

Charaka samhita 549
Chelating agents 536
Chemoprophylaxis 429
Chemoreceptor trigger zone 333
Chemotherapeutic agents 373
Chemotherapy 371
Chinese liver fluke 433
Chlamydia 379, 382, 384, 403, 404, 407, 408
 trachomatis 376, 404
 coinfection 421
 infection 422
Chlorambucil 495
Chloramphenicol 405
Chlorhexidine 541
Chlorine 541
Chloroprocaine 81, 83
Chloroquine 12, 440, 443, 448, 528
Chloroxylenol 540
Chlorpromazine 12, 24, 157, 158
Chlorthalidone 196
Cholecalciferol 311
Cholestyramine 244
Choline esters 33
Cholinergic alkaloids
 adverse effects of 35
 contraindications of 35
Cholinergics 33, 73
Cholinesterase enzyme, sites of 36
Ciclesonide 362
Ciclopirox olamine 456, 464
Cidofovir 469
Cinacalcet 316
Cinchonism 444
Ciprofibrate 246
Ciprofloxacin 382
Cisapride 354
Cisplatin 497
Citrate phosphate dextrose 249
Citrobacter 397
Cladribine 504
Clarithromycin 407-409, 429, 430, 432
Clavulanic acid 397

Clevidipine 175
Clindamycin 411
Clofazimine 430, 431, 504
Clofibrate 246
Clomiphene 293
Clonazepam 126
Clonidine 55, 204
Clopidogrel 238, 239
Clostridia 411, 447
Clostridium difficile 345, 349, 352, 392, 404, 448
Clostridium perfringens 407
Clostridium species 388
Clotrimazole 463
Cloxacillin 389, 390
Clozapine 159, 160
Coagulants 223
Cocaine 81, 82, 143, 166
Coccidioides species 457, 458
Coccidioidomycosis 465
Coffee ground vomiting 331
Colchicine 531
Colesevalam 244
Colestipol 244
Colistin 413
Colloidal bismuth subsalicylate 329, 345
Colloidal plasma expanders 251
Congestive glaucoma, acute 73
Congestive heart failure 188
  ace inhibitors in 189
  beta blockers in 191
  direct renin inhibitors in 190
  diuretics in 188
  dopaminergic drugs in 193
  hydralazine in 191
  nitrates in 191
  sodium nitroprusside in 191
  vasodilators in 189
  vasopressin antagonists in 190
Constipation
  agents in 342
  drugs in 338
Contraceptives, injectable 302

Corticosteroid 24, 278, 336, 362
  high dose 312
  types of 278
Corticotropin releasing hormone 278
Corynebacterium diphtheriae 407
Cotrimoxazole 15
Cough, drugs in 369
COX-2 inhibitors, selective 526
Coxiella 403
Crohn's disease 279, 351, 352, 516
Crotamiton 543
Cryptococcosis 465
Cryptococcus neoformans 457, 458
Cryptosporidium species 349
Crystalloid plasma expanders 253
Crystalluria 376
Cumulative toxicity 25
Cushing's syndrome 281
  treatment 282
Cutaneous candidiasis 466
Cyclizine 337
Cyclopentolate 43
Cyclophosphamide 493, 529
Cycloplegia 80
Cycloserine 426
Cyclospora 449
  infection 380
  species 349
Cyclosporine 515, 529
Cyproheptadine 92
Cytarabine 501
Cytolytic reaction, type II 22
Cytomegalovirus 471
Cytosine arabinoside 501

D

Dabigatran etexilate 234
Dacarbazine 496, 508
Daclizumab 516
Dactinomycin 507
Dalfopristin 412
Dalteparin 229
Danazol 306

Dapsone 430
Daptomycin 416
Darifenacin 44
Darunavir 484, 487
Daunorubicin 508
Deferasirox 539
Deferoxamine 538
Deflazacort 281
Dehydroemetine 447, 448
Delavirdine 483
Demecarium 38
Demelanizing agents 545
Denileukin diftitox 513
Deoxyribonucleic acid 257, 467
Depolarizing muscle relaxants 76
Depression and anxiety,
  pharmacotherapy of 151
Dermojet 9
Desflurane 108
Desirudin 231
Desmopressin
  adverse effects of 224
  uses of 225
Dexamethasone 280
Dexlansoprazole 325
Dexloxiglumide 355
Dexmedetomidine 115
Dexmethylphenidate 57
Dexpanthenol 343
Dextran 251
Dextrose 253
Diabetes
  insipidus, treatment of 187
    central 187
    nephrogenic 187
  mellitus 283
Diabetic ketoacidosis 290
Diarrhea 80, 338
  treatment of 349
Diazepam 126
Diazoxide 207
Diclofenac 524
Dicloxacillin 389, 390
Dicyclomine 43

Didanosine 479, 481
Diethyl ether 105
Diethylcarbamazine citrate 438
Diethylstilbestrol 292
Difenoxin 346, 347
Digitalis overdose, treatment of 192
Digitalization 192
Digoxin 12, 191, 218
  induced alterations in cardiac
    rhythm, treatment of 219
Dihydroergotamine 321
Dihydropyridine 171
  calcium channel blockers 174
Diiodohydroxyquin 447, 450
Dilling's formula 26
Diloxanide 447, 450
Diltiazem 173
Dimercaprol 536
  molecules of 536
Dinoprostone 96, 321
Dipeptidyl peptidase-4 inhibitor 288
Diphenhydramine 337
Diphenoxylate 143, 346, 347
Dipyridamole 238
Directly observed treatment short
  course 427
Disinfectants 540
Disopyramide 212
Disulfiram 102
Diuretics 180
  reduce edema 180
Dizziness 439
DNA gyrase, inhibition of 373
Dobutamine 50, 193
  actions 50
  adverse effects 51
  uses 51
Docosanol 472
Docusates, types of 339
Dofetilide 218
Domperidone 353, 354
Donepezil 38

Dopamine 49, 193, 263
  antagonists 333, 334, 353
  receptor agonists 134
Dopexamine 50
Dornase-α 368
Doxazosin 60, 310
Doxofylline 361
Doxorubicin 508
Doxycycline 446, 545
Dronabinol 336
Dronedarone 217
Drotrecogin α 231
Drug
  abuse 23
  action 16
    factors modifying 26
  addiction 23, 166
    treatment 166
  administration, routes of 4
    inhalational 6
    intra-arterial 8
    intradermal 7
    intramuscular 7
    intraosseous 9
    intraperitoneal 8
    intrathecal 8
    intravenous 7
    oral or enteric 4
    parenteral 6
    rectal 5
    subcutaneous 7
    sublingual 5
    transdermal 9
  allergy 21
    mechanisms of 21
  and Cosmetics Act 29
  and Magic Remedies Act 29
  antiarrhythmic 209
  anticancer 492
  anticholinergic 41, 136, 330, 333, 335, 363
  antiepileptic 121, 125
  antihypertensive 195
  anti-inflammatory 519
  antimalarial 440
  antimicrobial 374
  antipsychotic 157
  antipyretic 519
  antiretroviral 478
  antithyroid 271, 274
  combinations, preferred 490
  dependence 22
  fibrinolytic 235
  first-line 423
  habituation 23
  hypolipidemic 242
  induced diseases 24
  interaction 75, 155, 328
  metabolism, factors influencing 14
  miscellaneous 56, 176
  nonspecific 350
  overdose, treatment of 24
  regimen 490
  resistance, prevention of 374
  second line 423
  source of 3
    animal 3
    biological substances 3
    microorganisms 3
    natural products 3
    natural/plant 3
    oil 3
    oleoresin 3
    resin 3
    synthetic 3
  transport of 10
  withdrawal reaction 23
Dutasteride 308
Dwarf tapeworm 433
Dyclonine 81, 84
Dyes 542

E

East African (rhodesian)
  trypanosomiasis 452
Ecabet 330
Echinocandin 461, 505

Econazole 463
Ectoparasiticides 540, 542
Edematous states 180
Edrophonium 38
Efavirenz 482
Eflornithine 451
Electroconvulsive therapy 75
Electrolyte depletion 341
Emetine 12, 447, 448
Emtricitabine 479, 481
Enalapril 197, 198
Enema 343
Enflurane 107
Enfuvirtide 489
Enkephalinase inhibitor 347
Enoxaparin 229
Enprofylline 361
Entamoeba histolytica 349, 447, 449, 450
Entecavir 475
Enteric coated pills 5
Enterobacter 379, 381, 382, 397, 400
Enterobacteriaceae 392, 394, 395
Enterococci 390, 392
   infection 401
      treatment of 400
   species 399
Enterococcus 391
Entry inhibitors 488
Enzyme 505
   inhibition 14, 17
   linked receptors 18
Ephedrine 12, 58
Epidermophyton 462, 464
Epilepsy, therapy of 132
Epinephrine 46
Epipodophyllotoxins 505, 507
Epirubicin 5-8
Eplerenone 186
Epothilone 505, 507
Epstein-Barr virus 467
Eptifibatide 238, 240
Erectile dysfunction 97, 309
   therapy of 309

Ergocalciferol 313
Ergometrine 320
Ergonovine 320
Ergot alkaloids 63, 94, 320
Ergotamine 321
Erythema nodosum leprosum 432
Erythromycin 407, 408
Erythropoietin 258
Escherichia coli 349, 376, 379, 381, 400, 420, 424
   organisms 345
Esmolol 68, 215
Esomeprazole 325
Estradiol 292
Estradiol cypionate 292
Estradiol valerate 292
Estrogen receptor
   downregulators, selective 295
   modulators, selective 293
Estrogens 291
Estropipate 292
Eszopiclone 118
Etanercept 516
Ethambutol 425, 429
Ethamsylate 224
Ethanol 166
Ethinylestradiol 292
Ethionamide 426, 430, 432
Ethosuximide 124
Ethyl
   alcohol 101
   chloride 105
Ethylenediaminetetra-acetic acid 83
Ethyleneimines 493
Etodolac 523
Etomidate 112
Etoricoxib 527
Etravirine 483
Exemestane 295, 296, 510
Exfoliative dermatitis 387
Expectorants 368
Extracellular fluid 312
Ezetimibe 242, 247

F

Famciclovir 469
Familial adeno polyposis 523
Febuxostat 531, 533
Fedotozine 350
Felbamate 130
Felodipine 175
Fenofibrate 246
Fenoldopam 49
Fentanyl 143
Fetus 492
Fexofenadine 90
Fibrinogen and antihemophilic factor 224
Fibrinolysis, inhibitors of 237
Fibrinolytic drugs, action of 235
Filariasis 438
   chemotherapy of 438
Finasteride 308, 546
   inhibits 308
Fish tapeworm 433
Flecainide 214
Floxuridine 501
Fluconazole 459
Flucytosine 457
Fludarabine 503
Fludrocortisone 281
Flu-like syndrome 496
Flumazenil 119
Flunarizine 175
Fluoroquinolone 15, 381, 418, 427, 429
   first generation 382
   fourth generation 386
   mechanism of action of 381
   second generation 384
   third generation 385
Fluphenazine 157
Flutamide 307, 510
Fluticasone 362
Fluvastatin 243
Folic acid 257
   analogs 498
   deficiency 258

Follicle stimulating hormone 268, 291, 300, 305
Fomepizole 104
Fomivirsen 470
Fondaparinux 230
Formoterol 53, 360
Fosamprenavir 484, 486
Foscarnet 470
Fosinopril 197, 198
Fulvestrant 295, 510
Fungal infection 456, 462
   chemotherapy of 456
Furosemide 183
Fusion inhibitors 373, 478
Fusobacterium 411

G

Gabapentin 127
Gallstone dissolving drugs 355
Gametocidal 440
Gamma-aminobutyric acid 18, 101, 116, 121
   modulators 121
Ganciclovir 471
Ganglion blockers 79
Ganglionic stimulants 79
   and blockers 79
Ganirelix 270
Gas 105
Gastroesophageal reflux disease 326, 332
   drugs in 325
Gastrointestinal system 323
Gastrointestinal toxicity 492
Gastrointestinal tract 265, 141, 402, 521, 532
   bleeding 256
   conditions 338
   hormones 283
Gelatin polymers (haemacel) 252
Gemcitabine 502
Gemfibrozil 246
Gemifloxacin 386
Gemtuzumab 511
Genetic modifications 374

Index

Genital and anal warts 422
Genital herpes 422
Genitourinary tract 141
Gentamicin 400
Giardia lamblia 443, 449, 450
Glaucoma 72, 96
   drugs in open angle 73
Glucagon like peptide-1 analogs 289
Glucocorticoids 278, 352, 530
Glucose 348
   dependent insulinotropic polypeptide 289
Glycerin 343
Glyceryl trinitrate 170
Glycopeptides 414
Glycoprotein IIB/IIIA inhibitors 240
Glycopyrrolate 43
Gonadorelin 267
Gonadotropin-releasing hormone 291, 303
   agonists 263, 269
   antagonist 270, 308
Gonadotropins 263, 267
   diagnostic of 268
   therapeutic uses of 269
Gonads 492
Gonorrhea 421
Goserelin 269, 510
Gossypol 304
Gout, pharmacotherapy of 531
G-protein coupled receptors 18
Gram-negative bacilli 408
Gram-positive cocci and bacilli 408
Granulocytopenia 492
Graves' disease 274
Griseofulvin 462
Growth hormone 263
Guanabenz 56
Guanadrel 202
Guanfacine 56
Guanosine monophosphate 169
   cyclic 309, 361
Guinea worm 433

H

H_1 antihistamines 89
H_2 blockers 326
Haemophilus 382, 424
   ducreyi 376
   influenzae 376, 379, 380, 397, 406, 425
Halofantrine 440
Haloperidol 157, 159
Haloprogin 464
Halothane 106
Hamycin 465
Heart failure, drugs in 188
Helicobacter pylori 325, 330, 408, 447, 449
   organism 329
Hematopoietic growth factors 257, 258
Hematuria 376
Hemochromatosis 255
Hemolytic anemia 430
Hemolytic-uremic syndrome 508
Heparin 227
   overdose, treatment of 232
Hepatitis B virus, drugs in 475
Heroin 143
Herpes simplex virus 468
Herpes virus infection 467
Hexachlorophene 540
Histoplasma capsulatum 457, 458
Histoplasmosis 465
Histrelin 269
Hodgkin's lymphoma 496, 508
Homatropine 42
Homeopathy 549, 550
Hookworm 433
Hormonal contraceptives 300
Hormones 510
   and hormone antagonists 261
Human chorionic gonadotropin 268
Human immunodeficiency virus 264
   infection 478
   during pregnancy, therapy of 491
   tuberculosis in 428

Human serum albumin 251
Humoral mechanism 21
Huntington's disease, therapy of 137
Hydatid disease 433
Hydralazine 205
Hydrochlorothiazide 196
Hydrocortisone 280
Hydrogen peroxide 540
Hydroxy ethyl starches 252
Hydroxyurea 509
Hygroscopic, bulk forming agents 344
Hyperactivity disorder, deficit 56
Hypercalcemia 311
Hyperprolactinemia 158
Hypersensitivity reaction, type IV delayed 22
Hypertension 202
 alpha receptor blockers in 201
 direct renin inhibitor in 205
 diuretics in 195
 perioperative 208
 vasodilators in 205
Hypertensive emergency 208
Hypertensive urgency 208
Hyperthermia, malignant 77
Hyperthyroidism 273
 in pregnancy 277
Hypervitaminosis D 314
Hypocalcemia 312
Hypoglycemic agents 289
Hypogonadotropic hypogonadism, defects of 267
Hypoparathyroidism 314
Hypoprothrombinemia 519
Hypothyroidism 273

I

Ibuprofen 524
Ibutilide 218
Idarubicin 508

Idiosyncrasy 21
Idoxuridine 472
Idraparinux 230
Ifosfamide 494
Iloperidone 159, 162
Imidazoles 456, 458
Imipenem 395
Imiquimod 477
Immunosuppressants 352, 515
Important drug laws 29
In vitro fertilization 268
Inamrinone 194
Indacaterol 53
Indinavir 484, 487
Indomethacin 522
Indoramin 63
Inflammatory bowel disease, drugs in 351
Infliximab 516
Influenza
 prophylaxis in 374
 virus infection, drug for 472
Inhalational anesthetics 105
Inhalational steroids cause 363
Inhibit hormone
 release 274
 synthesis 274
Inhibiting cyclooxygenase enzyme 519
Insulin 283
 formulations 285
 long-acting 284, 285
 preparations 284
Integrase inhibitors 478, 489
Interferons 473
Interleukin-2 513
Intermediate acting
 insulin 284
 sulfonamide 377
Intravenous anesthetics 105
Intravenous infusion 311
Invasive aspergillosis 465
Iodide 275

Iodine 12, 541
Ion channel receptors 18
Ionic inhibitors 274, 275
Iron
   deficiency 254
      anemia 254
      dextran, infusion of 256
   toxicity
      acute 255
      chronic 255
Irritable bowel syndrome 349
Isavuconazole 461
Isoflurane 107
Isonicotinic acid hydrazide 423
Isoprenaline 50
Isosorbide dinitrate 171
Isosorbide mononitrate 171
Isradipine 175
Itopride 354
Itraconazole 459
Ivabradine 176, 178
Ivermectin 439, 543

J
JAK-STAT receptors 18
Jaundice 429

K
Kala azar 454
Kanamycin 402, 427
Katanserin 93
Ketamine 113
Ketoconazole 458
Ketolides 407
Ketorolac 523
Kinetics, first order 15
Klebsiella 379, 381, 382, 391, 392, 400, 419, 424

L
L. loa 438
Labetalol 70
Lacosamide 131
Lactulose 341

Lamivudine 476, 479, 480
Lamotrigine 128
Lanreotide 264
Lansoprazole 325
L-asparaginase 509
Laxatives 338
   act 338
   bulk forming 338
   stimulant 338, 340
   surfactant 338, 339
   types of 338
Leflunomide 529
Legionella 382, 384, 392, 403, 407
   infection 409
Leishmaniasis 454
Lepirudin 231
Lepra reaction 432
Leprosy 430
   chemotherapy of 430
Letrozole 295, 296, 510
Leukotriene antagonist 97, 364
Leuprolide 269, 510
Levalbuterol 359
Levamisole 436
Levetiracetam 128
Levodopa 133
Levofloxacin 384
Levonorgestrel 302
   and ethinylestradiol combination 301
Levothyroxine T_4 272
Lidocaine 81, 212
Lignocaine 81
Linaclotide 342
Lincosamide 411
Lindane 542
Linezolid 412
Liothyronine 272
Lipid derived autacoids 96
Lipopeptide 416
Lipoprotein cholesterol
   high-density 200, 292
   low-density 292
Liposomal amphotericin B 456

Lisinopril 197, 198
Listeria 391, 392, 407
Lithium 164, 276
Liver fluke 433
Lomefloxacin 384
Loop diuretics 182, 195, 196
Loperamide 143, 346
Lopinavir 484, 486
Lorazepam 126
Lovastatin 243
Low molecular weight heparin 228
Loxapine 157
Lubiprostone 342
Lugol's solution 276
Lumefantrine 440, 446
Luminal amebicides 447
Lung flukes 433
Luteinizing hormone 268, 291, 305
Lymphogranuloma venereum 422
Lysergic acid diethylamide 166

M

Macrolide 407
   antibiotic 354
Mafenide 379
Magaldrate 328
Magnesium 219
   citrate 341
   hydroxide 341
   salts 327
   sulfate 318, 341
Malaria 440
Male contraception 303
MAO-B inhibitors, selective 136
Maraviroc 489
Mast cell stabilizer 365
Mazzotti-like reaction 439
Mebendazole 433
Mechanical ventilation 120
Mechlorethamine 493
Meclizine 337
Medicine, alternative systems of 547
Mefenamic acid 525

Mefloquine 440, 444
Megakaryocyte growth factors 259
Megaloblastic anemia 257
Meglitinides 286
Melanin pigmentation of colon 340
Melanosis coli 340
Melarsoprol 453
Melatonin congener 119
Melphalan 494
Memantine 137
Meningococcal meningitis 374
Meningococcus 425
Menotropin 268
Menstrual cycle 291
Mephentermine 54
Mepivacaine 81, 83
Meropenem 396
Mesalamine 351
Messenger ribonucleic acid 467
Mestranol 292
Metabolism 12
   first pass 12
   phases of 13
Metal
   chelator 536
   salts of 542
Metaproterenol 51
Metaraminol 55
Metastatic carcinoid tumor 264
Methacholine 33
Methadone 144
Methamphetamine 57
Methenamine 420
Methicillin 389
Methicillin-resistant
   Staphylococcus aureus 392
Methimazole 275
Methotrexate 499, 528
Methyl alcohol poisoning,
   treatment of 103
Methyl hydrazine 493
Methyldopa 203
Methylergometrine 320
Methylnaltrexone 342, 343

Methylphenidate 57
Methylprednisolone 280
Methylxanthines 360
   common uses of 361
Methysergide 92
Metoclopramide 353
Metolazone 196
Metoprolol 67
Metrifonate 437
Metronidazole 15, 447
Mexiletine 213
Mianserin 153
Miconazole 463
Microsporum 462
   infection 464
Midodrine 55
Mifepristone 298
Migraine 95
   therapy of acute 95
Milrinone 194
Miltefosine 455
Mineralocorticoids 281
Minocycline 430, 432, 545
Minoxidil 206, 546
Mirtazapine 153
Misoprostol 96, 321
Mitotane 509
Moexipril 197, 198
Moguisteine 369
Molindone 157
Mometasone 362
Monoamine oxidase inhibitors 47, 155
Monobenzone destroys melanocytes 545
Monoclonal antibody 352, 364, 516
   in cancer 511
Montelukast 364
Moraxella catarrhalis 394
Morphine 140
   dose of 28
Mosapride 354
Motilides 353, 354, 355
Motion sickness, treatment of 337
Moxifloxacin 386, 430

mTOR inhibitors 513, 515
Mucolytics 367
Multibacillary leprosy, regime for 432
Multidrug resistant TB regime 428
Mupirocin 416
Muromonab 516
Muscle relaxants 115
   centrally acting 78
Myasthenia gravis 38
Mycobacteria 401, 403
   atypical 403
Mycobacterial cell wall 423
Mycobacterium 382, 425
   avium complex infection 429
   leprae 430, 432
      antigens 432
   tuberculosis 423, 424, 427
Mycoplasma 382, 384, 403, 404
   pneumoniae 407
Mycosis
   deep 465
   superficial 465
Mydriasis 80
Myeloid growth factors 258
Myelosuppression 497
Myocardial infarction
   nursing responsibilities in 179
   therapy of 179
Myxoedema coma 273

N

Nabilone 336
Nabumetone 524
N-acetylcysteine 368
N-acetyl-para-benzoquinone imine 521
Nadolol 66
Nadroparin 229
Nafarelin 269
Nafcillin 389
Naftifine 456, 464
Nalbuphine 145
Nalidixic acid 381

Nalorphine 146
Naloxone 146
Naltrexone 103, 146
Naproxen 525
Narcotic and Psychotropic
    Substances Act 29
Natural alkaloids 34, 41
    arecoline 35
    cevimeline 35
    muscarine 35
    pilocarpine 35
Natural opioids 139
Natural products 505
Naturopathy 552
Nebivolol 71
Necator americanus infestation 435
Nefazodone 153
Neisseria 379, 382, 407
    gonorrhoeae 421
    meningitidis 376, 406, 424
Nelarabine 504
Nelfinavir 484, 488
Nematodes 433
Neomycin 401
Neostigmine 37
Netilmicin 401
Neuraminidase inhibitors 373
Neurodegenerative disorders, drugs
    in 133
Neuroendocrine function 140
Neuroleptic malignant syndrome
    134
Neuromuscular blockers 74
Neurosyphilis lesion 421
Neutral protamine hagedorn 284
Nevirapine 482
Newer drugs 241
Newer insulin delivery devices 285
Niacin 242, 245
Nicardipine 175
Niclosamide 436
Nicorandil 177
Nicotine 166
Nifedipine 174, 318

Nifurtimox 454
Nilutamide 510
Nimodipine 175
Nitazoxanide 447, 449
Nitrates 169
Nitrofurantoin 419
Nitrogen mustards 493
Nitrosoureas 493, 496
Nitrous oxide 109
Nocardia 376, 379, 380, 411
Nocturnal angina 178
Non-edematous states 180
Nongonococcal urethritis 422
Non-nucleoside reverse
    transcriptase inhibitors 478,
    482
Non-opioid analgesics 139
Nonselective adrenergic agonists
    72
Nonselective alpha blockers 62
Nonsteriodal anti-inflammatory
    drugs 326, 519, 525, 528, 530,
    534, 535
    therapy, nursing responsibilities
    in 527
Non-systemic antacids 327
Noradrenaline 48, 253
Norepinephrine 48
Norfloxacin 383
Novel benzodiazepine receptor
    agonists 118
Nucleoside reverse transcriptase
    inhibitors 478, 484
Nursing practice, legal aspects in 28
Nutritional rickets 314
Nystatin 465

O

Obsessive compulsive disorder 156
Obstructive pulmonary disease,
    chronic 367
Octreotide 264, 347
Ofloxacin 383, 430, 431
Olanzapine 159, 160
Olsalazine 352

Omeprazole 325
Onapristone 299
Opioid 166, 346
　analgesics 139
　antagonists 146
　induced constipation 342
　induced postoperative paralytic ileus 343
　management of 342
　poisoning 142
　therapy, nursing responsibilities in 146
Opium Act 29
Oral
　agents 227
　anticoagulants 232
　contraceptive
　　combination 300
　　pills 122, 304
　hypoglycemic drugs 283, 285
　iron therapy 254
　sodium phosphate 312
　steroids cause 363
Orciprenaline 51
Organophosphorus compound poisoning 40
Ormeloxifene 303
Ornidazole 447
Oropharyngeal candidiasis 465
Orthostatic hypotension 158, 208
Oseltamivir 473
Osmotic diuretics 181
Osmotic laxatives 341
Osteomalacia 314
Osteoporosis 316
Otilonium bromide blocks neurokinin 350
Oxacillin 389, 390
Oxaliplatin 498
Oxandrolone 306
Oxazolidinone 412
Oxcarbazepine 124
Oxiconazole 464
Oximes 40
Oxybutynin 44
Oxytocics 319
Oxytocin 319
　receptors, number of 319

P

Paget's disease 314, 316
Paliperidone 159, 162
Panchabhuta 549
Pancreatitis, drugs in 355
Panitumumab 511, 512
Pantoprazole 325
Para-aminobenzoic acid 376, 426
Paracetamol toxicity 521
Paracoccidioides 457
　brasiliensis 458
Parathormone 311, 312
Parecoxib 526
Parenteral agents 227
Parenteral anticoagulants 230
Parenteral iron therapy 255
Parkinsonism
　drugs in 136
　therapy of 133
Paromomycin 402, 447, 449, 455
Pasteurella 379
　multocida 407
Patent ductus arteriosus, maintenance of patency of 96
Paucibacillary leprosy, regime for 432
Pectin-kaolin mixture 344
Pefloxacin 384
Pegvisomant 265
Pemetrexed 500
Penciclovir 468
Penicillamine 537
Penicillin 387, 418, 419
　common properties of 387
　G 388
　V 388
Penicillinase resistant penicillins 389
Pentamidine 452

Pentazocine 145
Pentostatin 505
Peptic ulcer 96
  drugs in 325
Peptococcus 411
Peptostreptococcus 411
Pergolide 267
Perindopril 197, 198
Peripherally acting antitussives 369
Permethrin 542
Perphenazine 157
Pethidine (meperidine) 142
Pharmacodynamics 17
Pharmacokinetics 10
Phenazopyridine 420
Phenol 540
Phenolphthalein 341
Phenothiazines 334
Phenoxybenzamine 62
Phentolamine 62
Phenylalkylamine 171
Phenylephrine 54
Phenytoin 121
Phosphate 312
Phosphodiesterase inhibitors 193
Photosensitivity reaction 22
Physostigmine 36
Pindolol 67
Pinworm 433
Piperazine citrate 435
Pirenzepine 44
Piroxicam 526
Pityrosporum folliculitis 464
Plasma 250
  concentration, monitoring of 15
  estradiol levels 267
  half-life 15
Plasminogen 235, 236
  inactivators 235
Plasmodia 403
Plasmodium 445
  falciparum 430, 442, 445
  knowlesi malaria 440
  malariae 440

ovale 440
species 440, 442, 445, 446
vivax 440, 445
Platelet-activating factor 21
Platinum complexes 493, 497
Plicamycin 312
Pneumocystis
  carinii pneumonia 279
  jirovecii 379, 380, 411, 430
  pneumonia 452
Poisons Act 29
Polyethylene glycol 24
  solution 341
Polymyxin B 413
Polymyxin B_1 and B_2 413
Polyvinyl pyrolidine 252
Pork tapeworm 433
Posaconazole 460
Postcoital contraceptive 301
Potassium
  channel openers in angina 177
  chloride 348
  permanganate 540
  sparing diuretics 184, 195, 196
Pramipexole 134
Pramoxine 81, 85
Pranlukast 364
Prasugrel 238, 239
Pravastatin 243
Praziquantel 437
Prazosin 59
Prednisolone 280
Pregabalin 127
Premoline 57
Price control/drug order 29
Prilocaine 81, 83
Primaquine 445
Prinzmetal angina 169
Probenecid 531, 534
Probiotics 346
Procainamide 211
Procaine 81, 84
Procarbazine 498
Prodrug 12

Index

Progestin 291, 297
　alone preparation 302
　only contraceptive 301
Proguanil 440, 442
Prokinetic agents 353
　in constipation 342
Prolactin 263, 265
Propafenone 214
Proparacaine 81, 85
Prophylactic agents
　causal 440
　suppressive 440
Propionic acid derivatives 524
Propofol 112
Propoxyphene 143
Propranolol 65, 215
Propylthiouracil 274
Prostaglandins 72, 321, 329
　uses of 96
Prostatic hypertrophy, therapy of
　benign 310
Protamine sulfate 232
Protease inhibitors 373, 478, 484
Proteasome inhibitors 513
Protein tyrosine kinase inhibitors
　511
Proteus 379, 381
Proton pump inhibitors 325
Protozoal diarrhea 349
Protozoal infection 451
Prucalopride 342, 354
Prulifloxacin 385
Pseudomonas 379, 382, 391, 392,
　395, 400, 402, 419
　infection 391, 401
Psoralen ultraviolet A 545
Psoriasis
　treatment of 545
　vulgaris 314
Psychopharmacology 149
Psychosis and mania,
　　pharmacotherapy of 157
Pulmonary hypertension 97
Pulmonary tuberculosis, regimes
　for 427

Purine analogs 502
Pyrantel pamoate 435
Pyrazinamide 425
Pyridostigmine 38
Pyrimethamine 440, 442
Pyrimidine analogs 500

Q

Quetiapine 159, 161
Quinagolide 266
Quinapril 197, 198
Quinidine 210
Quinine 440, 444
Quiniodochlor 447, 450, 456
Quinolones 381
Quinupristin 412

R

Rabeprazole 325
Radioactive iodine 276
Raloxifene 294
Raltegravir 490
Raltitrexed 500
Ramelteon 119
Ramipril 197, 198
Ranolazine 176, 177
Rasburicase 531, 534
Reactive oxygen species 445
Rebamipide 330
Reboxetine 153
Receptors regulating gene
　transcription 18
Recombinant human growth
　hormone 263
Red blood cell 442
Red cells, packed 250
Reductase inhibitors 308
Rehydration 348
Remifentanil 144
Renal osteodystrophy 314
Reserpine 202
Respiration 140
Respiratory alkalosis 520
Respiratory distress syndrome,
　acute 249

Respiratory system 357
Respiratory tract 79
Reteplase 235, 236
Reverse transcriptase enzyme inhibitors 373
Reversible anticholinesterases 36
 uses of 39
Reviparin 229
Reye's syndrome 520
Rheumatoid arthritis 520
 pharmacotherapy of 528
Ribavirin 474
Ribonucleic acid 467
Ricinus communis 340
Rickettsia 403
Rifabutin 429
Rifampin 424, 430, 431
Riluzole 138
Rimantadine 472
Ringworm 466
Risperidone 159, 161
Ritodrine 54
Ritonavir 484, 485
Rituximab 511
Rivaroxaban 234
Rivastigmine 38
Ropinirole 134
Ropivacaine 81, 84
Rosuvastatin 244
Roundworm 433
Roxithromycin 407, 409
Rufinamide 131
Rutin 224

S

Salicylates 24, 520
Saline, normal 253
Salmeterol 360
Salmon calcitonin 315
Salmonella 379, 382
 species 349
Saquinavir 484, 485
Scabies and pediculosis, drugs in 542

Schizophrenia 163
Sclerosing agents 226
Scopolamine 42, 335
Secnidazole 447
Sedatives and hypnotics 116
Semisynthetic derivatives of atropine 42
Semisynthetic opioids 139
Senna 340
Serotonin agonists 92, 93, 353, 354
Serotonin antagonists 92, 333
Serotonin noradrenaline reuptake inhibitors 152
Serotonin reuptake inhibitor, selective 151, 350
Serratia 379, 400
Sertaconazole 464
Sertindole 159
Serum sickness 387
Sevoflurane 109
Sexually transmitted diseases, chemotherapy of 421
Shigella 376, 379, 381
 species 349
Shock
 anaphylactic 248
 cardiogenic 248, 249
 hypovolemic 248
 management of 248
 neurogenic 248
 septic 248
 treatment of 248
 types of 248
Short acting β_2 adrenergic receptors, selective 51
Short-acting insulin 284
 analogs 284
Short-acting sulfonamides 377
Short-acting β_2 agonists 359
Siddha 549, 550
Sildenafil 309
Silodosin 61
Silver sulfadiazine 378

Simethicone 356
Simvastatin 243
Sincalide 355
Skeletal muscle relaxant 74
　directly acting 77
Skin 141, 492
　and mucous membrane, drugs acting on 544
Sodium
　channel blockers 209
　channel modulator 121
　chloride 348
　nitroprusside 207
　phosphate 341
　stibogluconate 454
　valproate 125
Solifenacin 44
Somatostatin 264, 347
Somatropin 263
Sotalol 215
Sparfloxacin 385
Spectinomycin 413
Spectrum penicillins
　extended 390
　narrow 388
Spironolactone 185
Sporothrix species 457
Sporotrichosis 465
Stable exertional angina, typical 169
Stanozolol 306
Staphylococcus 397
　aureus 379, 389, 391, 393, 397, 404, 420, 424
　epidermidis 379, 420
Statins 242
Status asthmaticus
　nursing responsibilities in 365
　therapy of 366
　treatment 366
Status epilepticus 132
Stavudine 478, 480
Steatorrhea, drugs in 355
Steroidal hormones 278
Stevens-Johnson syndrome 387

Streptococcus pneumoniae 376, 379, 380, 389, 406
Streptococcus pyogenes 376, 379, 389
Streptococcus viridans 379, 389
Streptogramins 412
Streptokinase 235, 236
Streptomycin 399, 425
Styptics 225
Subdermal implants 303
Succimer 537
Succinylcholine apnea 26
Sucralfate 328
Sufentanil 144
Sugammadex 76
Sulbactam 397
Sulconazole 464
Sulfacetamide 378
Sulfadiazine 377
Sulfadoxine 378, 446
Sulfamethoxazole 377
Sulfamethoxazole-trimethoprim 418
Sulfasalazine 351, 378, 528
Sulfisoxazole 377
Sulfonamide 24, 373, 376, 418, 440, 445, 446
　common properties of 376
　locally acting 378
　long-acting 378
　topical acting 378
Sulfone syndrome 430
Sulfonylureas 286
　first generation 286
　second generation 286
Sulindac 523
Sulpiride 159
Suprainfection 374
Suramin 452
Sympatholytic drugs 200
Synthetic derivatives of atropine 43
Synthetic opioids 139
　agonists-antagonists 139
　antagonists 140

lacking analgesic action 139
morphine analogs 139
with other actions 139
Synthetic progesterone derivatives 298
Syphilis 421
Systemic antacid 327
Systolic heart failure 188

T

Tachycardia 272
Tachyphylaxis 27
Tacrine 38
Tacrolimus 515
Tadalafil 309
Taenia solium 437
Tamoxifen 293, 510
Tamsulosin 61, 310
Tardive dyskinesia 158
Taxanes 505, 506
Tazarotene 544
Tazobactam 398
Tegaserod 350
Teicoplanin 415
Telbivudine 476
Telenzepine 44
Telithromycin 410
Tenecteplase 235, 236
Tenofovir 476, 484
Teratogenicity 23
Terazosin 60, 310
Terbinafine 456, 462
Terconazole 464
Teriparatide 313
Terizodine 427
Terlipressin
　adverse effects of 225
　uses of 225
Testosterone 305
　cypionate 305
　enanthate 305
　undecanoate 305
Tetrabenazine 138
Tetracaine 81, 84

Tetracyclines 12, 403, 440, 447, 450
Tetrahydrogestrinone 306
Theophylline 360, 361
Therapeutic drug monitoring 15
Thiacetazone 427
Thiazide
　adverse effects of 196
　diuretics 183, 195
Thiazolidinediones 287
Thiopentone 12
　sodium 111
Thioridazine 157
Thiotepa 495
Thioureylene derivatives 274
Threadworm 433
Thrombin inhibitors, direct 230
Thrombocytopenia 492, 497
　secondary prevention of 259
Thyroid
　hormone 271, 272
　actions of 271
　synthesis of 271
　tissue, destruction of 274
Tiagabine 129
Tibolone 295
Ticagrelor 238, 241
Ticlopidine 238
Timolol 66
Tinea infection 464
Tinidazole 447
Tinzaparin 229
Tioconazole 464
Tipranavir 484, 488
Tirofiban 238, 241
Tissue
　amebicides 447
　plasminogen activator 235, 236
　storage 12
Tizanidine 56
Tobramycin 399, 400
Tocolytics 318
Tolerance 26
　acquired 26
　acute 27

conditioned 27
cross 27
innate 26
types 26
Tolmetin 523
Tolnaftate 456, 464
Tolterodine 44
Topiramate 129
Toremifene 294, 510
Torsades de pointes 210, 219
Torsemide 183
Toxic effects 20
Toxicity profile 479
Toxoplasma gondii 430
Tramadol 143
Trandolapril 197, 198
Tranexamic acid 237
Transudate (hydrocele) 438
Trastuzumab 511
Traveler's diarrhea 347, 349
Trazodone 153
Trematodes 433
Treponema 403
 pallidum 388, 421
Tretinoin 544
Triamcinolone 280
 acetonide 362
Triamterene 185
Triazenes 493, 496, 456
Triazoles 458
Trichloroethylene 106
Trichomonas vaginalis 449, 450
Trichomoniasis 422
Trichophyton 462, 464
Tricyclic antidepressant 47, 154, 225
Trientine 538
Trifluoperazine 157
Trifluridine 472
Trihexyphenidyl 44
Trimetazidine 176, 178
Trimethoprim 376, 379
Trimethoprim-sulfamethoxazole
 (co-trimoxazole) 379
Trimetrexate 500

Triptans 93
Triptorelin 269
Trisodium citrate 348
Tropicamide 43
Trospium 44
Trypanosoma brucei
 gambiense 451
 rhodesiense 451, 452
Trypanosoma cruzi 453
Tuberculosis
 chemotherapy of 423
 corticosteroids in 429
 in pregnancy 428
Tumor necrosis factor 529
Typhoid carrier 380

U

Ulcer protective 328
Ulipristal 299, 302
Unani medicine 549
Unani system 551
Undecylenic acid 456, 465
Unstable angina 169, 179
Ureaplasma 403
Urinary analgesic 420
Urinary antiseptics 418, 419
Urinary tract infection,
 chemotherapy of 418
Urine
 alkalinization of 120
 depending, alkalinization of 24
Ursodeoxycholic acid 356
Uterine
 relaxants 318
 stimulants 319
 and relaxants 318

V

Valacyclovir 468
Valganciclovir 471
Vancomycin 414
Vardenafil 309
Variant angina 179
Varicella-zoster virus 467

Vasculitis 387
Vasopressin
  adverse effects of 225
  agonists 224
  analogs 186
  antagonists 187
Veno-occlusive disease 496
Verapamil 173
Vernakalant 219
Vibrio cholerae 345, 349
Vigabatrin 127
Vinblastine 506, 508
Vinca alkaloids 505
Vincristine 505
Vinorelbine 506
Viral hepatitis, drugs in 473
Viral replication, suppression of 373
Vitamin
  B_{12} 257
    deficiency of 257
  D 311, 313
  D_2 313
  D_3 311, 313
  K 223
    deficiency 519
Volatile liquids 105
Volume expanders 249
Voriconazole 460
Vulvovaginal candidiasis 465

W
Warfarin 232
Water 348

Wegener's granulomatosis 279
West African (gambian) trypanosomiasis 451
Whipworm 433
Whitfield's ointment 465
Whole blood 249
Wilms' tumor 506
Worm infestation, chemotherapy of 433
Wuchereria bancrofti 438, 439

X
Xenon 110
Xerostomia 80

Y
Yersinia enterocolitica 379
Yoga 552
Yohimbine 62
Yondelis (trabectedin) 509

Z
Zafirlukast 364
Zaleplon 118
Zanamivir 473
Zero order kinetics 15
Zidovudine 478, 479
Zileuton 364
Ziprasidone 159, 162
Zoledronate 315
Zollinger-Ellison syndrome 326, 332
Zolpidem 118
Zonisamide 130